An Atlas of
Human Blastocysts

THE ENCYCLOPEDIA OF VISUAL MEDICINE SERIES

An Atlas of
Human Blastocysts

Lucinda L. Veeck, MLT, hDSc

Assistant Professor of Embryology in Obstetrics and Gynecology
Assistant Professor of Reproductive Medicine
Director, Embryology Laboratories
The Center for Reproductive Medicine and Infertility
Weill Medical College of Cornell University, New York

and

Nikica Zaninović, MS

Supervisor, Embryology Laboratories
The Center for Reproductive Medicine and Infertility
Weill Medical College of Cornell University, New York

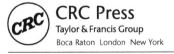

CRC Press
Taylor & Francis Group
Boca Raton London New York

CRC Press is an imprint of the
Taylor & Francis Group, an **informa** business

CRC Press
Taylor & Francis Group
6000 Broken Sound Parkway NW, Suite 300
Boca Raton, FL 33487-2742

First issued in paperback 2019

© 2003 by Taylor & Francis Group, LLC
CRC Press is an imprint of Taylor & Francis Group, an Informa business

No claim to original U.S. Government works

ISBN-13: 978-1-84214-169-4 (hbk)
ISBN-13: 978-0-367-39528-5 (pbk)

A CIP record for this book is available from the British Library.

Library of Congress Cataloging-in-Publication Data available on application

**Visit the Taylor & Francis Web site at
http://www.taylorandfrancis.com**

**and the CRC Press Web site at
http://www.crcpress.com**

Contents

List of contributing authors

Michal Amit
Department of Obstetrics and Gynecology
Rambam Medical Center
PO Box 9602
Haifa 31096
Israel

David L. Becker
Department of Anatomy and Developmental Biology
University College London
Gower Street
London WC1 6BT
UK

Owen Davis
Center for Reproductive Medicine and Infertility
Weill Medical College of Cornell University
New York
USA

Kate Hardy
Institute of Reproductive and Developmental Biology
Imperial College
Hammersmith Hospital
Du Cane Road
London W12 0NN
UK

Joseph Itskovitz-Eldor
Department of Obstetrics and Gynecology
Rambam Medical Center
PO Box 9602
Haifa 31096
Israel

David K. Gardner
Colorado Center for Reproductive Medicine
Englewood
Colorado 80110
USA

Howard W. Jones, Jr
Jones Institute for Reproductive Medicine
610 Colley Avenue
Norfolk
Virginia 23507
USA

Hung-Chih Kuo
Oregon National Primate Research Center
505 NW 185th Avenue
Beaverton
Oregon 97006
USA

Michelle Lane
Colorado Center for Reproductive Medicine
Englewood
Colorado 80110
USA

Shoukhrat M. Mitalipov
Oregon National Primate Research Center
505 NW 185th Avenue
Beaverton
Oregon 97006
USA

Zev Rosenwaks
Center for Reproductive Medicine and Infertility
Weill Medical College of Cornell University
New York
USA

Sophie Spanos
Institute of Reproductive and Developmental Biology
Imperial College
Hammersmith Hospital
Du Cane Road
London W12 0NN
UK

Don P. Wolf
Oregon National Primate Research Center
505 NW 185th Avenue
Beaverton
Oregon 97006
and
Departments of Obstetrics and Gynecology, and
   Physiology and Pharmacology
Oregon Health and Science University
Portland
Oregon 97201
USA

Foreword

Assisted reproductive technology has many intriguing aspects, but two are of surpassing fascination. First is the breathlessness of clinical result. With success, there is elation and presumed understanding of the physiological process; with failure, there is a frustration that leads the scientific community to strive for better understanding and more satisfactory results. Second is the moving experience of viewing microscopically the morphological processes that lead to an independent being – in this case a human being. The enigma is to distinguish the potential for viability from the many observed variations, which, according to our present understanding, are often expressions of the genetic misfits and misfires that are characteristic of human reproduction. Are we having a glimpse of the evolutionary process?

From its microscopic origin, the preembryo blooms into the human form, a process both wondrous and scientifically intriguing. Heeding biological commands, cells grow purposefully according to a predefined plan, endowing the new genetic entity with viability and function. Now, there is even more, as our experience extends beyond morphology. We are beginning to understand something about genes, gene products, enzymes, and proteins which drive these morphological characteristics.

The excitement and reality of clinical and laboratory work are captured by Lucinda Veeck, Nikica Zaninović, and their collaborators in *An Atlas of Human Blastocysts*. This is a book for those who wish to experience the satisfaction of being certain that they are up to date regarding extended culture procedures and the complexities of blastocyst development, considered key to achieving high pregnancy rates while minimizing the troublesome complication of multiple pregnancies.

In the following pages, the reader is given an opportunity to study the human, rhesus and murine blastocyst under optimal clinical and research conditions. The blastocyst's nutrient requirements during culture, its growth through various key stages, and its ability to survive freezing and thawing are all examined. We are guided through the early aspects of cell allocation and differentiation and are enlightened to the processes of hatching and programmed cell death. In sum, the reproductive process is demonstrated photographically from fertilization through to completion of implantation. Additionally, and of great interest, current scientific research applications are included.

Leaders in various clinical and scientific fields have come together to create this superb volume. *An Atlas of Human Blastocysts* is a dynamic and authoritative collection of microanatomical examples and definitively captures the earliest events of mammalian development *in vitro*. It is an absolute 'must-read' for clinicians and scientists working in the field of assisted reproduction.

Howard W. Jones, Jr, MD

Georgeanna Seegar Jones, MD

Preface

Why have those of us working in assisted reproductive laboratories become so suddenly fascinated with blastocysts? The answers are simple. First and foremost, never before in history have we had the opportunity to study closely human blastocyst development *in vitro*. Early descriptions of human morulae and blastocysts often relied on studying discarded material grown under suboptimal culture conditions after *in vitro* fertilization (IVF) trials. Investigating morphology, growth rate, metabolic requirements and genetic factors under these conditions probably led us to many misleading conclusions. Only with the development of sequential media have we been able routinely to grow viable blastocysts in our laboratories with some measure of confidence. Without doubt, *in vitro* culture techniques will continue to improve as additional knowledge is gained, enabling us to understand better the human reproductive process and ultimately provide our patients with tremendous benefit.

Second, we recognize that, through *in vitro* developmental investigations involving extended culture, we have been given the opportunity to offer a much improved and safer service to our patients by reducing the number of preembryos for transfer. How often in the past have we observed patients desperately desiring a healthy child, anxious to receive three or more preembryos for transfer, and then watched them agonize guiltily when forced to reduce selectively a high-order multiple pregnancy? This sad treatment option is all too often necessary because higher-order gestations, those involving more than two fetal hearts on ultrasound examination, are the largest single cause of poor obstetric outcome and subsequent neonatal difficulties. Triplet and quadruplet pregnancies are associated with high incidences of preeclampsia, gestational diabetes, pregnancy-induced hypertension, preterm labor, low birth weight and extensive neonatal care[1]. Although multifetal pregnancy reduction to twins is an option, the procedure itself carries medical and emotional risks[2,3].

Clearly, the most efficient way to avoid any form of multiple pregnancy is to limit the number of preembryos for intrauterine transfer to a single conceptus. While straightforward in theory, the reality of this approach leaves much to be desired. Indeed, most IVF programs experience no greater than a 20–30% clinical pregnancy rate per transfer when a single 4–8-cell conceptus is replaced. With treatment costs of $5000–$15 000 per IVF attempt in the United States, often not covered by insurance, this figure is too low to be cost-effective or desirable to the couple being treated. For this reason, more than one, and frequently more than three, day-2 or day-3 preembryos have been routinely replaced in an effort to optimize the chances for pregnancy. Therein lies the problem: *multiple transfer of early developing preembryos carries the risk of plural gestation, a risk that, until recently, could not be fully eliminated without decreasing the overall likelihood of pregnancy*. In the Cornell program, one in three young women under the age of 34 years will establish a multiple pregnancy if three preembryos are replaced on day 3, and 20% of women aged 34–39 years old will follow the same pattern. Because this trend is seen world-wide, it has become the recommended policy of many IVF centers to replace no more than two conceptuses whenever possible, many countries mandating this by law.

The incidence of multiple pregnancy has risen throughout the world as a consequence of assisted reproductive technologies. It has been reported that the rate of triplet and higher-order gestation infants per 100 000 Caucasian live births in the United States increased by 191% between 1972 and 1991, with 38% due to assisted conceptions and 30% to increased child-bearing among older women[4]. Another negative aspect to the rising rate of multiple pregnancy involves the associated economic burden resulting from preterm birth and increased hospital stays. Analysis of births at Brigham and Women's Hospital in Boston between 1986 and 1991 revealed that assisted reproductive technologies accounted for 2% of single, 35% of twin and 77% of triplet deliveries in that particular unit. Hospital charges per single baby averaged $9845, for twins they averaged $37 947 ($18 974 per baby) and for triplets they averaged $109 765 ($36 588 per baby)[5]. Since these figures are more than a decade old, one may assume that hospital costs are even higher today for couples experiencing multiple births.

Unfortunately, early demise of the human conceptus is a common event. Approximately 73% of *natural* single conceptions are lost before reaching 6 weeks of gestation, and, of the remainder, roughly 90% survive to term[6]. Although conceptions from IVF do nearly as well as natural pregnancies after clinical recognition, they result in higher losses between the onset of fertilization and completion of implantation, presumably due to developmental arrest or unrecognized abnormalities. Realization of this shortcoming prompts patients to ask for the replacement of multiple preembryos and allows us to agree in an effort to optimize ongoing pregnancy rates. Nevertheless, the necessity of replacing more than a single preembryo in order to establish good pregnancy rates would be moot if one could appropriately choose for transfer the healthiest and most viable conceptus from a cohort of growing preembryos. Imagine one day in the future when our patients will receive a single, healthy hatched blastocyst while having all other potentially viable ones frozen. The incidence of twin and greater gestations would be effectively eradicated!

It is not only reasonable, but prudent, to enquire which factors contribute to preembryo viability. Certainly, genetic stability is a major prerequisite for the implantation and delivery of a healthy child. At present, we know little about the genetic make-up of the preembryos within our incubators unless they are biopsied and examined, hardly a practical screening modality for every preembryo growing in the laboratory. Yet, when these examinations are performed, evidence comes to light that chromosomal abnormalities, both numerical and structural, are often associated with fragmented, multinucleated or poorly developing preembryos, and, conversely, many preembryos presenting good morphology possess lethal genetic aberrations. This leads us to recognize that, although morphological evaluations may furnish clues that minimally enhance our proficiency at choosing the best preembryos for transfer, these systems are severely limited in their ability to provide rock-hard evidence for subsequent normal development. Only by using new and very exciting non-invasive methods of assessment, such as amino acid profiling, will we enter a new era for diagnostic preembryo selection[7].

In further support of blastocyst transfer, it has been observed that genetically unhealthy preembryos often cease growth at very early cleavage stages. Almeida and Bolton proposed that there is a progressive loss of chromosomally abnormal preembryos after pronuclear development to at least the 8-cell stage[8]. When preembryos of varying morphological grades were studied cytogenetically, these investigators found a 65% incidence of abnormality at the pronuclear stage, a 55% incidence at the 2–4-cell stage and a 27% incidence at the 5–8-cell stage. Preembryos with poor morphology demonstrated almost a three-fold increase in chromosomal anomalies as compared to those with good morphology. From these data, it is logical to deduce that some form of natural selection continues beyond the 8-cell stage, perhaps through early fetal development. Might we not expect progressive natural selection to occur if we extend culture times beyond the standard 2 or 3 days? Will blastocyst transfer allow us successfully to replace a single conceptus? The purpose of the following text and photographic collection is to demonstrate to the reader that extended culture to blastocyst stages of development is now indeed an achievable option in our laboratories.

Lucinda L. Veeck

'Faith' is a fine invention when Gentlemen can see.
But Microscopes are prudent in an emergency

Emily Dickinson (contributed by Helen Maloney)

Nikica Zaninović

It will be found that everything depends on the
composition of the forces with which these particles
of matter act upon one another: and from these
forces, as a matter of fact, all phenomena of
Nature take their origin

Ruđer Bošković, Croatian scientist
(The Theory of Natural Philosophy, 1758)

References

1. Skupski DW, Nelson S, Kowalik A, *et al*. Multiple gestations from *in vitro* fertilization: successful implantation alone is not associated with subsequent preeclampsia. *Am J Obstet Gynecol* 1996;175:1029–32

2. Melgar CA, Rosenfeld DL, Rawlinson K, Greenberg M. Perinatal outcome after multifetal reduction to twins compared with nonreduced multiple gestations. *Obstet Gynecol* 1991;78:763–7

3. Groutz A, Yovel I, Amit A, Yaron Y, Azem F, Lessing JB. Pregnancy outcome after multifetal pregnancy reduction to twins compared with spontaneously conceived twins. *Hum Reprod* 1996;11:1334–6

4. Wilcox LS, Kiely JL, Melvin CL, Martin MC. Assisted reproductive technologies: estimates of their contribution to multiple births and newborn hospital days in the United States. *Fertil Steril* 1996;65:361–6

5. Callahan TL, Hall JE, Ettner SL, Christiansen CL, Greene MF, Crowley WF Jr. The economic impact of multiple-gestation pregnancies and the contribution of assisted-reproduction techniques to their incidence. *N Engl J Med* 1994;331:244–9

6. Boklage CE. Survival probability of human conceptions from fertilization to term. *Int J Fertil* 1990;35:75, 79–80, 81–94

7. Houghton FD, Hawkhead JA, Humpherson PG, *et al*. Non-invasive amino acid turnover predicts human embryo developmental capacity. *Hum Reprod* 2002;17:999–1005

8. Almeida PA, Bolton VN. The relationship between chro mosomal abnormality in the human preimplantation embryo and development *in vitro*. *Reprod Fertil Dev* 1996;8:235–41

Acknowledgements

Sincere appreciation is extended to the physicians, nurses and support staff of the Institute for Reproductive Medicine of Weill Medical College of Cornell University/New York Hospital for their direct or indirect contribution to the work detailed in this book. Very special acknowledgement is given to the many hard-working embryologists and laboratory support staff at Cornell who make up a quite dedicated and unique team of professionals: Rosemary Berrios, Richard Bodine, Jose Bustamante, Robert Clarke, Carol Ann Cook, Margarita Fienco, June Hariprashad, Myriam Jackson, Deborah Liotta, Rose Moschini, Gianpiero Palermo, Jason Park, Patricia Pascal Roy, Takumi Takeuchi, Kangpu Xu and Zhen Ye, and our sadly missed friends, David Travassos and Eric Urcia.

We also thank Dr Michael Bedford and Mrs Pamela Sully of Weill Medical College for editorial assistance, and offer extreme gratitude to those who contributed photographic material or text: Dr Michal Amit, Dr David Becker, Dr Owen Davis, Dr David Gardner, Dr Kate Hardy, Drs Howard and Georgeanna Jones, Dr Hung-Chi Kuo, Dr Joseph Itskovitz-Eldor, Dr Michelle Lane, Dr Shoukhrat Mitalipov, Dr Zev Rosenwaks, Dr Sophie Spanos and Dr Don Wolf.

Most figures were photographed using a Nikon Diaphot TE300 microscope equipped with a Sony CatsEye DKC-5000 camera. Parthenon Publishing is responsible for the color matching and placement of selected photographs.

1 Overview of early human preimplantation development *in vitro*

Ovulation induction for assisted reproductive procedures

The cornerstone of successful assisted reproductive technology (ART) has been the ability to replace several selected preembryos from a larger cohort obtained following recruitment, harvest and fertilization of multiple oocytes. Thus, although the first successful human *in vitro* fertilization (IVF) pregnancy followed the retrieval of a single oocyte in a spontaneous menstrual cycle[1], current standard practice in ART programs worldwide entails the use of controlled ovarian hyperstimulation in order to maximize pregnancy rates. This strategy, while maximizing pregnancy rates, has also been associated with the inherent increased risks of multiple pregnancies. A wide variety of ovulation-inducing agents have been employed in the practice of ART, including clomiphene citrate, human menopausal gonadotropins (hMG), and recombinant gonadotropin preparations, with and without the adjunctive use of gonadotropin releasing hormone (GnRH) agonists and antagonists. Currently, the dominant approach to ovulation induction for IVF combines exogenous gonadotropins (hMG, purified follicle stimulating hormone (FSH) and recombinant FSH) with GnRH agonists.

Although clomiphene citrate was once extensively employed for ART, either as a single agent or in combination with gonadotropins, the current dominance of pure gonadotropin-based protocols was spurred by the premise that this approach is more physiological and might avoid the potentially detrimental effects of clomiphene on the oocytes and endometrium. Commercially available gonadotropin preparations include: hMG, formulated in ampules containing 75 IU each of FSH and luteinizing hormone (LH); purified FSH, containing 75 IU of FSH with less than 1 IU of LH and, more recently, recombinant FSH. Urinary-derived gonadotropins are heterogeneous with respect to glycosylation and the presence of degraded fragments, which can lead to varying biopotency among batches, whereas recombinant gonadotropins are uniform.

Over 2000 different GnRH agonists have been synthesized. Endogenous GnRH is rapidly degraded by cleavage at the Gly^6–Leu^7 and Pro^9–Gly^{10} positions, with a resultant half-life of less than 10 min. The selective substitution of amino acids at positions 6 and 10 of the GnRH molecule leads both to enhanced binding affinity to the GnRH receptor and decreased susceptibility to degradation by endopeptidases, thus prolonging the half-life and enhancing the biological activity of these agents. The pharmacological response to GnRH agonist administration is biphasic, with an initial surge of gonadotropin release from the adenohypophysis, but prolonged GnRH receptor occupancy results in desensitization and down-regulation of the gonadotropes, thus effecting reversible hypogonadism. The adjunctive use of GnRH agonists in IVF has several apparent advantages, including a reduction in the incidence of untimely LH surges and premature luteinization, the ability to program the initiation of stimulations so as to permit a more even distribution of a clinic's workload, and, most significantly, an overall improvement in IVF success rates, a finding confirmed by a published meta-analysis of randomized, controlled trials[2].

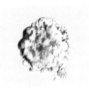

When applied to IVF, GnRH agonists may be administered either in a long or a short protocol. In the long protocol, currently favored by most centers, GnRH agonist treatment is initiated in the mid-luteal phase of the preceding menstrual cycle; pituitary down-regulation ensues within 5–10 days, and is indicated by the onset of menses. Gonadotropin therapy is then undertaken concurrently, typically commencing on cycle day 3 or once adequate suppression of estradiol is documented. The dosage of gonadotropins ranges from two to four ampules per day, with higher doses occasionally employed in patients predicted to have a poor response. The cycle is monitored with daily estradiol determinations commencing after 2–3 days of therapy; serial sonographic follicular measurements are performed once the estradiol exceeds a threshold level, generally by the sixth or seventh day of the cycle. The daily dosage of gonadotropins may be adjusted according to the individual patient's response, e.g. with a step-down once follicular recruitment has been achieved, in an effort to attain greater synchronization of follicular maturation and a reduced risk for the development of ovarian hyperstimulation syndrome. Appropriate timing of the ovulatory dose of human chorionic gonadotropin (hCG) is critical for the retrieval of an adequate number of optimally mature oocytes, and is determined by parameters including the mean diameter of the lead follicles (typically > 16 mm), the absolute estradiol level (e.g. > 500 pg/ml) and the pattern of estradiol rise and follicular growth. The GnRH agonist is discontinued on the day of hCG administration. The oocyte retrieval procedure, performed transvaginally with ultrasound guidance, is typically undertaken 34–36 h following the administration of hCG.

In the short or 'flare' GnRH agonist protocols, the agonist is initiated in the early follicular phase, usually on cycle day 2 or 3. Concurrent therapy with gonadotropins commences 1–3 days later. This approach exploits the agonist phase of GnRH agonist treatment, thus reducing the total dosage requirement for gonadotropins and shortening the duration of stimulation. Although both long and short protocols have their adherents, the former approach is more prevalent. More recently, GnRH antagonists have been introduced, which allow for late follicular suppression of the LH surge, eliminating the need for prolonged pretreatment down-regulation.

The goal of all ovulation induction protocols for ART is to permit the recruitment and harvest of an optimal number of preovulatory oocytes, so as to maximize clinical efficiency. Pregnancy rates may thus be optimized through the selection and transfer of a few of the 'best quality' preembryos, with the option of cryopreserving potentially viable conceptuses in excess of that number.

Gametes

In most species, there are just two types of gametes, and they are radically different. Apart from motor neurons with their remarkably long axons, the oocyte is among the largest cells of the human organism. Conversely, spermatozoa and red blood cells are two of the smallest.

The diameter of the mature human oocyte is approximately 110–115 μm, and it is bounded by a plasma membrane called the *oolemma*. Surrounding the oocyte/oolemma is a glycoprotein envelope called the *zona pellucida*, a structure approximately 15–20 μm wide (becoming a bit thinner after fertilization) that protects the oocyte during transport and fertilization. Between the oolemma and the zona pellucida is the fluid-filled *perivitelline space*. The use of this term persists despite its inaccuracy when describing the oocytes of humans or most other mammals; it acknowledges the word *vitellus*, a term traditionally used to describe the yolky substance of a hen's egg, which contains abundant nutrient reserves. The cytoplasm of the mammalian oocyte is usually referred to as the *ooplasm*, a more appropriate term for describing the living portion of the human gamete. The main organelles of the ooplasm are the mitochondria, the endoplasmic reticulum and the Golgi system.

When fully capable of undergoing a normal fertilization process, the secondary oocyte is briefly arrested in its course of maturation at metaphase II of meiosis. Nuclear maturation is usually closely attended by a general maturation of the cytoplasm, and is characterized by an increase in the number of organelles scattered throughout the ooplasm. The presence of a first polar body conveys that nuclear maturation has reached this stage. Along with the zona pellucida and perivitelline space, the total diameter of the mature human oocyte is approximately 150 μm.

An oocyte incubated with spermatozoa before reaching metaphase II may incorporate a spermatozoon into its ooplasm and yet fail to initiate events leading to sperm decondensation; such an oocyte ultimately lacks a functional male pronucleus[3]. One study examining 518 non-fertilized oocytes demonstrated that 22% had actually been penetrated by sperm, but without oocyte activation or pronuclear formation[4]. Many of these oocytes may have been immature when combined with spermatozoa.

Besides the requirement for nuclear maturation, it is believed that a brief period is necessary after extrusion of the first polar body for the oocyte to gain full cytoplasmic competence. An oocyte that is meiotically mature but slightly underdeveloped or overdeveloped with regard to its cytoplasm may be more apt to display one, three or more pronuclei. With immature cytoplasm, the cortical granule numbers and response may be inadequate; with postmature cytoplasm, cortical granule release may be inhibited owing to the inward migration of the granules towards the interior of the cell. In either instance, there is evidence that the zona reaction is also often poorly functional when the sperm–oocyte interaction is not appropriately timed with regard to oocyte nuclear and cytoplasmic maturity[5].

Oocytes collected for IVF are generally surrounded by several layers of cells, which define the *cumulus oophorus*. Cells of the cumulus are instrumental, via gap junctions, in nurturing the oocyte during growth and possibly in passing inhibiting factors (e.g. cyclic adenosine monophosphate (cAMP)) necessary for deterring the resumption of meiosis[6]. The innermost layer of cells is called the *corona* or *coronal layer*. This layer expands and presents a radiant pattern as oocytes mature in response to exogenous hCG or a mid-cycle surge of LH. Near ovulation, as they loosen and expand, cumulus cells are observed to retract from the zona pellucida of the oocyte, presumably cutting off the previously important cellular–oocyte communication. It has been proposed that oocytes not associated with proliferative cellular changes near ovulation have very limited potential for implantation, despite fertilization and apparently normal development *in vitro*[7].

In most mammalian species studied *in vivo*, the oocyte arrives at the site of fertilization in the ampulla of the Fallopian tube still surrounded by the cumulus mass. The cumulus may play a role in assisting transport of the oocyte into the Fallopian tube through fimbrial cilia–cumulus cell contact. Another possible use of the cumulus after oocyte maturation is that its radially arranged cells help to guide spermatozoa towards the oocyte just before fertilization; however, there is no hard evidence for this speculation. Break-up of the cumulus mass is brought about by dissolution of its mucoid

hyaluronic acid matrix by enzymes released by the spermatozoa.

Follicular *membrana granulosa cells* disassociated from cumulus cells are found in follicular aspirates collected for IVF. The number of cells collected will vary from follicle to follicle according to the extent of negative pressure exerted during suction, the size of the needle and the overall maturity of the follicle. As with cumulus cells, the correlation between morphological aspects of free granulosa cells and oocyte nuclear maturity is not exact, but mature-appearing cells (large, well-dispersed cells) are generally collected along with mature oocytes, and immature-appearing cells (smaller, tightly packed cells) along with immature oocytes. Follicular membrana granulosa cells may be assessed at the time of oocyte harvest to aid in the evaluation of follicular maturity. They are subsequently often used during *in vitro* studies to examine metabolic activity or steroid synthesis.

The oocyte observed while its chromosomes are at metaphase I of maturation requires some time in culture before attaining full meiotic competence[8]. More than 98% of these oocytes will complete their journey towards metaphase II and first polar body extrusion. Oocytes with chromosomes at prophase I of maturation are truly immature; more than 80% of these will continue through metaphase I to metaphase II if isolated and incubated in an appropriate medium for 24 h.

Assessment of maturity

Traditionally, evaluation of oocyte maturity has been based upon the expansion and radiance of the cumulus–corona complex which surrounds the harvested oocyte[9,10]. With this assessment, oocytes are rapidly categorized as mature (correlated to metaphase II of maturation) when they possess an expanded and luteinized cumulus matrix and a radiant or *sun-burst* corona radiata. A less-expanded cumulus–corona complex denotes an intermediate stage of maturity (correlated to metaphase I of maturation), and absence of expanded cumulus is generally associated with immaturity (correlated to prophase I of maturation). While this type of analysis usually closely approximates the true nuclear status of the oocyte, it is too often imprecise, and may lead to subsequent laboratory errors in the handling of gametes. In fact, nuclear maturation of the oocyte and cellular maturation of the cumulus are frequently disparate[11-15]. When disparity occurs,

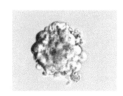

immature oocytes may be inseminated prematurely, and fail to produce a favorable outcome. As well as fertilization failure, other detrimental side-effects accompany combining sperm and eggs at suboptimal times; ovulation-induction protocols may not be suitably appraised and male factor issues become difficult to interpret, based on poor fertilization results.

Because of these pitfalls, techniques have been developed to assess more accurately the meiotic status of the oocyte. A systematic approach can be used to produce a *maturation score* by grading the size of the follicle, expansion of the cumulus mass, radiance of the corona cells, size/cohesiveness of associated membrana granulosa cells and shape/color of the oocyte itself, if visible within the mass of surrounding cellular investments. Alternatively, frank visualization of the oocyte and its germinal vesicle or first polar body can be attempted by spreading out the cumulus mass, or by removing it altogether with the aid of enzymes.

If clearly visible or denuded of cells, oocytes are classified according to the presence or absence of first polar bodies/germinal vesicles, and are inseminated/injected accordingly:

Metaphase II (MII) First polar body present, no germinal vesicle; inseminated or injected 3–5 h after collection;

Metaphase I (MI) No first polar body, no germinal vesicle; inseminated or injected 1–5 h after extrusion of the first polar body;

Prophase I (PI) Germinal vesicle present; inseminated or injected 26–29 h after collection.

Our experience has been that oocytes collected at more advanced stages of *in vivo* maturation demonstrate the greatest ability to form two pronuclei after insemination[8,9,11]. Fertilization rates drop only slightly when oocytes require a period of 5–15 h in culture before extruding the first polar body, but fertilization is markedly reduced when more than 15 h pass before the maturational process is completed. The reason for this is probably related to sperm functionality as well as oocyte maturity, since processed sperm may be more than 24 h old before being placed with an early MI or PI oocyte. Under these conditions, the precise cause of the lower incidence of fertilization of very immature oocytes is difficult to interpret[8].

If small follicles are punctured, approximately 20–30% of oocytes collected for IVF are meiotically immature at the time of harvest from the ovary. This is undoubtedly due to the stimulation of multiple follicles during clinical ovulation induction, some large and well-vascularized, and some small with late recruitment: If all oocytes are placed with sperm at the same time, a proportion slightly higher than this percentage will fail to become fertilized normally. Logically enough, when oocytes are placed with sperm only as they have reached full maturity, far better fertilization results are attained.

The incidence of abnormal fertilization (one pronucleus, three or more pronuclei) is not different between MII oocytes and MI or PI oocytes that have matured in culture before insemination or injection[8-10]. Pregnancy potential after the transfer of preembryos developed from MII and MI oocytes is similar, regardless of whether 0 or 20 h has been required for maturation before insemination or injection[16]. Only preembryos developing from PI oocytes demonstrate a significantly reduced potential for implantation and live birth, although such births are certainly within the realm of possibility[17-20].

Metaphase II oocyte

The MII oocyte (Figure 1.1) is often termed *mature*, *ripened* or *preovulatory*, vague descriptions that fail to specify the exact meiotic status of the gamete. This oocyte is at a resting stage of meiosis II after extrusion of the first polar body and direct passage to MII. Chromosomes are divided between the oocyte and the polar body (23 chromosomes, 46 chromatids, 2n DNA in each), those in the oocyte being attached to spindle microtubules[3] (Figure 1.2).

For a while after its formation, the first polar body remains connected to the oocyte by the meiotic spindle, forming a cytoplasmic bridge. Chromosomes within the first polar body may remain clumped together, may undergo a second meiotic division or may scatter within the cytoplasm; generally a nucleus is not formed[3,21]. The first polar body contains cortical granules because of its extrusion before sperm penetration and cortical granule release; in the oocyte, 1–3 layers of cortical granules are present at the periphery. Under the microscope, the oocyte is characterized by its round, even shape and displays an ooplasm of light color and homogeneous granularity. It is usually associated with an expanded, luteinized cumulus and a *sun-burst* corona radiata. Membrana granulosa cells harvested along with the MII oocyte are loosely aggregated, with mature features[8,10,14,20].

Metaphase I oocyte

The MI oocyte (Figure 1.3) is considered *nearly mature* or *intermediate* in maturation. The oocyte has completed prophase of meiosis I; the germinal vesicle and its nucleolus have faded and disappeared. During this stage a spindle forms, and recombined maternal and paternal chromosomes line up randomly towards the poles. Later, at telophase, whole chromosomes sort independently to oocyte or first polar body.

An MI oocyte requires 1–24 h in culture before reaching full maturity. Those needing less than 15 h are considered *late* in maturity, while those requiring more than 15 h are defined as early[8–11,14,15].

Under the microscope, the MI oocyte is characterized by the absence of both germinal vesicle and first polar body. A late MI oocyte is round and even in form, with homogeneously granular and light-colored ooplasm. Early MI oocytes may display minor central granularity. Mature-appearing cumulus cells are usually associated with late stages.

Because first polar body extrusion can occur at any time after harvest, it is necessary to examine the oocyte at regular intervals to determine the correct timing for insemination. If sperm are placed with the oocyte before nuclear and cytoplasmic maturation are complete, they generally fail to decondense within the ooplasm, or abnormal fertilization occurs. If insemination is delayed too long, *in vitro* aging may follow, with similar undesired consequences[3,8] (Figures 1.4 and 1.5).

Prophase I oocyte

The PI oocyte (Figure 1.6) is often termed *immature* or *unripened*. It possesses a tetraploid amount of DNA owing to the presence of 46 double-stranded chromosomes. This oocyte begins to mature in response to gonadotropin surges and reduction in follicular maturation-inhibiting factors. The germinal vesicle, which persisted throughout earlier growth phases, begins its progression to germinal vesicle breakdown (GVBD) and the oocyte enlarges. Most PI oocytes collected for IVF have been stimulated to resume meiosis, are in the final stages of the first meiotic prophase and have already reached full size. If a spermatozoon penetrates this immature oocyte, it will fail to promote activation since the oocyte is not meiotically mature, and its chromosomes will undergo

premature condensation[22]. GVBD may occur within minutes or require up to several hours after harvest; the length of time appears to depend on how far maturational events have progressed within the follicle before collection. More than 80% will succeed in passing through MI of maturation, ultimately to reach MII.

The germinal vesicle, or nucleus, of the human oocyte is spherical and contains a large, refractile, exocentric nucleolus. Upon close examination, a second smaller nucleolus may be detected. The germinal vesicle is centrally located within the ooplasm of young PI oocytes and in those that exhibit developmental arrest. It migrates to a more cortical position in healthy oocytes before GVBD. The dissolution of the germinal vesicle marks the first practical microscopic indication that meiosis has resumed. As the oocyte matures, defenses against polyspermy are established in the form of cortical granule accumulation and alignment at the oocyte periphery. These granules are sparse and discontinuous in immature oocytes[3].

Under the microscope, the PI oocyte is characterized by its distinct germinal vesicle and refractile nucleolus. An irregular shape, darkened center and granular ooplasm are almost always displayed. Attached cumulus cells are usually compact and multilayered, but may be proliferative. Free follicular membrana granulosa cells within the immature follicle are usually small and appear in compact masses. PI oocytes with very mature characteristics of the cumulus (expanded appearance and very radiant corona) generally fail to undergo GVBD.

The sperm-penetrated human oocyte

Fertilization process

Human fertilization begins when a spermatozoon, with its haploid number of chromosomes, passes through oocyte cellular investments and makes contact with the protective zona pellucida that surrounds the oocyte. This contact induces an acrosomal reaction whereby the spermatozoon releases the contents of its acrosomal vesicle, including enzymes that aid the sperm in digesting its way through the zona to the oocyte plasma membrane. The equatorial segment of the sperm head attaches to the plasma membrane of the oocyte, and sperm incorporation occurs through a process similar to phagocytosis. Only acrosome-reacted sperm are believed

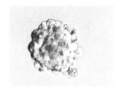

to be capable of fusing with the oolemma of the oocyte. Spermatozoon–oolemma fusion is bypassed when performing intracytoplasmic sperm injection (ICSI) to assist the fertilization process.

It has been reported that, under *in vitro* insemination conditions, spermatozoa transverse oocyte cellular investments by 3 h, and first appear in the oocyte cortex by 4 h. Of interest is that oocytes need to be incubated with spermatozoa for only 1 h to achieve fertilization outcomes similar to 16-h controls[23].

Fusion of gametes invokes a cascade of events that are initiated by the hydrolysis of phosphatidylinositol biphosphate in the oolemma[24]. Electrical changes occur on the oolemma, and intracellular calcium levels rise in the oocyte. Cortical granule exocytosis from the ooplasmic periphery causes a chemical alteration of the zona pellucida, which generally renders it impermeable to other sperm. Thus, the oocyte is said to become *activated* by its fusion with the spermatozoon. It completes its second meiotic division; 23 double-stranded chromosomes split at their centromeres, and chromatids separate to oocyte or second polar body. In this manner, a haploid number of chromosomes and a haploid amount of DNA are contributed by the oocyte. Activation does not necessarily require the stimulus of a spermatozoon. Oocytes can be activated through mechanical trauma, temperature shock, chemical stimulus or electrical signals. Oocytes are commonly activated during ICSI procedures by simply piercing the oolemma, or by aggressively disturbing the ooplasm.

Within a few hours, male and female pronuclei are formed from the sperm and oocyte chromatin (Figure 1.7). The stage at which pronuclei are visible is termed the *pronuclear stage*, and the specimen is defined as a *prezygote* or *ootid*. Technically, the *zygote* has not yet formed (*see* Glossary). During pronuclear formation, the zygotic centrosome is assembled; centrosomal proteins and sperm aster microtubules gather around the sperm centriole. This assembly of the zygotic centrosome is a crucial step for subsequent pronuclear apposition and genomic union[25]. Pronuclei come in close contact, eventually lose their apposed pronuclear membranes and enter into syngamy (Figure 1.8).

This final event of the fertilization process involves the reorganization and pairing of maternal and paternal chromosomes and formation of the zygote. Recall that the mixing of maternal and paternal gamete chromosomes during meiosis I results in a mathematical probability of more than eight million possible chromosome combinations (2^{23}) for each gamete. If each parent has this many combinations possible, a couple could produce more than 7×10^{13} offspring with different combinations of parental chromosomes. This astronomic number does not take into consideration the additional genetic variability generated by crossing-over events that occur during meiosis I. Without crossing-over, gene combinations on a given chromosome would remain coupled indefinitely. With crossing-over, the theoretical possibility of creating genetically different offspring after fertilization reaches 80^{23}. This is why it is impossible, or nearly so, for any two individuals apart from monozygotic twins (or, in this age, clones) to be genetically identical.

There is a brief period after pronuclei breakdown during which the zygote remains single-celled. In the human, the nearly 24-h long fertilization process is completed with the initiation of the first (mitotic) cleavage.

Block to polyspermy

One consequence of sperm–oolemma fusion is the exocytosis of cortical granules from the oocyte periphery. This release, occurring within minutes of fusion, is a key component of the oocyte's strategy for preventing polyspermy. The dispersal of cortical granule contents into the perivitelline space is followed by a chemical alteration of the zona pellucida, an event often termed *zona hardening* or the *zona reaction*. Before fusion, the zona exhibits a porous appearance, and comprises a large number of ring-shaped structures called *hoops*, randomly superimposed in several layers; pore diameters decrease in size towards the inside of the zona. After fusion, the zona is observed to be more compact and its diameter decreases slightly; hoops are not distinguished and pores are obliterated by an amorphous material emerging from the inner zona[26]. The zona reaction may render the zona pellucida impenetrable by other sperm, or may cause secondary sperm to become entrapped in its altered matrix, unable to pass the highly condensed inner layer of the zona. A slow or incomplete cortical granule exocytosis and zona reaction may represent the most common causes of polyspermic fertilization. Premature or failed cortical granule discharge may be responsible for some instances of failed fertilization after standard insemination.

It has been postulated that human oocytes do not possess a true block to polyspermy at the level of the oolemma[27]. This theory is supported by a study that retrospectively examined the polyspermy rate in over 3000 human oocytes subjected to subzonal insemination techniques (SUZI) when 1–20 sperm were placed under their zonae. The authors concluded that all sperm possessing fertilizing ability were indeed capable of fusing with the oocyte cell membrane, indicating the absence of a polyspermic block at this level[28]. However, in another experiment where zona-free human oocytes were exposed to high concentrations of sperm, it appeared that sperm were not able to penetrate oocytes indiscriminately at rates that would be expected[29]. At 30 min, an average of 1.3 sperm had penetrated the oocytes, and, at 60 min, 2.9 had been successful. The number of penetrating sperm peaked at 2 h, regardless of sperm concentration. In addition, sperm demonstrated a reduced ability to bind to membranes of previously fertilized oocytes, few or none binding to the membranes of 4-cell preembryos. These authors concluded that the oolemma does, in fact, play a role in preventing polyspermy and that a plasma membrane block may involve permanent changes to sperm binding/fusion ability. Based on these and other conflicting reports[30], one can only conclude that, for the time being, the question of a membrane block in the human remains unresolved.

Commonly, 5–10% of oocytes cultured *in vitro* are observed to incorporate more than one spermatozoon, as evidenced by the subsequent development of three or more pronuclei. The reported frequency in the literature ranges from as low as 1–2% after inseminating mature oocytes[23,31] to greater than 30% after inseminating immature oocytes[32]. Some investigators have found a high correlation between triploidy and inseminating sperm concentration; as early as 1986, one such study reported a tripling of polyspermy with increasing sperm concentrations[33]. Others have reported that the incidence of abnormal fertilization is no higher when oocytes are exposed to large numbers of sperm[15,34]. Although it is tempting to try to correlate polyspermic fertilization to the unnaturally high numbers of spermatozoa used for standard insemination *in vitro*, it has been our observation that this incidence is better correlated to oocyte maturity and viability than to gross numbers of inseminating spermatozoa. Approximately 4–5% of mature oocytes exhibit three pronuclei after the injection of a single sperm during ICSI procedures (they are largely *digynic*), indicating a relatively high occurrence of second polar body suppression at meiosis II. Although one cannot dismiss the possibility that the ICSI procedure itself is instrumental in causing this, and

although the possibility exists that a sperm possessing two nuclei was injected, digynic fertilization has been noted often enough after natural intercourse and *in vitro* insemination to suggest that it is not restricted to assisted fertilization techniques. Most late-term triploid fetuses and live-born triploid children have been shown to have developed from digynic preembryos[35,36]. Moreover, recent studies confirm that digyny is clearly the most common origin of triploidy in the human[37]. These studies indicate that oocyte factors are commonly accountable for triploid fertilization.

Which oocyte factors might this include? Certainly, oocyte aging has been shown to be associated with an increased incidence of spindle defects; retention of chromosomes within the ooplasm after suppression of first or second polar body extrusion may represent one possible mechanism for digyny. Oocytes that are postmature (aged) have been shown to exhibit a centripetal migration of their cortical granules when analyzed under the electron microscope[3,38]. These would trigger a retarded zona reaction at best, which could result in multiple sperm fusion during fertilization. Conversely, oocyte immaturity has been implicated in contributing to polyspermic fertilization, presumably due to delayed cortical granule release[39]. Poor *in vitro* culture conditions may be implicated in some cases of spindle damage if oocytes are allowed to chill for long periods[40], or overheat. Additionally, mature oocytes may develop from binucleate primary oocytes.

In all probability, polyspermy results from different mechanisms, or combinations of different mechanisms, in different oocytes. In some oocytes, immaturity or postmaturity may be implicated, or oocytes may be intrinsically abnormal. In others, minute cracks may be present in the zona pellucida after oocyte harvest procedures, allowing for multiple sperm entry. In others still, entry of two sperm may simply be a random event that occurs when two sperm simultaneously make their way through the zona and concurrently fuse with the oolemma; whether the odds for this happening increase in the presence of high numbers of motile spermatozoa remains to be elucidated.

Male and female pronuclei

Male and female pronuclei (Figure 1.9) are usually formed simultaneously; the male pronucleus forms near the site of sperm entry, and the female originates at the ooplasmic pole of the meiotic spindle[41]. These structures,

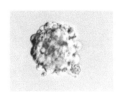

although small and faint, may be visualized as early as 4 h after ICSI or 5–6 h after insemination. The male pronucleus may be somewhat larger in humans[5], but the difference in some specimens is difficult, if not impossible, to discern under the light microscope. When one group of investigators attempted to distinguish pronuclear gender by using morphological criteria under the light microscope, they observed sperm tail remnants in only 3/342 pronucleate oocytes; furthermore, pronuclear diameter and position within the ooplasm failed to yield any informative distinctions between male and female pronuclei[42].

Early in their formation, pronuclei may be seen at a distance from each other; later, they migrate together towards the center of the cell. By 15 h after insemination, pronuclei are most often observed lying close to one another; they may present a 'figure of 8' appearance if viewed in an overlapping position. Although they appear to contact or fuse, transmission electron microscopy has demonstrated that they remain separated by a narrow strip of ooplasm that may contain mitochondria and elements of smooth endoplasmic reticulum, or be altogether absent of organelles[27,38,43]. As male and female pronuclei become closely associated, adjacent areas of each appear to flatten out. During the same time, nucleoli move from random locations within each pronucleus to line up at the regions of juxtaposition. One to nine nucleoli can be observed in each structure, the smaller pronucleus often demonstrating a lower number.

Pronuclei are surrounded by a dense aggregation of cellular organelles, which may appear granular or even darkened under the light microscope. The female pronucleus often dismantles its envelope and undergoes membrane breakdown slightly ahead of the male[44]. During the human pronuclear phase, DNA synthesis within male and female pronuclei begins synchronously at about 12 h after sperm–oocyte fusion. Errors of DNA synthesis may be responsible for developmental arrest at the pronuclear stage; it may be that pronuclear membranes require signalling of DNA replication before dismantling.

In one elegant study, oocytes in the process of fertilization were monitored for up to 20 h by time-lapse video cinematography following ICSI[45]. Fertilization patterns in 50 oocytes followed a defined course of events, but varied markedly in timing between individual prezygotes. The investigators described a circular wave of granulation moving throughout the cytoplasm that

lasted for approximately 20–53 min. Granulation occurred in cortical regions of the oocyte and moved in 2–10 full circular rotations, some clockwise, and some counter-clockwise. During this active phase, the sperm head decondensed. This was followed by extrusion of the second polar body and central development of the male pronucleus. After polar body extrusion (mean time from injection, 2.5 h), the granulation wave ceased in all oocytes. At the same time, or just after male pronucleus formation, the female pronucleus was seen to form near the site of second polar body extrusion, which was not always near the site of first polar body extrusion; it was gradually drawn towards the male pronucleus until the two abutted. Both pronuclei were then observed to increase in size and to contain moving nucleoli, some of which coalesced over time. During the period of pronuclear growth, cytoplasmic organelles were seen to migrate inwardly to the center of the oocyte, leaving a clear zone at the cortex. Measurements confirmed that the female pronucleus was indeed smaller than the male pronucleus in these specimens (22.4 μm vs. 24.1 μm, respectively), and possessed fewer nucleoli (4.2 vs. 7.0). It was discovered that subsequent preembryo quality, as judged by morphology and developmental rate, was correlated to sequential timing of events and duration of the cytoplasmic granulation wave, good preembryos showing uniform (though not necessarily more rapid) progression and longer granulation waves. It was interesting to note in this series that pronuclei could be identified as early as 3 h post-injection and that, by 5 h, over half of the oocytes possessed visible, small pronuclear structures. In this fascinating study, the existence of the cytoplasmic granulation wave proved to be a novel and unique finding.

Without video cinematography, the embryologist must rely on the presence and number of pronuclei, assessed during one or two brief examinations, to determine whether or not normal fertilization is ongoing. Practical criteria for sperm penetration in living material include first, observation of two pronuclei at 10–18 h post-insemination, and second, visualization of two polar bodies in the perivitelline space. Assessment of these two parameters is rapid and simple. Unfortunately, the identification of two pronuclei cannot ensure a normal fertilization process and does not guarantee that one pronucleus is of paternal, and one is of maternal, origin. Evaluating second polar bodies is also potentially misleading because of first polar body fragmentation. Yet another serious drawback to using a single observation to assess pronuclear number lies in the fact that counts have been observed to change during the pronuclear period; most embryologists can relate instances of visualizing two pronuclei in an oocyte at an initial observation and one pronucleus (or three pronuclei) during a follow-up evaluation, or vice versa. While pronuclear and polar body determination is not ideal for the assessment of sperm penetration, it does provide the most useful and least time consuming means of clinical evaluation. Perhaps one day we will be evaluating all fertilized oocytes as described by Dianna Payne's time-lapse video study[45]; until then, less informative methods will have to suffice.

Chromosomes and fertilization

Fusion between male and female gametes is not always successful, even under optimal conditions. When investigating causes of fertilization failure, gamete maturity and genetic health emerge as two important factors related to fertilizing potential. In one study carried out to examine fertilization failure in 293 oocytes inseminated *in vitro*, it was discovered that 30% of the oocytes were not fully mature at the time of sperm–oocyte interaction (chromosomes at MI or PI of maturation), and a full 59% were chromosomally abnormal[46]. Figures like these are often reported in the scientific literature, making it evident that a large proportion of human gametes are genetically incompetent to generate normal offspring.

Gamete immaturity represents less of a problem now than it did when we began trying to optimize our IVF techniques many years ago. Certainly, ovarian stimulation regimes have been refined in the past 20 years, so that virtually all our patients produce healthy, mature oocytes. We have also been mildly successful in clinically applying *in vitro* maturation methods. Healthy babies have been generated from germinal vesicle-bearing immature oocytes collected from stimulated cycles[20,47] and unstimulated cycles[17,18]. Unfortunately, implantation rates are not in the range expected from *in vivo* matured oocytes.

Immature spermatozoa have generated considerable interest in recent years as well. Almost unthinkable two decades ago, the time has arrived when investigators are reporting the use of haploid round and elongated spermatids in the clinical treatment of azoospermia[48,49], and healthy children have been conceived[50–52]. It now appears, based on experiments in the mouse, that injecting secondary spermatocytes will prove to be a future treatment modality; incredibly, normal offspring have been reported as being born after these cells completed meiosis II within oocytes, following injection and electroactivation. The extra set of chromosomes was extruded into the perivitelline space as an extra (male) polar body[53].

The fact that many gametes are genetically abnormal must account for much of the failed fertilization we observe in our programs. If we are to accept earnestly the many reports describing very high percentages of chromosome abnormalities in sperm, eggs and developing preembryos, it seems a wonder that we are managing so well to overpopulate the earth. It is well documented that chromosomal abnormalities among first-trimester spontaneous abortions occur at a rate of about 60%[54]. As well, it has been estimated that more than one-quarter of oocytes that fail fertilization[55,56] and up to 10% of spermatozoa carry a chromosomal aberration[57]. A review of the literature led one investigator to conclude that at least 50% of conceptuses developing after natural conception are chromosomally abnormal[58].

Males with non-mosaic Klinefelter's syndrome (47,XXY) are now capable of fathering children if even one or two mature or maturing sperm cells can be isolated from testicular tissue and used in assisted fertilization procedures. Whether the very presence of spermatozoa or spermatids in the testicular tissue indicates mosaicism in germ cell-lines must be investigated further. Several cases have been reported thus far showing normal karyotypes of preembryos generated from men without evidence of mosaicism in peripheral blood cells. In one report, after performing preimplantation genetic diagnosis on five preembryos from three Klinefelter's individuals, all were found to be chromosomally normal[59]. In our own program, the first report of a Klinefelter's birth was presented in 1998[60]. A healthy, unaffected male child was delivered in this instance. Since then, seven other ongoing clinical pregnancies have been established using testicular spermatozoa from husbands with presumed non-mosaic Klinefelter's syndrome. Three additional male children and seven female children have been delivered, inclusive of three twin sets. All of the children are healthy and perfectly normal in regard to their karyotypes. Through efforts such as these, we are continually learning more about the complex stages of reproduction. Perhaps no other branch of science is quite so interesting as the exploration of this fundamental life-generating process.

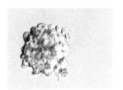

The cleaving human preembryo: 2-cell to 16-cell stage

Cytokinesis

Cytoplasmic division following nuclear replication and segregation is a universal characteristic of all cells. Cleavage of the human preembryo involves a series of mitotic divisions of the cytoplasm, every 12–18 h, without any discernible increase in its overall size (Figure 1.10). Failing to progress to the first cleavage after forming two pronuclei is relatively uncommon, occurring in less than or equal to 5% of normally fertilized oocytes[61]. As in most mammals, other than some rodents, the human sperm centrosome controls the first mitotic divisions after fertilization has taken place[62].

As the first cleavage mitosis reaches telophase, the cytoplasm of the zygote elongates and the surface contracts around the lesser circumference. This constriction continues until the zygote is divided into two blastomeres. The same process continues throughout all subsequent mitotic cell divisions[21] (Figures 1.11 and 1.12). It has been estimated that mean blastomere volume is reduced by approximately 28.5% per division through the first three cleavages, and that some diversity normally exists between the volumes of sister blastomeres[63]. The 2–8-cell conceptus depends largely on the translation of stored maternal RNA for cleavage.

Morphology

The quality of 2–16-cell preembryos produced after IVF is variable. Many contain multiple cellular fragments or unequally sized blastomeres, or exhibit slow cell-doubling times. Fragments arise because blastomeres constantly change shape, making and breaking cell contacts during cleavage; in doing so they can leave behind cellular debris[3]. This constant, living motion is particularly apparent when specimens are viewed under time-lapse cinematography where continuous pulsing, formation of fragments and blebs, and cytoplasmic reorganization is noted (personal observation). Human and primate preembryos may be more disposed to these actions, since fragments are rarely seen in the conceptuses of other mammals. Because preembryos flushed from the uterine cavity after fertilization *in vivo* also exhibit fragments, it can be deduced that *in vitro* culture methods are not solely responsible for aberrant development. We certainly observe in our laboratories that preembryos exhibiting large numbers of anucleate fragments tend to implant less frequently. This may be the result of a reduction in the available cytoplasm for normal cell division that subsequently leads to reduced cell numbers in the blastocyst. Alternatively, numerous fragments may interfere with the process of *compaction* by making intimate cell-to-cell contact difficult.

Cytoplasmic fragments often arise during the first cleavage. In studying the frequency of this observation at 24 h post-insemination, we found that when excessive numbers of fragments form so early, subsequent development of the preembryo is generally impaired. On the other hand, the development of small fragments after the first division usually has no detrimental effect on the cleaving conceptus.

Extensive cytoplasmic fragmentation has been associated with impending preembryo death. After studying fragmented preembryos and comparing them to non-fragmented controls, Jurisicova and colleagues concluded that the high incidence of condensed chromatin, degraded DNA, cell corpses and apoptotic bodies commonly found in fragmented conceptuses almost certainly indicate a reduced potential for continued growth[64]. This contention is supported by the experience of most embryologists and physicians working in assisted reproduction programs, who observe lower implantation rates associated with irregular blastomeres and excessive fragmentation, although some preembryos with these qualities retain the capacity for implanting normally[65]. Shulman and co-workers reported that the implantation potential of transferred day-2 or -3 preembryos can be directly correlated to morphological parameters, and suggested that the number of preembryos replaced be balanced against their grade to reduce multiple gestation[66].

Rates of cleavage

Many reports have linked normal cell-doubling times to preembryo viability, finding that slowly growing conceptuses demonstrate a markedly impaired capacity to implant after intrauterine transfer. The cell-doubling time in human preembryos between days 2 and 6 has been reported to be 31 h, with accelerated doubling noted after the first two divisions[67]. At first glance, these rates seem quite slow. During IVF treatment, one generally sees doubling in well under 24 h (2-cell stage by 24 h, 4-cell stage before 48 h, and 8-cell stage or more before 72 h), perhaps averaging every 18–20 h in healthy preembryos. However, it is not unreasonable to conclude that 31 h might represent the average doubling time if poor-quality and slowly growing and arrested preembryos are also calculated into the mean.

In 1987, Claman and associates reported that 21/23 ongoing IVF pregnancies arose from transfers where at least one preembryo had reached the 4-cell stage by 40 h post-insemination[68]. Other reports have similarly concluded that preembryos with slow cleavage (fewer than four blastomeres at 42–44 h post-insemination) were less likely to produce a pregnancy[69,70]. McKiernan and Bavister demonstrated in the hamster that faster-cleaving preembryos not only lead to more morulae and blastocysts in culture, but that subsequent *in vivo* development of faster-growing conceptuses is associated with a higher incidence of viable fetuses[71]. These last authors suggest that the timely completion of the third cell cycle (8-cell stage) is a critical and favorable factor for predicting successful embryogenesis in the hamster. Regular cleavage to the 8-cell stage has also been noted as being a favorable observation in the human, but often proves to be an inexact tool for predicting implantation success when used as a single analytical parameter. Despite this, it has been proposed that developmental rate may be more important than morphology when weighing individual factors for human intrauterine transfer[72]. Some groups report that accelerated preembryonic growth combined with minimal fragmentation leads to increased pregnancy[73]. Yet other studies associate the occurrence of a timely first cleavage (before 25 h post-insemination) with enhanced pregnancy outcome[74].

Factors other than fragmentation and growth rate have also been associated with the implantation potential of human preembryos. These include zona pellucida thickness and/or variation in thickness, thin and variable being better[75–77], adequate blastomere expansion[76] and absence of multinucleation[78]. In addition, studies on follicular blood flow have demonstrated a high correlation between dissolved oxygen content in the follicle (greater than or equal to 3%) and subsequent normal development of the oocyte/preembryo[79–81].

On a practical basis, 2-cell conceptuses are observed any time after 20 h post-insemination, usually around 24 h, and may persist until 42 h post-insemination. Viable 4-cell preembryos are observed between 36 and 60 h post-insemination. Eight-cell stages are not generally seen until after 54 h, but usually before 72 h. In the human, seeing 3-, 5- and 7-cell preembryos is not uncommon, particularly when the examination is carried out during mitotic cell division. This sometimes asynchronous division persists throughout cleavage of the early conceptus, and any number of blastomeres can be noted in a given observation. Interestingly, in some strains of mice and cows, male preembryos cleave faster than female ones[82]. There have been reports that this may be true for human preembryos as well[83], although not all investigators have confirmed this finding[84].

In normally fertilized specimens, retarded growth (no doubling in 24 h) often indicates reduced viability, but accelerated cleavage (doubling in 12 h) may not necessarily reflect a healthier conceptus[9]. Occasionally, pregnancies are established with slowly growing preembryos, even those found to possess only 6–8 blastomeres at 96 h. In the Cornell program, intrauterine transfer is usually postponed for 1 day whenever preembryos are observed to possess fewer than five blastomeres on day 3. If any further cleavage occurs over the next 24 h, transfer is carried out; if no further cleavage occurs, transfer is cancelled. It has been surprising to note the number of pregnancies resulting from the transfer of 6- or 8-celled preembryos on day 4.

A conceptus exhibiting three pronuclei may appear to cleave at an accelerated rate to the morula stage, at which time its development is usually arrested[61]. This is because many triploid zygotes split directly into three cells at the first cleavage because they possess a tripolar spindle; subsequent divisions reflect the higher overall cell number in the conceptus, not more rapid growth.

Preembryo grading schemes (days 2–3 post-insemination)

As a result of the reported correlations between morphology and pregnancy, embryologists generally use some sort of grading scheme to document the presumptive quality of transferred preembryos. Most of these schemes are related to the extent of observed cytoplasmic fragmentation and growth rate, but some include other factors such as zona pellucida thickness or blastomere size and regularity. Usually, a grade is assigned to the transfer based on the morphology of the highest-grade preembryo in the group, with additional fractions added or subtracted for appropriate growth or for the concurrent transfer of other exceptional conceptuses. Some groups will attempt to calculate an

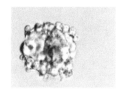

average score for the cohort of transferred preembryos, based on the assigned grades of each individual preembryo, but these systems tend to be less informative when wide disparity exists between conceptuses, distorting the meaningfulness of an averaged final figure.

In one early scoring system, a morphological grade of 1–4 was given to each preembryo and then combined with a grade developed from direct comparison to ideal growth rate. Using this two-stage system, the scores proved to be of value in predicting clinical success[85]. Similarly, in 1987, Puissant and colleagues published the results of grading preembryos based on their number of anucleate fragments and rate of division[86]. It was found that those preembryos endowed with high grades contributed more often to pregnancy and multiple pregnancy. These authors recommended that, if grading scores are high in conjunction with optimal clinical parameters, fewer preembryos should be transferred to offset high multiple pregnancy rates.

A three-grade scoring system was evaluated by Erenus and associates in 1991[87]. Grade 1 preembryos represented those with equal-sized blastomeres and no fragmentation, grade 2 included preembryos with unequal-sized blastomeres and grade 3 included preembryos associated with cytoplasmic fragments. In cycles where the best preembryo transferred was grade 1, 22% achieved clinical pregnancy. This was compared to grades 2 and 3, where pregnancy rates were 13% and 0%, respectively. Additionally, pregnancy rates increased with the transfer of multiple grade 1 preembryos (40% with three grade 1 preembryos).

In 1992, Steer and co-workers developed a cumulative grading system in an effort not only to predict pregnancy outcome, but also potentially to reduce high-order gestation in the Bourne Hall and Hallam programs[88]. With this system, the morphological grade of each preembryo (1–4; larger number associated with better morphology) was multiplied by the preembryo's number of blastomeres. The sum of grades from all conceptuses transferred on day 2 after insemination represented the final score. It was retrospectively analyzed that pregnancy rates in women under age 36 years rose as the cumulative score increased to a maximum of 42. A continued increase above this number did not contribute further to establishing pregnancy, but did impact upon the multiple pregnancy rate. They estimated that, using this system prospectively, 78% of triplet and 100% of quadruplet pregnancies could have been predicted and avoided.

Using this same system, Visser and Fourie reported pregnancy rates of only 4% associated with scores of 1–10, but greater than 35% with scores between 41 and 50[89]. They also found more biochemical pregnancies, but not clinical pregnancy losses, occurring with low-end scores. All triplet and quadruplet pregnancies were associated with scores above 40.

Giorgetti and associates[90] devised a system whereby preembryos were assigned one point for each of the following parameters: cleavage, no fragmentation, no irregular cells and four blastomeres on day 2. The idea for this system arose from the previous evaluation of 957 single preembryo transfers where no ongoing pregnancies were established from the transfer of uncleaved preembryos or after delayed fertilization (99 transfers), and where higher pregnancy rates were found to be associated with regular blastomeres and absence of fragmentation (858 transfers). Applying their four-point scoring system retrospectively, they discovered that both clinical pregnancy rates and delivery rates correlated significantly to a higher score after single preembryo transfer, and that each point corresponded to a 4% increase in pregnancy. Only female age (over 38 years) had as great an impact as the simple morphological assessment.

Tasdemir and co-workers developed a system in which the degree of preembryo fragmentation and general morphology were assessed as being either good (A) or poor (B)[91]. They then examined the outcomes of transfers with AA, BB and AB double transfers, or AAA, BBB, AAB and ABB triple transfers. When only good-quality preembryos were transferred, the pregnancy rates in double (AA) and triple (AAA) transfers were 41% and 43%, respectively. When only poor-quality preembryos (BB and BBB) were transferred, rates were 11% and 23%. AB transfers resulted in a 37% pregnancy rate, and AAB/ABB transfers resulted in a 40% incidence. The authors concluded that if at least one good-quality preembryo was available for transfer, then double, rather than triple, transfer should be carried out; higher numbers should be considered only in cases of poor preembryo quality. After applying this policy for 1 year in patients under the age of 37, they compared their results to previous data generated from triple transfers. Although this prospective trial demonstrated a slightly lower pregnancy rate in the study group as compared to the control group, the authors believe that the lower incidence of triplet gestations provides a practical compromise between high pregnancy rates and high-order gestation[92].

At Cornell, a system is used first to grade the morphology of cleaving preembryos and second, to classify transfers according to the highest score in the cohort of conceptuses being replaced:

Grade 1 preembryo with blastomeres of equal size; no cytoplasmic fragmentation;

Grade 2 preembryo with blastomeres of equal size; minor cytoplasmic fragmentation covering less than or equal to 15% of the preembryo surface;

Grade 3 preembryo with blastomeres of distinctly unequal size; variable fragmentation;

Grade 4 preembryo with blastomeres of equal or unequal size; moderate to significant cytoplasmic fragmentation covering greater than or equal to 20% of the preembryo surface;

Grade 5 preembryo with few blastomeres of any size; severe fragmentation covering greater than or equal to 50% of the preembryo surface.

We have observed that transfers with at least one grade 1 or grade 2 preembryo possess a greater potential for establishing pregnancy[93]. When data are normalized for the number of preembryos transferred, this trend still exists for all groups except single preembryo transfer, where the number of replacements is too low for comparison and the group is highly represented by patients with poor ovarian response. Clearly, transferring three or four preembryos of good quality produces the best clinical pregnancy rates, albeit with a concurrent increase in multiple implantations. Although a higher score (lower number) is favorable, pregnancy is quite possible even in cycles with grade 4 or 5 morphology demonstrating unequal-sized blastomeres and moderate to severe cytoplasmic fragmentation. Of interest is that scores are remarkably repetitive for the same patient in succeeding cycles.

In the Cornell program, two or three day-3 (6-cell to 10-cell) preembryos are replaced in women under the age of 34; three or four are recommended for women between the ages of 34 and 39; five are often replaced in women over the age of 40 when and if they are available; more may be considered in special circumstances over the age of 43 years. This strategy is based on the obstetrical outcomes of more than 7000 IVF deliveries.

While the multiple pregnancy rate is high when more than two are replaced, particularly in young women, the vast majority are twin gestations, suitable to most infertile couples. An attractive alternative is to replace one less preembryo than described above in cycles producing adequate numbers of preembryos with grade 1 or 2 morphology. Doing so may result in continued acceptable pregnancy rates while reducing the occurrence of multiples (*see* Chapter 6).

It has been reported that the concept of older women establishing multiple pregnancy at lower rates than younger women is a fallacy[94]. In this report, the authors suggest limiting the number of preembryos for transfer to three, regardless of age. Our own data do not support reducing transfer numbers in this particular population. After examining replacement outcomes during 6 years for 1876 cycles involving women over age 40, we find a significantly higher clinical pregnancy rate per transfer when four or more preembryos are replaced as compared to three (43% vs. 28%, respectively; $p < 0.0001$), as well as a significant difference in the incidence of multiple pregnancy per transfer (11% vs. 6%). One could argue that, since the policy exists to replace more than three preembryos in older women whenever possible, those receiving three represent women with poor ovarian response or limited oocyte reserve; this is quite true and should be overlooked when weighing the comparisons. Nevertheless, transferring more than three preembryos to older patients does not appear to expose these women to excessively or unacceptably high rates of multiple pregnancy, and does not lead to the multiple pregnancy rates seen after transfer of three or more preembryos to younger women (three replaced under age 40, 61% clinical pregnancy and 28% multiple pregnancy; more than three replaced under age 40, 58% clinical pregnancy and 27% multiple pregnancy).

The selection of viable preembryos for intrauterine transfer is considered an important factor in establishing pregnancy; it is assumed that overall morphology and cleavage rate will, at least to some extent, reflect a preembryo's potential for continued growth and implantation (*see* Chapter 6). In deciding how many preembryos to transfer to a given individual on day 2 or 3, it seems most reasonable to weigh the risks of multiple pregnancy against age, previous history, preembryo morphology and development, desires of the couple, and the delivery rates of a given clinic.

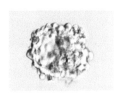

Totipotency

As discussed in later chapters, individual blastomeres remain distinct, and are totipotent (capable of developing independently to form a new organism) until about the 8-cell stage, when changes occur in the structure and properties of their plasma membranes and cytoplasm. Cells at this point become less distinct as they adhere more tightly to one another during the process of compaction. After compaction, they begin to commit themselves to becoming either inner cell mass or trophectoderm, and thus, lose this totipotency.

References

1. Steptoe PC, Edwards RG. Birth after the reimplantation of a human embryo. *Lancet* 1978;2:366

2. Hughes EG, Fedorkow DM, Daya S, Sagle MA, Van de Koppel P, Collins JA. The routine use of gonadotropin-releasing hormone agonists prior to *in vitro* fertilization and gamete intrafallopian transfer: a meta-analysis of randomized controlled trials. *Fertil Steril* 1992;58:888–96

3. Sathananthan AH, Trounson A, Wood C, eds. *Atlas of Fine Structure of Human Sperm Penetration, Eggs, and Embryos Cultured In Vitro*. New York: Praeger, 1986:2 (penetration of immature oocytes), 4 (chromosomes and spindle microtubules), 10 (cortical granules), 42, 126 (oocyte aging), 90 (polar body nucleus)

4. Van Blerkom J, Davis PW, Merriam J. A retrospective analysis of unfertilized and presumed parthenogentically activated human oocytes demonstrates a high frequency of sperm penetration. *Hum Reprod* 1994;9:2381–8

5. Edwards RG. Fertilization. In Edwards RG, ed. *Conception in the Human Female*. New York: Academic Press, 1980:604 (zona reaction), 617 (male pronucleus)

6. Dekel N, Beers WH. Development of the rat oocyte *in vitro*: inhibition and induction of maturation in the presence or absence of the cumulus oophorus. *Dev Biol* 1980;75:247–54

7. Gregory L, Booth AD, Wells C, Walker SM. A study of the cumulus–corona cell complex in *in-vitro* fertilization and embryo transfer; a prognostic indicator of the failure of implantation. *Hum Reprod* 1994;9:1308–17

8. Veeck LL. Oocyte assessment and biological performance. *Ann NY Acad Sci* 1988;541:259–74

9. Veeck LL. The morphological assessment of human oocytes and early concepti. In Keel BA, Webster BW, eds. *Handbook of the Laboratory Diagnosis and Treatment of Infertility*. Boca Raton: CRC Press, 1990:353

10. Veeck LL. The morphological estimation of mature oocytes and their preparation for insemination. In Jones HW Jr, Jones GS, Hodgen GD, Rosenwaks Z, eds. *In Vitro Fertilization – Norfolk*. Baltimore: Williams & Wilkins, 1986:81

11. Veeck LL. Pregnancy rate and pregnancy outcome associated with laboratory evaluation of spermatozoa, oocytes, and preembryos. In Mashiach S, Ben-Rafael Z, Laufer N, Schenker JG, eds. *Advances in Assisted Reproductive Technologies*. New York: Plenum Press, 1990:745

12. Hammitt DG, Syrop CH, Van Voorhis BJ, Walker DL, Miller TM, Barud KM. Maturational asynchrony between oocyte cumulus–coronal morphology and nuclear maturity in gonadotropin-releasing hormone agonist stimulations. *Fertil Steril* 1993;59:375–81

13. Laufer N, Tarlatzis BC, DeCherney AH, *et al*. Asynchrony between human cumulus–corona cell complex and oocyte maturation after human menopausal gonadotropin treatment for *in vitro* fertilization. *Fertil Steril* 1984;42:366–72

14. Veeck LL. *Atlas of the Human Oocyte and Early Conceptus*, 1st edn. Baltimore: Williams & Wilkins; 1986:7,

127 (mature granulosa), 57, 68 (oocyte classification), 74 (disparity cumulus and nucleus), 142 (fertilization)

15. Veeck LL. *Atlas of the Human Oocyte and Early Conceptus*, 2nd edn. Baltimore: Williams & Wilkins, 1991:3, 13, 27 (granulosa), 13 (oocyte classification), 27 (disparity cumulus and nucleus, 218 (spermatozoa)

16. Coetzee K, Windt ML. Fertilization and pregnancy using metaphase I oocytes in an intracytoplasmic sperm injection program. *J Assist Reprod Genet* 1996;13:768–71

17. Barnes FL, Crombie A, Gardner DK, *et al*. Blastocyst development and birth after *in-vitro* maturation of human primary oocytes, intracytoplasmic sperm injection and assisted hatching. *Hum Reprod* 1995;10:3243–7

18. Cha KY, Koo JJ, Ko JJ, Choi DH, Han SY, Yoon TK. Pregnancy after *in vitro* fertilization of human follicular oocytes collected from nonstimulated cycles, their culture *in vitro* and their transfer in a donor oocyte program. *Fertil Steril* 1991;55:109–13

19. Liu J, Katz E, Garcia JE, Compton G, Baramki TA. Successful *in vitro* maturation of human oocytes not exposed to human chorionic gonadotropin during ovulation induction, resulting in pregnancy. *Fertil Steril* 1997;67:566–8

20. Veeck LL, Wortham JW Jr, Witmyer J, *et al*. Maturation and fertilization of morphologically immature human oocytes in a program of in vitro fertilization. *Fertil Steril* 1983;39:594–602

21. Austin CR. *The Mammalian Egg*. Oxford: Blackwell Scientific Publications, 1961:75, 78

22. Plachot M, Crozet N. Fertilization abnormalities in human *in-vitro* fertilization. *Hum Reprod* 1992;7(Suppl 1):89–94

23. Gianaroli L, Cristina Magli M, Ferraretti AP, *et al*. Reducing the time of sperm–oocyte interaction in human *in-vitro* fertilization improves the implantation rate. *Hum Reprod* 1996;11:166–71

24. Alberts B, Bray D, Lewis J, Raff M, Roberts K, Watson JD, eds. Germ cells and fertilization. In *Molecular Biology of the Cell*, 2nd edn. New York: Garland Publishing, 1989:877

25. Sutovsky P, Hewitson L, Simerly C, Schatten G. Molecular medical approaches for alleviating infertility and under standing assisted reproductive technologies. *Proc Assoc Am Physicians* 1996;108:432–43

26. Nikas G, Paraschos T, Psychoyos A, Handyside AH. The zona reaction in human oocytes as seen with scanning electron microscopy. *Hum Reprod* 1994;9:2135–8

27. Soupart P, Strong PA. Ultrastructural observations on human oocytes fertilized *in vitro*. *Fertil Steril* 1974;25:11–44

28. Wolf JP, Ducot B, Aymar C, *et al*. Absence of block to polyspermy at the human oolemma. *Fertil Steril* 1997;67:1095–102

29. Sengoku K, Tamate K, Horikawa M, Takaoka Y, Ishikawa M, Dukelow WR. Plasma membrane block to polyspermy in human oocytes and preimplantation embryos. *J Reprod Fertil* 1995;105:85–90

30. Van Blerkom J, Davis PW, Merriam J. The developmental ability of human oocytes penetrated at the germinal vesicle stage after insemination *in vitro*. *Hum Reprod* 1994;9:697–708

31. Van Blerkom J, Henry G, Porreco R. Preimplantation human embryonic development from polypronuclear eggs after *in vitro* fertilization. *Fertil Steril* 1984;41:686–96

32. van der Ven HH, Al-Hasani S, Diedrich K, Hamerich U, Lehmann F, Krebs D. Polyspermy in *in vitro* fertilization of human oocytes: frequency and possible causes. *Ann NY Acad Sci* 1985;442:88–95

33. Englert Y, Puissant F, Camus M, Degueldre M, Leroy F. Factors leading to tripronucleate eggs during human *in-vitro* fertilization. *Hum Reprod* 1986;1:117–19

34. Diamond MP, Rogers BJ, Webster BW, Vaughn WK, Wentz AC. Polyspermy: effect of varying stimulation protocols and inseminating sperm concentrations. *Fertil Steril* 1985;43:777–80

35. Dietzsch E, Ramsay M, Christianson AL, Henderson BD, de Ravel TJ. Maternal origin of extra haploid set of chromosomes in third trimester triploid fetuses. *Am J Med Genet* 1995;58:360–4

36. Miny P, Koppers B, Dworniczak B, *et al*. Parental origin of the extra haploid chromosome set in triploidies diagnosed prenatally. *Am J Med Genet* 1995;57:102–6

37. McFadden DE, Pantzar JT. Placental pathology of triploidy. *Hum Pathol* 1996;27:1018–20

38. Sathananthan AH. Ultrastructural morphology of fertilization and early cleavage in the human. In Trounson AO, Wood C, eds. *In Vitro Fertilization and Embryo Transfer*. London: Churchill Livingstone, 1984:110 (pronuclei), 131 (cortical granules)

39. Sathananthan AH, Trounson AO. Ultrastructure of cortical granule release and zona interaction in monospermic and polyspermic human ova fertilized *in vitro*. *Gamete Res* 1982;6:225

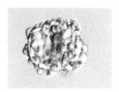

40. Almeida PA, Bolton VN. The effect of temperature fluctuations on the cytoskeletal organisation and chromosomal constitution of the human oocyte. *Zygote* 1995;3:357–65

41. Wright G, Wiker S, Elsner C, *et al*. Observations on the morphology of pronuclei and nucleoli in human zygotes and implications for cryopreservation. *Hum Reprod* 1990;5:109–15

42. Wiker S, Malter H, Wright G, Cohen J. Recognition of paternal pronuclei in human zygotes. *J In Vitro Fertil Embryo Transf* 1990;7:33–7

43. Zamboni L. In *Fine Morphology of Mammalian Fertilization*, 1st edn. New York: Medical Department, Harper & Row, 1971

44. Sathananthan AH, Trounson AO. The human pronuclear ovum: fine structure of monospermic and polyspspermic fertilization *in vitro*. *Gamete Res* 1985;12:385

45. Payne D, Flaherty SP, Barry MF, Matthews CD. Preliminary observations on polar body extrusion and pronuclear formation in human oocytes using time-lapse video cinematography. *Hum Reprod* 1997;12:532–41

46. Almeida PA, Bolton VN. Immaturity and chromosomal abnormalities in oocytes that fail to develop pronuclei following insemination *in vitro*. *Hum Reprod* 1993;8:229–32

47. Nagy ZP, Cecile J, Liu J, Loccufier A, Devroey P, Van Steirteghem A. Pregnancy and birth after intracytoplasmic sperm injection of *in vitro* matured germinal-vesicle stage oocytes: case report. *Fertil Steril* 1996;65:1047–50

48. Chen SU, Ho HN, Chen HF, Tsai TC, Lee TY, Yang YS. Fertilization and embryo cleavage after intracytoplasmic spermatid injection in an obstructive azoospermic patient with defective spermiogenesis. *Fertil Steril* 1996;66:157–60

49. Vanderzwalmen P, Lejeune B, Nijs M, Segal-Bertin G, Vandamme B, Schoysman R. Fertilization of an oocyte microinseminated with a spermatid in an *in-vitro* fertilization programme. *Hum Reprod* 1995;10:502–3

50. Fishel S, Green S, Bishop M, *et al*. Pregnancy after intra-cytoplasmic injection of spermatid. *Lancet* 1995;345:1641–2

51. Tesarik J, Mendoza C, Testart J. Viable embryos from injection of round spermatids into oocytes. *N Engl J Med* 1995;333:525

52. Antinori S, Versaci C, Dani G, Antinori M, Pozza D, Selman HA. Fertilization with human testicular spermatids:

four successful pregnancies. *Hum Reprod* 1997;12:286–91

53. Kimura Y, Yanagimachi R. Development of normal mice from oocytes injected with secondary spermatocyte nuclei. *Biol Reprod* 1995;53:855–62

54. Boue J, Bou A, Lazar P. Retrospective and prospective epidemiological studies of 1500 karyotyped spontaneous human abortions. *Teratology* 1975;12:11–26

55. Plachot M. Cytogenetic analysis of oocytes and embryos. *Ann Acad Med Singapore* 1992;21:538–44

56. Plachot M. The human oocyte. Genetic aspects. *Ann Genet* 1997;40:115–20

57. Martin RH, Balkan W, Burns K, Rademaker AW, Lin CC, Rudd NL. The chromosome constitution of 1000 human spermatozoa. *Hum Genet* 1983;63:305–9

58. Schulman JD, Dorfmann A, Evans MI. Genetic aspects of *in vitro* fertilization. *Ann NY Acad Sci* 1985;442:466–75

59. Staessen C, Coonen E, Van Assche E, *et al*. Preimplantation diagnosis for X and Y normality in embryos from three Klinefelter patients. *Hum Reprod* 1996;11:1650–3

60. Palermo GD, Schlegel PN, Sills ES, *et al*. Births after intra-cytoplasmic injection of sperm obtained by testicular extraction from men with nonmosaic Klinefelter's syndrome. *N Engl J Med* 1998;338:588–90

61. Van Blerkom J. Developmental failure in human reproduction associated with preovulatory oogenesis and preimplantation embryogenesis. In Van Blerkom J, Motta PM, eds. *Ultrastructure of Human Gametogenesis and Early Embryogenesis; Electron Microscopy in Biology and Medicine 5*. Boston: Kluwer Academic Publishers, 1989:125

62. Palermo G, Munne S, Cohen J. The human zygote inherits its mitotic potential from the male gamete. *Hum Reprod* 1994;9:1220–5

63. Goyanes VJ, Ron-Corzo A, Costas E, Maneiro E. Morphometric categorization of the human oocyte and early conceptus. *Hum Reprod* 1990;5:613–18

64. Jurisicova A, Varmuza S, Casper RF. Programmed cell death and human embryo fragmentation. *Mol Hum Reprod* 1996;2:93–8

65. Grillo JM, Gamerre M, Lacroix O, Noizet A, Vitry G. Influence of the morphological aspect of embryos obtained by *in vitro* fertilization on their implantation rate. *J In Vitro Fertil Embryo Transf* 1991;8:317–21

66. Shulman A, Ben-Nun I, Ghetler Y, Kaneti H, Shilon M, Beyth Y. Relationship between embryo morphology and implantation rate after *in vitro* fertilization treatment in conception cycles. *Fertil Steril* 1993;60:123–6

67. Herbert M, Wolstenholme J, Murdoch AP, Butler TJ. Mitotic activity during preimplantation development of human embryos. *J Reprod Fertil* 1995;103:209–14

68. Claman P, Armant DR, Seibel MM, Wang TA, Oskowitz SP, Taymor ML. The impact of embryo quality and quantity on implantation and the establishment of viable pregnancies. *J In Vitro Fertil Embryo Transf* 1987;4:218–22

69. Lewin A, Schenker JG, Safran A, *et al.* Embryo growth rate *in vitro* as an indicator of embryo quality in IVF cycles. *J Assist Reprod Genet* 1994;11:500–3

70. Zhu J, Meniru GI, Craft IL. Embryo developmental stage at transfer influences outcome of treatment with intracytoplasmic sperm injection. *J Assist Reprod Genet* 1997;14:245–9

71. McKiernan SH, Bavister BD. Timing of development is a critical parameter for predicting successful embryogenesis. *Hum Reprod* 1994;9:2123–9

72. Ziebe S, Petersen K, Lindenberg S, Andersen AG, Gabrielsen A, Andersen AN. Embryo morphology or cleavage stage: how to select the best embryos for transfer after *in-vitro* fertilization. *Hum Reprod* 1997;12:1545–9

73. Wiemer KE, Dale B, Hu Y, Steuerwald N, Maxson WS, Hoffman DI. Blastocyst development in co-culture: development and morphological aspects. *Hum Reprod* 1995;10:3226–32

74. Shoukir Y, Campana A, Farley T, Sakkas D. Early cleavage of *in-vitro* fertilized human embryos to the 2-cell stage: a novel indicator of embryo quality and viability. *Hum Reprod* 1997;12:1531–6

75. Cohen J, Inge KL, Suzman M, Wiker SR, Wright G. Videocinematography of fresh and cryopreserved embryos: a retrospective analysis of embryonic morphology and implantation. *Fertil Steril* 1989;51:820–7

76. Morgan K, Wiemer K, Steuerwald N, Hoffman D, Maxson W, Godke R. Use of videocinematography to assess morphological qualities of conventionally cultured and cocultured embryos. *Hum Reprod* 1995;10:2371–6

77. Garside WT, Loret de Mola JR, Bucci JA, Tureck RW, Heyner S. Sequential analysis of zona thickness during *in vitro* culture of human zygotes: correlation with embryo quality, age, and implantation. *Mol Reprod Dev* 1997;47:99–104

78. Kligman I, Benadiva C, Alikani M, Munne S. The presence of multinucleated blastomeres in human embryos is correlated with chromosomal abnormalities. *Hum Reprod* 1996;11:1492–8

79. Nargund G, Bourne T, Doyle P, *et al.* Associations between ultrasound indices of follicular blood flow, oocyte recovery and preimplantation embryo quality. *Hum Reprod* 1996;11:109–13

80. Chui DK, Pugh ND, Walker SM, Gregory L, Shaw RW. Follicular vascularity – the predictive value of transvaginal power Doppler ultrasonography in an *in-vitro* fertilization programme: a preliminary study. *Hum Reprod* 1997;12:191–6

81. Van Blerkom J. Can the developmental competence of early human embryos be predicted effectively in the clinical IVF laboratory? *Hum Reprod* 1997;12:1610–14

82. Leese HJ, Edwards RG. The potential for preimplantation diagnosis by non-invasive methods. In Edwards RG, ed. *Preconception and Preimplantation Diagnosis.* Cambridge: Cambridge University Press, 1993:299

83. Ray PF, Conaghan J, Winston RM, Handyside AH. Increased number of cells and metabolic activity in male human preimplantation embryos following *in vitro* fertilization. *J Reprod Fertil* 1995;104:165–71

84. Ng E, Claman P, Leveille MC, *et al.* Sex ratio of babies is unchanged after transfer of fast- versus slow-cleaving embryos. *J Assist Reprod Genet* 1995;12:566–8

85. Cummins JM, Breen TM, Harrison KL, Shaw JM, Wilson LM, Hennessey JF. A formula for scoring human embryo growth rates in *in vitro* fertilization: its value in predicting pregnancy and in comparison with visual estimates of embryo quality. *J In Vitro Fertil Embryo Transf* 1986;3:284–95

86. Puissant F, Van Rysselberge M, Barlow P, Deweze J, Leroy F. Embryo scoring as a prognostic tool in IVF treatment. *Hum Reprod* 1987;2:705–8

87. Erenus M, Zouves C, Rajamahendran P, Leung S, Fluker M, Gomel V. The effect of embryo quality on subsequent pregnancy rates after *in vitro* fertilization. *Fertil Steril* 1991;56:707–10

88. Steer CV, Mills CL, Tan SL, Campbell S, Edwards RG. The cumulative embryo score: a predictive embryo scoring technique to select the optimal number of embryos to transfer in an *in-vitro* fertilization and embryo transfer programme. *Hum Reprod* 1992;7:117–19

89. Visser DS, Fourie FR. The applicability of the cumulative embryo score system for embryo selection and quality

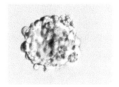

control in an *in-vitro* fertilization/embryo transfer programme. *Hum Reprod* 1993;8:1719–22

90. Giorgetti C, Terriou P, Auquier P, *et al*. Embryo score to predict implantation after *in-vitro* fertilization: based on 957 single embryo transfers. *Hum Reprod* 1995;10:2427–31

91. Tasdemir M, Tasdemir I, Kodama H, Fukuda J, Tanaka T. Two instead of three embryo transfer in *in-vitro* fertilization. *Hum Reprod* 1995;10:2155–8

92. Kodama H, Fukuda J, Karube H, *et al*. Prospective evaluation of simple morphological criteria for embryo

selection in double embryo transfer cycles. *Hum Reprod* 1995;10:2999–3003

93. Veeck LL. *An Atlas of Human Gametes and Conceptuses: an Illustrated Reference for Assisted Reproductive Technology*. Carnforth, UK: Parthenon Publishing Group, 1999

94. Senoz S, Ben-Chetrit A, Casper RF. An IVF fallacy: multiple pregnancy risk is lower for older women. *J Assist Reprod Genet* 1997;14:192–8

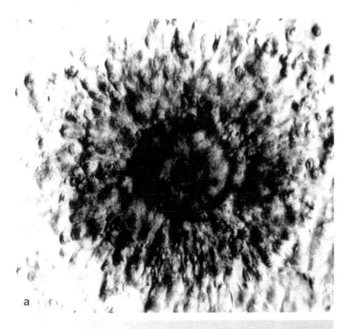

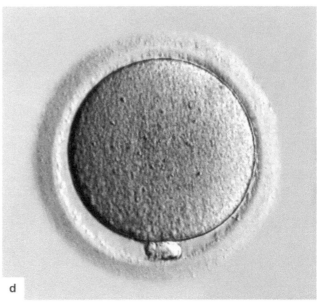

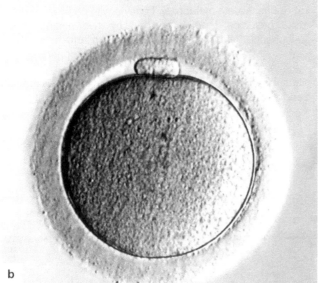

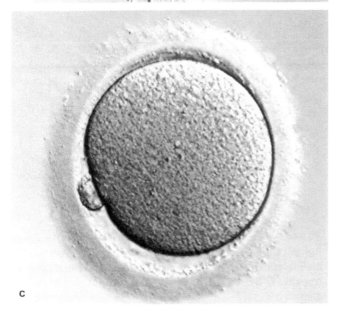

Figure 1.1 Mature oocytes at metaphase II of maturation. (a) A mature oocyte in its natural state near the time of ovulation. At x 100, the oocyte is surrounded by both an expanded corona radiata which is many layers thick, and a dense outer cumulus oophorus. Under the cover of obscuring cells, the oocyte itself is somewhat difficult to visualize; nonetheless, a first polar body was confirmed after enzymatic removal of cells; (b) MII oocyte exhibiting spherical shape and first polar body at a 12-o'clock position; (c) MII oocyte possessing minor perivitelline debris; first polar body at 8-o'clock position; (d) MII oocyte; first polar body at 6-o'clock position

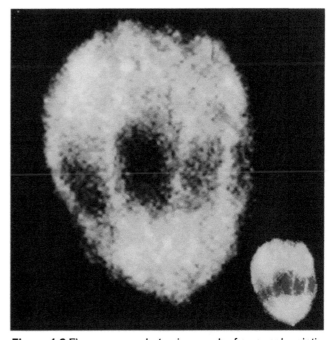

Figure 1.2 Fluorescence photomicrograph of a normal meiotic spindle of an oocyte with chromosomes at metaphase II of maturation; stained with α-tubulin-FITC (green); small insert to bottom right shows DNA lined up on the equatorial plane, stained with DAPI (blue)

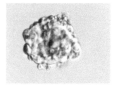

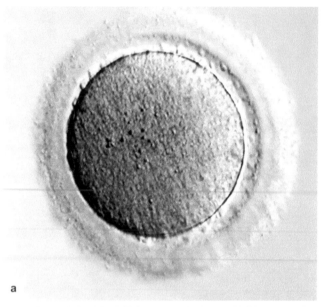

a

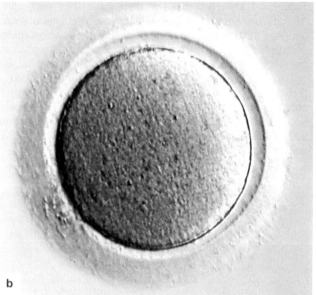

b

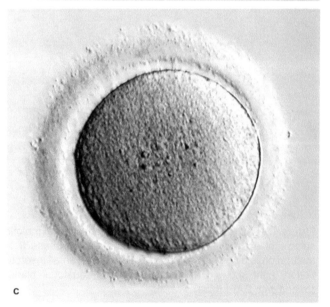

c

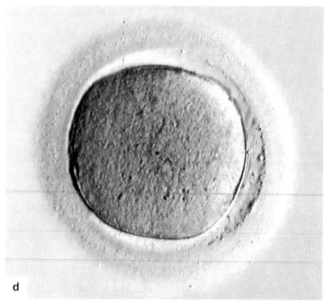

d

Figure 1.3 Oocytes at metaphase I of maturation. (a) Spherical, late metaphase I oocyte with perivitelline debris; zona pellucida is distinguished by two distinct layers; (b) spherical, late metaphase I oocyte with zona pellucida that demonstrates variable thickness; (c) spherical, late metaphase I oocyte; large perivitelline space; (d) earlier metaphase I oocyte as compared to (a)–(c); shape is irregular; zona pellucida demonstrates bilayering defect at right

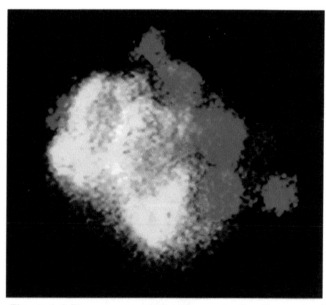

Figure 1.4 Fluorescence photomicrograph of a disorganized meiotic spindle of an aged oocyte; stained with α-tubulin-FITC (green). DNA, stained with DAPI (blue), is scattered and chaotic

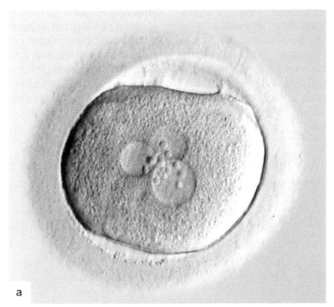
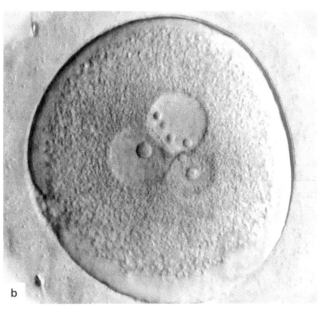

Figure 1.5 Oocytes exhibiting a triploid condition after *in vitro* aging. (a) Oocyte after ICSI displaying three pronuclei; the fact that one pronucleus is large and two are smaller suggests that retention of polar body chromosomes may be the cause of abnormal fertilization (digyny). In fact, polar bodies cannot be identified clearly; (b) inseminated oocyte with three pronuclei; the fact that two pronuclei are large and one is smaller suggests that penetration by more than one spermatozoon or penetration by a binucleate spermatozoon may be the cause of abnormal fertilization (diandry). Nucleoli in the bottom pronucleus and the one to the left appear abnormal in regard to number

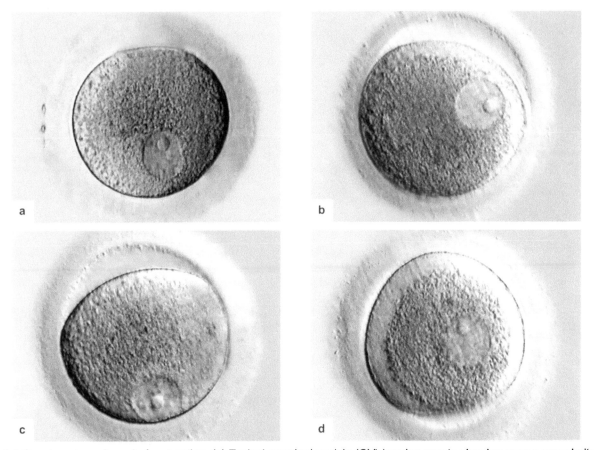

Figure 1.6 Oocytes at prophase I of maturation. (a) Typical germinal-vesicle (GV)-bearing oocyte showing coarse granularity, exocentric GV, and extremely thick zona pellucida; (b) immature oocyte with irregular shape and a clear peripheral zone; germinal vesicle is located at 3-o'clock; (c) immature oocyte with exocentric germinal vesicle; (d) oocyte with centrally located germinal vesicle displaying extreme granularity and exaggerated clear peripheral zone

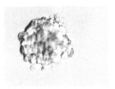

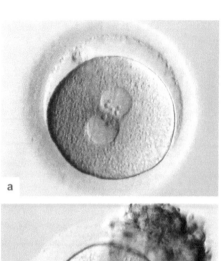

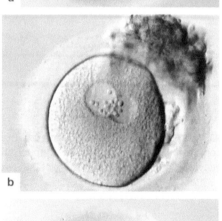

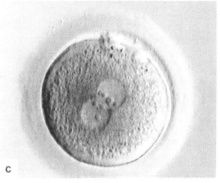

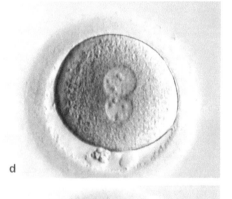

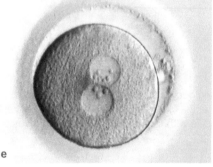

Figure 1.7 Sperm-penetrated oocytes displaying two pronuclei. (a) Pronuclei of approximately equal size; nucleoli beginning to align at adjacent areas within pronuclei; (b) smallest pronucleus nearest polar bodies; female pronucleus has aligning nucleoli while male pronucleus retains scattered nucleoli; zona pellucida thick; (c) clear cortical zone and coarse granularity of cytoplasm; pronuclei of approximately equal size and shape; (d) clear cortical zone; female pronucleus nearest two polar bodies, one of which has fragmented; (e) female pronucleus nearest polar bodies and contains a larger number of smaller nucleoli; male pronucleus contains three nucleoli

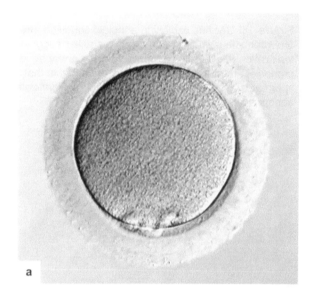

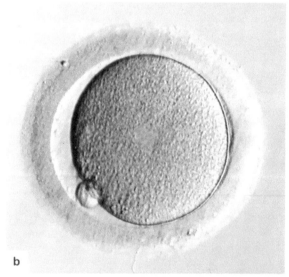

Figure 1.8 Fertilized oocytes in syngamy. (a) At 20 hours post-insemination, pronuclei have disappeared entirely; (b) at 20 hours post-insemination, a faint remnant of one central pronucleus is still seen

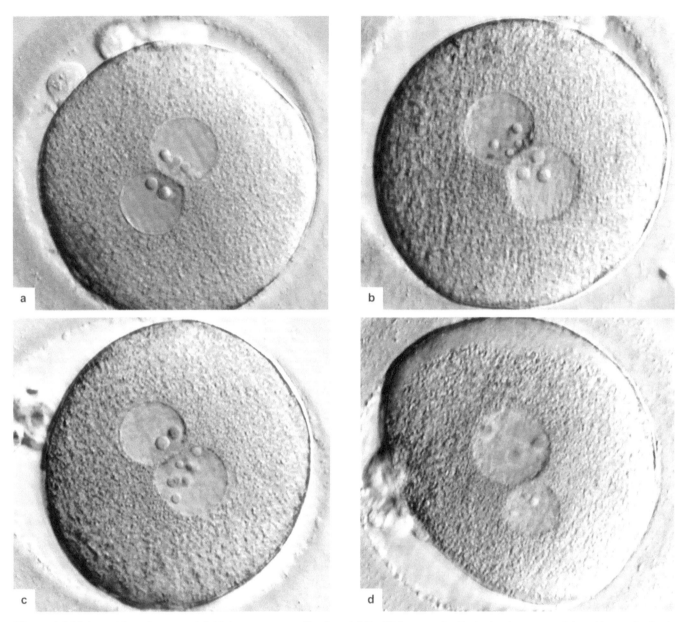

Figure 1.9 Male and female pronuclei; high-power magnification. (a) Fertilizing oocyte displaying two pronuclei and two polar bodies; nucleoli are aligned at adjacent pronuclear interfaces; (b) pronuclear oocyte; non-aligned nucleoli of differing sizes; (c) pronuclear oocyte; female pronucleus nearest polar bodies and differing nucleoli sizes; (d) pronuclear oocyte with pronuclei of distinctly different sizes; clear cortical zone

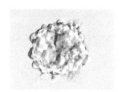

Figure 1.10 Preeembryos after the first cleavage (2-cell stage of development). (a) First cleavage in progress; (b)–(e) two-cell stages

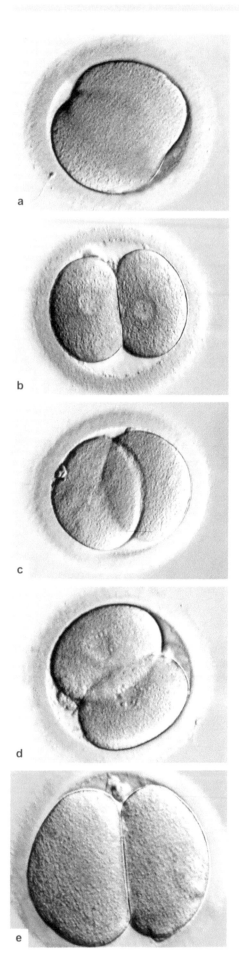

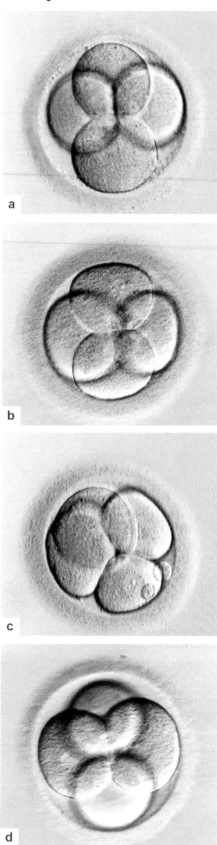

Figure 1.11 Preembryos after the second cleavage (4-cell stage of development)

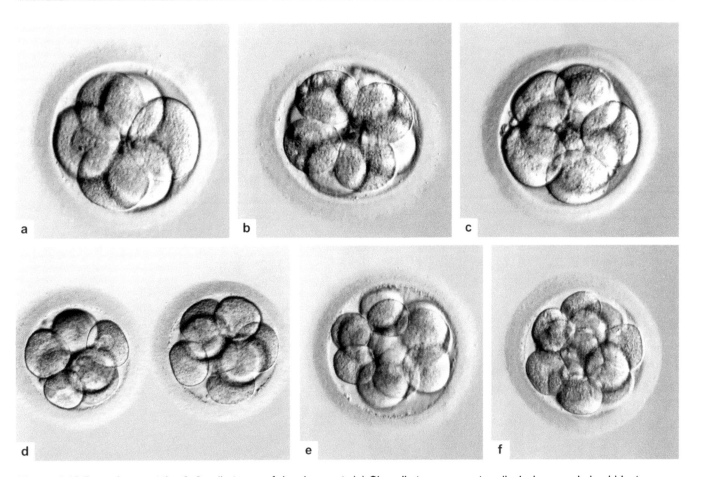

Figure 1.12 Preembryos at the 6–8-cell stages of development. (a) Six-cell stage conceptus displaying equal-sized blastomeres and healthy appearance; (b) 8-cell stage; very minor fragmentation along periphery; (c) 8-cell stage; thin zona pellucida; no fragmentation; (d) two preembryos before transfer, 7-cell stage to left and 8-cell to right; (e) and (f) preembryos with 12 blastomeres

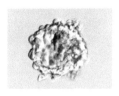

2 Metabolic requirements during preimplantation development and the formulation of culture media

David K. Gardner and Michelle Lane

Introduction

Conventional culture conditions for the preimplantation mammalian embryo induce a considerable amount of cellular stress within the blastomeres of the embryo. Manifestations of such stress are retarded rates of cleavage, cleavage arrest, cytoplasmic blebbing, abnormal genome activation and gene transcription, and abnormal patterns of energy metabolism. All of these manifestations of culture-induced stress culminate in a loss of viability. It is therefore paramount that culture media minimize such stress within the embryo and facilitate normal cell function, and hence maintain embryo viability[1-3]. One of the cellular processes affected by suboptimal culture conditions, energy metabolism, has been shown to be a useful marker of embryo normalcy *in vitro*. Furthermore, energy metabolism may also be used to identify the most viable embryo from within a given cohort for transfer. It is therefore the aim of this chapter not only to review the nutrient requirements and energy metabolism of the mammalian preimplantation embryo, but also to put energy metabolism into a meaningful context with regard to embryo development, culture and viability assessment.

Nutrient requirements of the embryo

The preimplantation period of human embryo development is highly dynamic and takes place in a changing environment *in vivo*[4]. Table 2.1 highlights some of the major differences in the embryo before and after compaction. With regard to carbohydrate utilization, the zygote and cleavage-stage embryo consume pyruvate

Table 2.1 Differences in embryo physiology pre- and post-compaction

Pre-compaction	Post-compaction
Low biosynthetic activity	high biosynthetic activity
Low QO_2	high QO_2
Pyruvate preferred nutrient	glucose preferred nutrient
Non-essential amino acids	non-essential + essential amino acids
Maternal genome	embryonic genome
Individual cells	transporting epithelium
One cell type	two distinct cell types: ICM and trophectoderm

QO_2, oxygen consumption/mg protein; ICM, inner cell mass

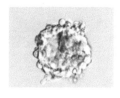

and lactate preferentially[5,6], while post-compaction the embryo switches to a more glucose-based metabolism[5-7]. The reasons and mechanisms underlying this biphasic metabolism are described in detail below.

Along with changes in carbohydrate utilization, the preimplantation embryo also undergoes changes in its requirements for amino acids[8,9]. Prior to compaction, embryo development is highest in the presence of alanine, aspartate, asparagine, glutamate, glutamine, glycine, proline, serine and taurine[10], while after compaction the embryo's requirements for amino acids increase, and development and differentiation are supported by a wider array of amino acids[8]. The roles of amino acids in embryo development are listed in Table 2.2. It is proposed that amino acids are among the most important regulators of gamete and embryo function, and the use of any culture medium lacking amino acids will confer significant trauma to the embryo[3].

Table 2.2 Functions of amino acids during preimplantation mammalian embryo development

Function	Reference
Biosynthetic precursors	11
Sources of energy	12
Regulators of energy metabolism	13
Osmolytes	14
Buffers of intracellular pH	15
Antioxidants	16
Chelators	17

Energy metabolism during the preimplantation period

The mammalian preimplantation embryo undergoes significant changes in the way in which it generates its cellular energy as it develops from the zygote to the blastocyst stage[1,18-20]. During development, the relative activities of the two major energy-generating pathways, glycolysis and the tricarboxylic acid (TCA) cycle, change dramatically, to the extent that the zygote and blastocyst are metabolically analogous to two totally different somatic cell types. The zygote, and the oocyte from

which it was derived, have a relatively low oxygen consumption[21-23], and depend on low levels of oxidation of pyruvate and/or lactate[20,24]. The zygote cannot use glucose as the sole energy source[25]. In contrast, the blastocyst exhibits a large capacity to utilize glucose both oxidatively[26] and through aerobic glycolysis[27] (aerobic glycolysis is here defined as the conversion of glucose to lactate even in the presence of adequate levels of oxygen for oxidative metabolism). As such, the zygote can be likened to a quiescent tissue such as bone, while the blastocyst to an invasive tumor. The significance of these similarities to other tissues is reflected in the physiology of the embryos at these given times. Whereas the oocyte remains relatively dormant in the ovary for a significant percentage of the female's life, the blastocyst not only has to proliferate and differentiate, but also has to maintain the blastocoel and subsequently invade the endometrium.

Of significance is that the levels of nutrients available to the human embryo as it develops mirror the changing requirements of the embryo[4]. At the time when the cleavage-stage embryo is present in the oviduct, the fluid is characterized by relatively high levels of pyruvate and lactate and low levels of glucose. In contrast, the fluid within the uterus is characterized by relatively high levels of glucose and low levels of pyruvate and lactate (Table 2.3).

Furthermore, the cumulus cells surrounding the oocyte, zygote and early cleavage stage embryo readily consume glucose and convert it to both pyruvate and lactate[4,28]. Subsequently the human embryo will be exposed to a declining pyruvate and lactate gradient, but an increasing glucose gradient, as it develops.

Understanding the change in carbohydrate preference and utilization

The change in carbohydrate utilization can be explained in terms of the changing physiology of the embryo as it develops. The oocyte, and hence the zygote, exhibit relatively low levels of biosynthesis prior to embryonic genome activation and expression. As a direct result of this there is a high adenosine triphosphate/adenosine diphosphate (ATP/ADP) ratio within the embryo, which in turn will allosterically inhibit the flux of glucose through the glycolytic pathway[19,29,30]. As the embryo becomes increasingly transcriptionally active[31], protein synthesis increases[32], and as the blastocoel is formed

Table 2.3 Concentration of carbohydrates in the human oviduct and uterus. Data from reference 4

	Pyruvate (mmol/l)	Lactate* (mmol/l)	Glucose (mmol/l)
Oviduct (mid-cycle)	0.32	10.50	0.50
Uterus	0.10	5.87	3.15

*Lactate measured as the biologically active L-isoform

through the action of the basolateral ATPases[33,34], there will be an increasing demand for energy (ATP). Consequently, the ATP/ADP ratio in the later-stage embryo will fall[35,36], and an increased glycolytic flux will become possible. Indeed, glucose metabolism by the mammalian embryo increases with development, with the highest rates of utilization occurring at the blastocyst stage[12,37–40].

Alternative explanations proposed for the observed switch in carbohydrate utilization are the lack of glucose carriers on the plasma membrane of the early embryo and/or the synthesis of sufficient enzymes for glucose metabolism by the later stages[41]. However, it is unlikely that these are the underlying mechanisms involved in the switch, as a carrier for glucose appears to present at all stages of development[42–45], and there appears to be more than sufficient total enzyme activity present to accommodate glucose metabolism through glycolysis[46,47]. What is probably more important than total enzyme activity is the appearance of new isoforms of enzymes as development proceeds. The significance of enzyme isoforms and their relative changes in abundance in terms of embryo physiology/metabolism has not been fully determined, although it is evident that the isoforms of key enzymes do change during the pre- and peri-implantation period[1,48,49]. Different isoforms vary in their response to specific regulators of enzyme function, and could therefore help to explain the observed metabolic responses of different stages of development to their environment in culture[3].

Is glucose toxic to the embryo?

In simple embryo culture media lacking amino acids, such as human tubal fluid (HTF)[50], and Earle's[51], high concentrations of glucose have been shown to impair human embryo development in culture[52,53]. An explanation for this observation has been derived from work on embryos from other mammalian species. Although glucose is not the preferred energy substrate of the cleavage-stage embryo, its uptake and utilization in a medium lacking amino acids is driven by its concentration in the culture medium[54]. As glycolysis is far less efficient in terms of energy production than oxidation, it is proposed that the premature utilization of glucose via glycolysis will culminate in inadequate energy production and hence impaired embryo development. This phenomenon is similar to that reported for certain types of tumor cell metabolism, and is known as the Crabtree effect[55]. The Crabtree effect, as described in tumor cells in culture, depends on the continued activity of hexokinase in the presence of increasing product, glucose-6-phosphate. The isoform of hexokinase present in these cells must therefore be a form of the enzyme that is not completely inhibited by glucose-6-phosphate. Kinetic analysis of hexokinase in preimplantation mouse embryos has revealed that there is a switch from isoform I at the zygote to isoform II at the blastocyst stage[56]. Indeed, these two isoforms have differing sensitivities to phosphate, with the inhibition of isoform I by glucose-6-phosphate being overcome by phosphate[57], thereby helping to explain the susceptibility of the cleavage-stage embryo to inhibition by glucose.

As a direct consequence of the inhibitory nature of glucose under certain culture conditions, there has been a trend to remove glucose from embryo culture media[53,58]. However, it is important to consider that glucose is actually present in the female reproductive tract[4], and that the oocyte and embryo possess a carrier mechanism for glucose entry into the cell[42–45]. Therefore, the inhibitory action of glucose in simple culture media should at best be considered as an *in vitro*-induced artifact. Importantly, the impairment of metabolic function in the embryo by glucose is not evident when specific amino acids[50] and the chelator ethylenediaminetetraacetic acid (EDTA) are present in

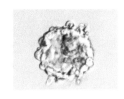

the culture medium[3]. When zygotes of CF1 mice are cultured in conventional culture media, which contain glucose but lack amino acids and EDTA, they arrest in development at the 2-cell stage. Such arrested embryos exhibit a significant increase in glycolysis with a concomitant decrease in pyruvate oxidation[13]. The addition of amino acids and EDTA to the culture medium alleviates developmental arrest at the 2-cell stage and facilitates growth to the blastocyst[59]. Analysis of embryo metabolism revealed that amino acids and EDTA act through independent mechanisms to suppress glycolytic activity in the early embryo while increasing the levels of oxidation within the embryo[1,13,60] (Figure 2.1a). Furthermore, amino acids and EDTA act in synergy to minimize the adverse metabolic effect of glucose on the cleavage-stage embryo, which is associated with an improvement in embryo development. Importantly, when zygotes from F1 mice were cultured to the 2-cell stage under the same conditions as those used for the CF1-derived embryos, their metabolism was unaffected by culture conditions (Figure 2.1b).

This therefore indicates that there are inherent differences between the embryos of different mouse strains in their ability to regulate their energy metabolism in culture, and that this in turn is related to their ability to develop in vitro. Indeed it does appear that 2-cell embryos from F1 mice can maintain a high ATP/ADP ratio in culture, thereby minimizing glucose flux through glycolysis[1]. In contrast, 2-cell embryos from CF1 mice cannot maintain a high ATP/ADP ratio in culture conditions which are associated with developmental arrest, i.e. medium containing glucose but lacking amino acids and EDTA. As a result of the fall in the ATP/ADP ratio in CF1 embryos, glycolytic activity increases (Figure 2.2)[61].

Thus, it would appear that high levels of glycolysis in the cleavage-stage embryo are not consistent with embryo development in culture, and that suppression of glycolysis culminates in increased embryo development. In further support of this hypothesis it has been shown that, under conditions that would otherwise result in developmental arrest, the inclusion of a specific inhibitor of the glycolytic enzyme phosphoglycerate kinase, cibacron blue, facilitates development of CF1 zygotes to the 2-cell stage[60]. So under the appropriate, more physiological, culture conditions glucose need not be removed from the medium. In light of its roles other than as an energy source (see below), it would appear prudent to keep glucose in the culture medium at low

levels initially, and then at increasing concentrations from the 8-cell stage onwards. Certainly, after the 8-cell stage the presence of glucose appears to be critical[59].

Significance of glucose to the embryo

The high levels of glycolysis exhibited by the mammalian blastocyst have been interpreted as the embryo's adaptation to its imminent invasion of the endometrium, which through histology has been shown to remain avascular for a period of up to 12 h, and will therefore be relatively anoxic[62,63]. Subsequently, glycolysis will be the sole means of generating energy at this time. However, this may not be the sole explanation for the high levels of glycolysis in the blastocyst. An alternative explanation for the metabolism of glucose by the blastocyst is that as well as being used to generate energy for blastocoel expansion and mitosis, glucose will be required for the synthesis of triacylglycerols and phospholipids, and as a precursor for complex sugars of mucopolysaccharides and glycoproteins. All of these are required by rapidly dividing cells[64-66]. Glucose metabolized by the pentose phosphate pathway (PPP) generates ribose moieties required for nucleic acid synthesis, and the NADPH (reduced nicotinamide–adenine dinucleotide phosphate) required for the biosynthesis of lipids and other complex molecules[65,67]. NADPH is also required for the reduction of intracellular glutathione, an important antioxidant for the embryo[68]. The synthesis of nucleic acids is therefore an important biosynthetic role for glucose in the blastocyst. It has been proposed that high levels of aerobic glycolysis, such as that observed in the mammalian blastocyst, will ensure that there is sufficient substrate available for biosynthetic pathways, such as DNA replication, RNA transcription and synthesis of new membranes, at the required times during cellular proliferation[69,70]. This in turn suggests that there are times within the cell cycle during which the PPP is more active then others. Interestingly, the work of Hewitson and Leese[71] indicates that the inner cell mass (ICM) generates its energy predominantly from glycolysis. An adequate supply of glucose may therefore be important for the optimal development of the ICM. In support of this, when mouse zygotes were cultured to the blastocyst in the absence of glucose, although resultant blastocysts implanted in the uterus after transfer, significantly more fetuses were lost compared with the control blastocysts which had developed in the presence of glucose[59], indicating impaired ICM development or function.

Significance of pyruvate and lactate to the embryo

Pyruvate enters the embryo both passively and by means of a facilitated carrier[28,44], and is the preferred nutrient of the cleavage stage embryo of several species, including the human[5]. Although lactate is readily taken up, and can be metabolized to some degree, it cannot support the first cleavage division in the mouse[18]. Inside the embryo, pyruvate and lactate are converted by the enzyme lactate dehydrogenase (LDH) through the following reaction:

$$\text{Pyruvate} + \text{NADH} + \text{H}^+ \xrightarrow{\text{Lactate dehydrogenase}} \text{Lactate} + \text{NAD}^+$$

A primary function of pyruvate and lactate in cells is to regenerate NAD$^+$ (oxidized nicotinamide–adenine dinucleotide) for subsequent use in glycolysis when under anaerobic conditions, and for the embryo this is of greatest significance at the blastocyst stage. Cytosolic regeneration of NAD$^+$ is required, as the cytoplasmic and mitochondrial pools of NADH (reduced NAD$^+$) are not shared. Rather, the reducing power between these two distinct cellular compartments is transferred through a specific system such as the malate/aspartate shuttle. It has been demonstrated that the malate/aspartate shuttle is involved in the metabolism of carboxylic acids and certain amino acids in the mouse zygote and cleavage-stage embryo. Significantly, a reduction of activity of this shuttle at the blastocyst stage may be responsible for aberrant levels of lactate production by blastocysts developed in vitro[72,73].

It has been shown that the mouse zygote and blastocyst differ in their ability to metabolize pyruvate and lactate, and that such differences can only be accounted for by a change in the intracellular NAD/NADH ratio, which in turn is affected by the ratio of pyruvate/lactate[74]. Therefore, by changing the ratio of certain medium components one can inadvertently change the ratio of important intracellular regulators. For example, changing the concentration of lactate in the culture medium can have a significant effect on mouse embryo viability[75]. This effect is stage-specific, with different stages of development having different requirements for lactate to maintain viability[75].

Different requirements of blastomeres after differentiation

As discussed, low levels of glycolysis are consistent with development of the cleavage-stage embryo in culture. However, as the later-stage embryo (morula and blastocyst) has a more glucose-dependent metabolism, this implies that different culture conditions will be required to support the changing metabolism of the embryo. For example, conditions which favor the development of the zygote, such as the limitation of glucose or the inhibition of a glycolytic enzyme (for example by EDTA), may well interfere with the development of the ICM, thereby affecting subsequent fetal development. Indeed this does appear to be the case. If mouse embryos are cultured to the blastocyst stage in the continual presence of EDTA, which inhibits glycolysis, then resultant fetal development is significantly lower than for those blastocysts which have been exposed to EDTA only for the first 48 h of culture from the zygote[59]. Similarly, the presence of EDTA in the culture medium for the first 72 h of culture significantly improved development of cattle embryos to the 8-cell stage. However, if the resultant 8-cell embryos were left in the presence of EDTA then the resultant blastocysts had a significantly smaller ICM, while the number of cells in the trophectoderm was unaffected[76] (Figure 2.3). Such data highlight the differing metabolism of the cleavage-stage and post-compaction embryo, and further support the hypothesis that different culture conditions are required at different stages of development in order to satisfy the changing requirements of the embryo[77–79].

'Metabolic control' hypothesis

In light of the inherent susceptibility of the mammalian embryo to culture-induced stress in vitro, the 'metabolic control' hypothesis has been developed[1]. Under suboptimal culture conditions the embryo exhibits abnormal energy metabolism, or expressed another way the embryo undergoes metabolic transformation. It is proposed that the ability of a given embryo to regulate against such metabolic transformation is related to its ability to develop in culture and ultimately to develop into a viable fetus after transfer. Interestingly, metabolic transformation is not restricted to the cleavage-stage embryo, but is also manifest at the blastocyst stage too. Menke and McLaren[80] were the first to report that mouse blastocysts cultured from the 8-cell stage in a balanced salt solution with added carbohydrates had an

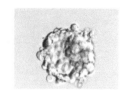

impaired oxidative ability, compared with blastocysts developed *in vivo*. Subsequently, Gardner and Leese[27] reported that culturing mouse morulae for around 12 h in medium MTF (mouse tubal fluid: balanced salt solution with carbohydrates but lacking amino acids) culminated in the production of blastocysts which exhibited very high levels of lactate production, inferring impaired oxidative capacity. Whereas a mouse blastocyst developed *in vivo* will convert around 40–50% of glucose consumed to lactate[26,27], those blastocysts obtained from cultured morulae converted almost 100% of the glucose consumed to lactate. Subsequently, Gardner and Sakkas[75] found that supplementing a culture medium based upon a simple balanced salt solution with amino acids and vitamins abolished this metabolic transformation. Lane and Gardner[81] then went on to investigate the timing of such metabolic transformation in the mouse blastocyst. It was observed that exposure to culture medium MTF for just 3 h resulted in an increase in lactate production, with maximum perturbation occurring after 6 h. Interestingly, the rate of glucose uptake was not affected by the incubation conditions, but rather its fate (Figure 2.4). Furthermore, the ability of blastocysts to oxidize pyruvate was significantly impaired after 6 h of culture in MTF. The addition of amino acids and vitamins to MTF independently decreased the excessive lactate production of blastocysts incubated for 6 h, and acted in synergy to reduce lactate production further. Moreover, the presence of both amino acids and vitamins in the incubation medium maintained the ability of the blastocyst to oxidize pyruvate.

Perhaps the more important finding from this work was that the impaired metabolism observed after just 6 h of culture was associated with a significant reduction in blastocyst implantation and subsequent fetal development after transfer, compared with blastocysts flushed from the uterus and transferred to a recipient, or compared with blastocysts maintained in culture for 6 h but in the presence of both amino acids and vitamins. Clearly then, metabolic transformation is associated with loss of viability. This therefore leads to the question whether assessment of an embryo's metabolism can be used to determine its viability before transfer, i.e. to select the most viable embryos from a given cohort.

Assessment of viability using metabolic criteria

Owing to the limited amount of material available for study of the preimplantation mammalian embryo,

miniaturizations of standard methods of biochemical analysis have to be employed. Two approaches have been used with great success: radiolabelled substrates in microincubation chambers, and ultramicrofluorescence. However, for the assessment of embryo viability prior to transfer, the former approach is not a realistic proposition, and so the latter approach is considered in detail here. Ultramicrofluorescence was developed by Mroz and Lechene and co-workers[35]. This technique was subsequently adapted[37,38] to determine the nutrient uptake of an individual embryo at each successive stage of development in culture. Ultramicrofluorescence is a totally non invasive approach, and is based upon placing an individual embryo in a known volume of defined culture medium and then removing serial samples of culture medium from around the embryo and analyzing them for nutrient composition (Figure 2.5).

The volumes of culture medium removed can be as small as nano- or picoliters. Such small volumes are manipulated with specially constructed micropipettes manufactured on a microforge and calibrated with tritiated water. These pipettes are manipulated using a micromanipulator, and the fluids taken up and expelled using an air-filled syringe. The sub-microliter samples of fluid are then analyzed fluorometrically (Figure 2.6) using a fluorescence microscope with photometry attachments.

In 1980, Renard and colleagues[86] observed that day-10 cattle blastocysts which had a glucose uptake higher than 5 µg/h developed better both in culture and *in vivo* after transfer than those blastocysts with a glucose uptake below this value. However, owing to the insensitivity of the spectrophotmetric method employed, they could not quantitate glucose uptake by younger embryos. Rieger[87] subsequently demonstrated that morphologically normal day-7 cattle blastocysts took up significantly more radiolabelled glucose than degenerating ones. In 1987, using the relatively new technique of non-invasive microfluorescence, Gardner and Leese[88] measured glucose uptake by individual day-4 mouse blastocysts prior to transfer to recipient females. Those embryos that went to term had a significantly higher glucose uptake in culture than those embryos that failed to develop after transfer. However, such studies were retrospective, and as such could not conclusively demonstrate whether it was possible to identify viable embryos prior to transfer using metabolism as a marker. Subsequently, a study of the metabolism of day-7 cattle blastocysts before and after cryopreservation showed that it was possible to identify those blastocysts capable of re-expansion in the hours immediately post-thaw[89]. Those blastocysts that survived the freeze–thaw procedure had a significantly higher glucose uptake and lactate production than those embryos that did not re-expand and subsequently died (Figure 2.7)[89]. Of greater significance, however, was the observation that there was no overlap in the distribution of glucose uptake by the viable and non-viable embryos, and very little overlap of lactate production, suggesting that it may therefore be possible to use metabolic criteria for prospective selection of viable embryos[89]. Interestingly, pyruvate uptake by blastocysts did not reflect their subsequent viability.

Therefore, in a prospective study, Lane and Gardner[90] used glucose uptake and lactate production to determine glycolytic activity in individual day-5 mouse blastocysts prior to transfer. Consistent with the metabolic control hypothesis, blastocysts were classified as viable or non-viable according to their rate of glucose uptake and lactate production. Mouse blastocysts of equal dimensions and morphology subsequently had their metabolism quantitated non-invasively and were then classified as either viable or non-viable. It was found that those blastocysts which exhibited a pattern of glycolytic utilization similar to that of embryos developed *in vivo* had a developmental potential of 80%, while those blastocysts which exhibited an excessive lactate production (i.e. aberrant glycolytic activity) had a developmental potential of only 6% (Figure 2.8). Interestingly, when a retrospective analysis of glucose uptakes was performed on the blastocysts transferred in this study, those blastocysts classified as viable has a significantly higher rate of glucose uptake than those blastocysts classified as non-viable. Therefore, it would appear that both the rate of nutrient uptake and its subsequent fate are important determinants of embryo viability.

Importantly, studies of nutrient uptake and subsequent viability have been performed on the human embryo. In a retrospective analysis, Conaghan and colleagues[91] observed an inverse relationship between pyruvate uptake by 2–8-cell embryos and subsequent pregnancy. However, it is important to note that such measurements were performed prior to human embryonic genome activation. It is therefore plausible that the observed differences in pyruvate uptake reported by Conaghan and colleagues[91] reflected differences inherited from the oocyte, and did not represent the true physiology of the later-stage embryo. Furthermore, the medium used to assess nutrient

consumption was a simple one, lacking amino acids and vitamins. In a study of human morulae and blastocysts of different degrees of expansion, no conclusive data were generated on the ability of nutrient consumption or utilization to predict pregnancy outcome[92]. Again, however, the medium used to assess embryo metabolism was a simple one, lacking pyruvate, lactate, amino acids and vitamins. Under such severe culture conditions, the resultant stress on the embryos would have been enormous, and therefore it is questionable whether any meaningful data could have been obtained. In fact, one would expect embryos undergoing such a treatment to be compromised. In contrast, Van den Bergh and associates[93] showed that, in patients who conceived following blastocyst transfer, embryos had a significantly lower glycolytic activity than those embryos which did not establish a pregnancy. Significantly, in the work of Van den Bergh and associates[93], a complete medium was used for the metabolic assessment, thereby alleviating the culture-induced stress associated with the work of Jones and colleagues[92].

More recently, two studies have determined the relationship between embryo nutrition and subsequent development *in vitro*[94,95]. Gardner and colleagues[94] determined that glucose consumption on day 4 by human embryos was twice as high in those embryos that went on to form blastocysts. Furthermore, it was determined that blastocyst quality affected glucose uptake. Poor-quality blastocysts consumed significantly less glucose than top-scoring embryos. Significantly, within a cohort of human blastocysts from the same patient with the same alpha-numeric score, i.e. 4AA, there existed a significant spread of metabolic activities. These embryos were cultured in sequential media G1 and G2, and their metabolism assessed in medium G2 in order to prevent metabolic transformation. Therefore, assessing metabolic activity and metabolic normality may prove to be a feasible way of determining embryonic 'health' (Figure 2.9). In a study of amino acids, Houghton and co-workers[95] determined that alanine release into the surrounding medium on day 2 and day 3 was highest in those embryos that did not form blastocysts.

Culture of the human embryo

Table 2.4 gives the compositions of the sequential media G1.2 and G2.2. The media were developed after taking into account the data described in this chapter. In G1.2, carbohydrates are present at concentrations measured in the human Fallopian tube at the time when the embryo

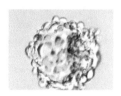

Table 2.4 Compositions of sequential culture media G1.2 and G2.2

Component	mmol/l	Component	mmol/l
G1.2 (cleavage-stage development)			
Sodium chloride	90.08	alanyl–glutamine	0.5
Potassium chloride	5.5	alanine	0.1
Sodium phosphate	0.25	aspartate	0.1
Magnesium sulfate	1.0	asparagine	0.1
Bicarbonate	25.0	glutamate	0.1
Calcium chloride	1.8	glycine	0.1
		proline	0.1
Glucose	0.5	serine	0.1
Lactate	10.5	taurine	0.1
Pyruvate	0.32	EDTA	0.01
G2.2 (blastocyst development)			
Sodium chloride	90.08	arginine	0.6
Potassium chloride	5.5	cystine	0.1
Sodium phosphate	0.25	histidine	0.2
Magnesium sulfate	1.0	isoleucine	0.4
Bicarbonate	25.0	leucine	0.4
Calcium chloride	1.8	lysine	0.4
		methionine	0.1
Glucose	3.15	phenylalanine	0.2
Lactate	5.87	threonine	0.4
Pyruvate	0.10	tryptophan	0.5
		tyrosine	0.2
Alanyl–glutamine	1.0	valine	0.4
Alanine	0.1		
Aspartate	0.1	choline chloride	0.0072
Asparagine	0.1	folic acid	0.0023
Glutamate	0.1	inositol	0.01
Glycine	0.1	nicotinamide	0.0082
Proline	0.1	pantothenate	0.0042
Serine	0.1	pyridoxal	0.0049
		riboflavin	0.00027

EDTA, ethylenediaminetetraacetic acid

is present. In contrast, in medium G2.2, concentrations of carbohydrates are those found in the human uterus. The amino acids present in medium G1.2 are those present at high levels in mammalian oviduct fluids, and have been shown to stimulate the cleavage-stage embryo[96,97] and minimize intracellular stress[1,15,13,98], while those in G2.2 are those needed for the development of both the ICM and trophectoderm, which have different nitrogen requirements[8]. EDTA is present in medium G1.2 for the reasons listed above, while it is absent from medium G2.2, to ensure optimal development of the ICM. Vitamins are absent from medium G1.2 but present in G2.2, to facilitate sufficient oxidation in the blastocyst[1,81].

Using such sequential media it is possible to culture the human embryo, along with those of several other species[97], to the blastocyst stage at high rates, culminating in a high implantation rate following transfer. Table 2.5 lists results of using these media in a clinical setting. Figure 2.10 shows the typical morphology of human blastocysts cultured in these sequential media.

As discussed, amino acids are among the most important regulators of mammalian embryo development in culture[1,3,97,102]. However, amino acids both are metabolized by the embryos and spontaneously break down at 37°C to produce ammonium[84], which impairs embryo development, ICM formation and fetal development[84,103,104]. The majority of ammonium released into the culture system comes from their spontaneous breakdown while at 37°C, which has profound implications for the storage and use of media containing them. Ideally, embryo culture media should be set up at least 4 h and no more than 18 h before use[105], and such media should be renewed at least every 48 h[84]. Of the amino acids present in culture media, glutamine is known to be the most labile, and contributes a disproportionate amount of ammonium to the system[84]. This particular problem can be alleviated by the substitution of glutamine with alanyl-glutamine[106], which does not readily deaminate at 37°C.

More recently, the concept of using sequential media has been challenged, and the use of one medium (KSOM[AA]) to support all the preimplantation stages has been proposed as an effective culture method[107]. It is evident that one culture medium will support blastocyst development in a number of mammalian species including the human[108]. However, as discussed at length above, there is considerable difference in the ability to culture blastocysts and the ability to culture viable blastocysts[78,79]. The question is, therefore, can one medium support the development of blastocysts with the same viability as those blastocysts developed in sequential media? The answer to this question, at least in animal models, is no[97]. The medium KSOM[AA] by default does not allow for any nutrient gradients, and therefore will induce some form of metabolic stress on the embryo as described in detail above. Furthermore, the medium KSOM[AA] contains EDTA. Subsequently, the embryo will be exposed to EDTA post-compaction, and this will have a negative effect on ICM development as discussed. Analysis of mouse and cow embryos cultured in either sequential media G1/G2 or KSOM[AA] have revealed that those embryos cultured in KSOM[AA] do indeed have reduced embryo development, reduced blastocyst cell number, impaired ICM development and lower viability after transfer[97]. These findings are consistent with the data presented in this chapter on nutrient requirements and metabolism of the embryo. Significantly, should KSOM[AA] be used, it is necessary to renew the medium every 48 h as it contains 1 mmol/l glutamine, and produces embryo toxic levels of ammonium within the duration of the culture period.

In an ideal world, rather than simply using two culture media in sequence, the embryo in culture could be exposed to any number of nutrient gradients, obtainable through a perfusion system[10]. Figure 2.11 shows the basic concept of such a system. Recently, with the introduction of microfluidic cells, the concept of perfusion culture in embryology is becoming a reality[109,110]. Embryo culture systems could be about to change in the clinical *in vitro* fertilization (IVF) laboratory.

Although this chapter endeavors to place the nutrition and metabolism of the embryo into a meaningful context, it would be remiss not to discuss, albeit briefly, the significance of macromolecules in the development of the embryo. Relative to other culture medium components, macromolecules have received relatively little attention. Recently, however, studies have demonstrated the benefit of the inclusion of the glycosaminoglycan hyaluronan in culture media on embryo development[111], cryosurvival[112–114] and transfer outcome[111,115]. Furthermore, recombinant albumin is now available, and not only has it been shown to be equally as effective in an IVF/embryo culture system as blood-derived human serum albumin[114,116–122], but it also increases embryo cyrosurvivability[113]. Significantly, the introduction of genetically engineered macromolecules

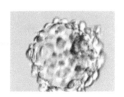

Table 2.5 Summary of blastocyst transfer data at the Colorado Center for Reproductive Medicine. From reference 99, with permission

	IVF patients*	Oocyte donors
Number of patients	401	211
Number of patients having embryo transfer	395	211
Mean age (± SEM) in years	33.4 ± 0.2	40.6 ± 0.3 recipients
Age range (years)	20–43	27–50
FSH (IU/l) (mean ± SEM)	6.7 ± 0.1	6.1 ± 0.1 donors
Patients with ICSI (%)	40.4	39.3
Number of pronucleate embryos (mean ± SEM)	14.5 ± 0.3	15.2 ± 0.4
Blastocyst development on day 5 (%)	44.1	51.7
Blastocyst development on day 6 (%)	8.1	8.3
Total blastocyst development (%)	52.2	60.0
Number of embryos transferred (mean ± SEM)	2.2 ± 0.03	2.1 ± 0.03
Patients with embryo freezing (%)[†]	75.3	85.3
Mean number of blastocysts frozen (mean ± SEM)	4.3 ± 0.2	5.6 ± 0.3
Implantation rate (fetal sac) (%)[‡]	50.1	62.1
Implantation rate (fetal heart) (%)[‡]	46.4	60.8
Clinical pregnancy rate (%)**	68.6	79.6

*In vitro fertilization (IVF) patients had at least ten follicles; [†]only blastocysts scoring 3BB or higher by the afternoon of day 6 were cryopreserved; [‡]implantation rates are expressed as fetal sac or heart/blastocyst transferred. The calculations included every patient who had an embryo transfer and not just those who subsequently became pregnant; **includes six patients in the blastocyst culture group who did not have an embryo transferred on day 5 owing to embryonic arrest at the cleavage stage. Clinical pregnancy was determined by the presence of a fetal heart beat; FSH, follicle stimulating hormone; ICSI, intracytoplasmic sperm injection

means that the potential transmission of blood-borne pathogens such as human immunodeficiency virus (HIV) and prions is effectively eliminated. Furthermore, the lot-to-lot variation associated with serum derived albumin[119,120] is also eliminated. Such changes have resulted in the development of new culture systems[97].

The adverse effects of whole serum on embryo development, metabolism and ultrastructure have been well documented. The use of serum in a clinical embryo culture system cannot be considered morally acceptable.

Conclusions

It is evident that suboptimal culture conditions induce a considerable degree of cellular stress in the preimplantation embryo. A key manifestation of such culture-induced stress is abnormal energy metabolism. Typically, under suboptimal conditions, glycolytic activity increases at the expense of oxidation, culminating in inadequate energy production and impaired embryo development. Culture conditions which increase embryo development *in vitro* appear to help the embryo maintain a more *in vivo*-like metabolism, i.e. low levels of glycolysis prior to compaction, while maintaining the embryo's ability to oxidize a percentage of the glucose consumed at the blastocyst stage. The normalcy of metabolic activity of an embryo appears to be related to both developmental capacity in culture and subsequent viability after transfer. Therefore, the non-invasive assessment of metabolism of an individual embryo within a given cohort prior to transfer may help identify those embryos most likely to give rise to a successful pregnancy.

By meeting the nutritional requirements of the embryo as it develops and differentiates (including carbohydrate and amino acid gradients), and by reducing stress, one can support the development of highly viable blastocysts in culture. By using sequential media it is now possible to obtain *in vivo* rates of embryo development *in vitro* in animal models[97,121].

References

1. Gardner DK. Changes in requirements and utilization of nutrients during mammalian preimplantation embryo development and their significance in embryo culture. *Theriogenology* 1998;49:83–102

2. Lane M, Gardner DK. Regulation of ionic homeostasis by mammalian embryos. *Semin Reprod Med* 2000;18:195–204

3. Gardner DK, Pool TB, Lane M. Embryo nutrition and energy metabolism and its relationship to embryo growth, differentiation, and viability. *Semin Reprod Med* 2000;18:205–18

4. Gardner DK, Lane M, Calderon I, Leeton J. Environment of the preimplantation human embryo *in vivo*: metabolite analysis of oviduct and uterine fluids and metabolism of cumulus cells. *Fertil Steril* 1996;65:349–53

5. Hardy K, Hooper MA, Handyside AH, Rutherford AJ, Winston RM, Leese HJ. Non-invasive measurement of glucose and pyruvate uptake by individual human oocytes and preimplantation embryos. *Hum Reprod* 1989;4:188–91

6. Gott AL, Hardy K, Winston RM, Leese HJ. Non-invasive measurement of pyruvate and glucose uptake and lactate production by single human preimplantation embryos. *Hum Reprod* 1990;5:104–8

7. Gardner DK, Lane M, Stevens J, Schoolcraft WB. Noninvasive assessment of human embryo nutrient consumption as a measure of developmental potential. *Fertil Steril* 2001;76:1175–80

8. Lane M, Gardner DK. Differential regulation of mouse embryo development and viability by amino acids. *J Reprod Fertil* 1997;109:153–64

9. Steeves TE, Gardner DK. Temporal and differential effects of amino acids on bovine embryo development in culture. *Biol Reprod* 1999;61:731–40

10. Gardner DK. Mammalian embryo culture in the absence of serum or somatic cell support. *Cell Biol Int* 1994;18:1163–79

11. Crosby IM, Gandolfi F, Moor RM. Control of protein synthesis during early cleavage of sheep embryos. *J Reprod Fertil* 1988;82:769–75

12. Rieger D, Loskutoff NM, Betteridge KJ. Developmentally related changes in the metabolism of glucose and glutamine by cattle embryos produced and co-cultured *in vitro*. *J Reprod Fertil* 1992;95:585–95

13. Gardner DK, Lane M. The 2-cell block in CF1 mouse embryos is associated with an increase in glycolysis and a decrease in tricarboxylic acid (TCA) cycle activity: alleviation of the 2-cell block is associated with the restoration of *in vivo* metabolic pathway activities. *Biol Reprod* 1993;48(Suppl 1):152

14. Van Winkle LJ, Haghighat N, Campione AL. Glycine protects preimplantation mouse conceptuses from a detrimental effect on development of the inorganic ions in oviductal fluid. *J Exp Zool* 1990;253:215–19

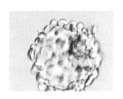

15. Edwards LJ, Williams DA, Gardner DK. Intracellular pH of the mouse preimplantation embryo: amino acids act as buffers of intracellular pH. *Hum Reprod* 1998;13:3441–8

16. Liu Z, Foote RH. Development of bovine embryos in KSOM with added superoxide dismutase and taurine and with five and twenty percent O_2. *Biol Reprod* 1995;53:786–90

17. Lindenbaum A. A survey of naturally occurring chelating ligands. *Adv Exp Med Biol* 1973;40:67–77

18. Biggers JD, Whittingham DG, Donahue RP. The pattern of energy metabolism in the mouse oocyte and zygote. *Proc Natl Acad Sci USA* 1967;58:560–7

19. Biggers JD, Gardner DK, Leese HJ. Control of carbohydrate metabolism in preimplantation mammalian embryos. In Rosenblum IY, Heyner S, eds. *Growth Factors in Mammalian Development*. Boca Raton: CRC Press, 1989:19–32

20. Leese HJ. Metabolism of the preimplantation mammalian embryo. *Oxf Rev Reprod Biol* 1991;13:35–72

21. Mills RM, Brinster RL. Oxygen consumption of preimplantation mouse embryos. *Exp Cell Res* 1967;47:337–44

22. Houghton FD, Thompson JG, Kennedy CJ, Leese HJ. Oxygen consumption and energy metabolism of the early mouse embryo. *Mol Reprod Dev* 1996;44:476–85

23. Thompson JG, Partridge RJ, Houghton FD, Cox CI, Leese HJ. Oxygen uptake and carbohydrate metabolism by *in vitro* derived bovine embryos. *J Reprod Fertil* 1996;106:299–306

24. Brinster RL. Studies on the development of mouse embryos *in vitro*. IV. Interaction of energy sources. *J Reprod Fertil* 1965;10:227–40

25. Brinster RL, Thomson JL. Development of eight-cell mouse embryos *in vitro*. *Exp Cell Res* 1966;42:308–15

26. Wales RG. Measurement of metabolic turnover in single mouse embryos. *J Reprod Fertil* 1986;76:717–25

27. Gardner DK, Leese HJ. Concentrations of nutrients in mouse oviduct fluid and their effects on embryo development and metabolism *in vitro*. *J Reprod Fertil* 1990;88:361–8

28. Leese HJ, Barton AM. Production of pyruvate by isolated mouse cumulus cells. *J Exp Zool* 1985;234:231–6

29. Barbehenn EK, Wales RG, Lowry OH. The explanation for the blockade of glycolysis in early mouse embryos. *Proc Natl Acad Sci USA* 1974;71:1056–60

30. Barbehenn EK, Wales RG, Lowry OH. Measurement of metabolites in single preimplantation embryos; a new means to study metabolic control in early embryos. *J Embryol Exp Morphol* 1978;43:29–46

31. Telford NA, Watson AJ, Schultz GA. Transition from maternal to embryonic control in early mammalian development: a comparison of several species. *Mol Reprod Dev* 1990;26:90–100

32. Epstein CJ, Smith SA. Amino acid uptake and protein synthesis in preimplantation mouse embryos. *Dev Biol* 1973;33:171–84

33. Benos D, Biggers JD. Blastocyst fluid formation. In Mastroianni LJ, Biggers JD, eds. *Fertilization and Embryonic Development In Vitro*. New York: Plenum Press, 1981:283–97

34. Biggers JD, Bell JE, Benos DJ. Mammalian blastocyst: transport functions in a developing epithelium. *Am J Physiol* 1988;255:C419–32

35. Leese HJ, Biggers JD, Mroz EA, Lechene C. Nucleotides in a single mammalian ovum or preimplantation embryo. *Anal Biochem* 1984;140:443–8

36. Rozell MD, Williams JE, Butler JE. Changes in concentration of adenosine triphosphate and adenosine diphosphate in individual preimplantation sheep embryos. *Biol Reprod* 1992;47:866–70

37. Gardner DK, Leese HJ. Non-invasive measurement of nutrient uptake by single cultured pre-implantation mouse embryos. *Hum Reprod* 1986;1:25–7

38. Gardner DK, Lane M, Batt P. Uptake and metabolism of pyruvate and glucose by individual sheep preattachment embryos developed *in vivo*. *Mol Reprod Dev* 1993;36:313–19

39. Leese HJ, Barton AM. Pyruvate and glucose uptake by mouse ova and preimplantation embryos. *J Reprod Fertil* 1984;72:9–13

40. Thompson JG, Simpson AC, Pugh PA, Tervit HR. Requirement for glucose during *in vitro* culture of sheep preimplantation embryos. *Mol Reprod Dev* 1992;31:253–7

41. Scott LA. Oocyte and embryo culture. In Keel BA, May JV, De Jonge CJ, eds. *Handbook of the Assisted Reproduction Laboratory*. Boca Raton: CRC Press, 2000:197–219

42. Aghayan M, Rao LV, Smith RM, *et al.* Developmental expression and cellular localization of glucose transporter molecules during mouse preimplantation development. *Development* 1992;115:305–12

43. Dan-Goor M, Sasson S, Davarashvili A, Almagor M. Expression of glucose transporter and glucose uptake in human oocytes and preimplantation embryos. *Hum Reprod* 1997;12:2508–10

44. Gardner DK, Leese HJ. The role of glucose and pyruvate transport in regulating nutrient utilization by preimplantation mouse embryos. *Development* 1988;104:423–9

45. Hogan A, Heyner S, Charron MJ, *et al*. Glucose transporter gene expression in early mouse embryos. *Development* 1991;113:363–72

46. Biggers JD, Stern S. Metabolism of the preimplantation mammalian embryo. *Adv Reprod Physiol* 1973;6:1–59

47. Martin KL, Hardy K, Winston RM, Leese HJ. Activity of enzymes of energy metabolism in single human preimplantation embryos. *J Reprod Fertil* 1993;99:259–66

48. Auerbach S, Brinster RL. Lactate dehydrogenase isozymes in mouse blastocyst cultures. *Exp Cell Res* 1968;53:313–15

49. Edwards LE, Gardner DK. Characterization of hexokinase kinetics in the preimplantation mouse embryo. *Proc Fertil Soc Aust* 1995;14:28

50. Quinn P, Kerin JF, Warnes GM. Improved pregnancy rate in human *in vitro* fertilization with the use of a medium based on the composition of human tubal fluid. *Fertil Steril* 1985;44:493–8

51. Edwards RG. Test-tube babies. *Nature (London)* 1981;293:253–6

52. Conaghan J, Handyside AH, Winston RM, Leese HJ. Effects of pyruvate and glucose on the development of human preimplantation embryos *in vitro*. *J Reprod Fertil* 1993;99:87–95

53. Quinn P. Enhanced results in mouse and human embryo culture using a modified human tubal fluid medium lacking glucose and phosphate. *J Assist Reprod Genet* 1995;12:97–105

54. Vella P, Lane M, Gardner DK. Induction of glycolysis in the day-3 mouse embryo by glucose. *Biol Reprod* 1997;57(Suppl 1):26

55. Koobs DH. Phospate mediation of the Crabtree and Pasteur effects. *Science* 1972;178:127–33

56. Edwards LE, Gardner DK. Characterisation of hexokinase kinetics in the preimplantation mouse embryo. *Proc Fertil Soc Aust* 1995;14:28

57. Wilson JE. Hexokinases. *Rev Physiol Biochem Pharmacol* 1995;126:65–198

58. Pool TB, Atiee SH, Martin JE. Oocyte and embryo culture: basic concepts and recent advances. *Infertil Reprod Med Clin North Am* 1998;9:181–203

59. Gardner DK, Lane M. Alleviation of the '2-cell block' and development to the blastocyst of CF1 mouse embryos: role of amino acids, EDTA and physical parameters. *Hum Reprod* 1996;11:2703–12

60. Lane M, Gardner DK. Inhibiting 3-phosphoglycerate kinase by EDTA stimulates the development of the cleavage stage mouse embryo. *Mol Reprod Dev* 2001;60:233–40

61. Gardner DK, Lane M. Alleviation of the 2 cell block in CF1 mouse embryos is associated with an increase in the ATP:ADP ratio and subsequent inhibition of PFK. *Biol Reprod* 1997;57(Suppl 1):216

62. Rogers PW, Murphy CR, Gannon BJ. Absence of capillaries in the endometrium surrounding the implanting rat blastocyst. *Micron* 1982;13:373–4

63. Rogers PW, Murphy CR, Gannon BJ. Changes in the spatial organization of the uterine vasculature during implantation in the rat. *J Reprod Fertil* 1982;65:211–14

64. Hume DA, Weidemann MJ. Role and regulation of glucose metabolism in proliferating cells. *J Natl Cancer Inst* 1979;62:3–8

65. Morgan MJ, Faik P. Carbohydrate metabolism in cultured animal cells. *Biosci Rep* 1981;1:669–86

66. Mandel LJ. Energy metabolism of cellular activation, growth, and transformation. *Curr Top Memb Trans* 1986;27:261–91

67. Reitzer LJ, Wice BM, Kennell D. The pentose cycle: control and essential function in HeLa cell nucleic acid synthesis. *J Biol Chem* 1980;255:5616–26

68. Rieger D. Relationship between energy metabolism and development of the early embryo. *Theriogenology* 1992;37:75–93

69. Newsholme EA, Crabtree B, Ardawi MS. The role of high rates of glycolysis and glutamine utilization in rapidly dividing cells. *Biosci Rep* 1985;5:393–400

70. Newsholme EA. Application of metabolic-control logic to the requirements for cell division. *Biochem Soc Trans* 1990;18:78–80

71. Hewitson LC, Leese HJ. Energy metabolism of the trophectoderm and inner cell mass of the mouse blastocyst. *J Exp Zool* 1993;267:337–43

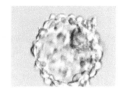

72. Gardner DK, Pool TB, Lane M. Embryo nutrition and energy metabolism and its relationship to embryo growth, differentiation, and viability. *Semin Reprod Med* 2000;18:205–18

73. Lane M, Gardner DK. Regulation of substrate utilization in mouse embryos by the malate–aspartate shuttle. *Biol Reprod* 2000;62(Suppl 1):371

74. Lane M, Gardner DK. Lactate regulates pyruvate uptake and metabolism in the preimplantation mouse embryo. *Biol Reprod* 2000;62:16–22

75. Gardner DK, Sakkas D. Mouse embryo cleavage, metabolism and viability: role of medium composition. *Hum Reprod* 1993;8:288–95

76. Gardner DK, Lane MW, Lane M. EDTA stimulates cleavage stage bovine embryo development in culture but inhibits blastocyst development and differentiation. *Mol Reprod Dev* 2000;57:256–61

77. Gardner DK, Lane M. Embryo culture systems. In Gardner DK, Trounson AO, eds. *Handbook of In Vitro Fertilization*. Boca Raton: CRC Press, 1993:85–114

78. Gardner DK, Lane M. Culture and selection of viable blastocysts: a feasible proposition for human IVF? *Hum Reprod Update* 1997;3:367–82

79. Gardner DK, Lane M. Culture of viable human blasto cysts in defined sequential serum-free media. *Hum Reprod* 1998;13(Suppl 3):148–59

80. Menke TM, McLaren A. Mouse blastocysts grown *in vivo* and *in vitro*: carbon dioxide production and trophoblast outgrowth. *J Reprod Fertil* 1970;23:117–27

81. Lane M, Gardner DK. Amino acids and vitamins prevent culture-induced metabolic perturbations and associated loss of viability of mouse blastocysts. *Hum Reprod* 1998;13:991–7

82. Gardner DK, Leese HJ. Assessment of embryo metabolism and viability. In Trounson AO, Gardner DK, eds. *Handbook of In Vitro Fertilization*, 2nd edn. Boca Raton: CRC Press, 1999:347–72

83. Gardner DK, Clarke RN, Lechene CP, Biggers JD. Development of a noninvasive ultramicrofluorometric method for measuring net uptake of glutamine by single preimplantation mouse embryos. *Gamete Res* 1989;24:427–38

84. Gardner DK, Lane M. Amino acids and ammonium regulate mouse embryo development in culture. *Biol Reprod* 1993;48:377–85

85. Johnson SK, Jordan JE, Dean RG, Page RD. The quantification of bovine embryo viability using a bioluminescent assay for lactate dehydrogenase. *Theriogenology* 1991;35:425–33

86. Renard JP, Philippon A, Menezo Y. *In-vitro* uptake of glucose by bovine blastocysts. *J Reprod Fertil* 1980;58:161–4

87. Rieger D. The measurement of metabolic activity as an approach to evaluating viability and diagnosing sex in early embryos. *Theriogenology* 1984;21:138–49

88. Gardner DK, Leese HJ. Assessment of embryo viability prior to transfer by the noninvasive measurement of glucose uptake. *J Exp Zool* 1987;242:103–5

89. Gardner DK, Pawelczynski M, Trounson AO. Nutrient uptake and utilization can be used to select viable day 7 bovine blastocysts after cryopreservation. *Mol Reprod Dev* 1996;44:472–5

90. Lane M, Gardner DK. Selection of viable mouse blastocysts prior to transfer using a metabolic criterion. *Hum Reprod* 1996;11:1975–8

91. Conaghan J, Hardy K, Handyside AH, Winston RM, Leese HJ. Selection criteria for human embryo transfer: a comparison of pyruvate uptake and morphology. *J Assist Reprod Genet* 1993;10:21–30

92. Jones G, Trounson A, Vella P, *et al.* Glucose metabolism of human morula and blastocyst stage embryos and its relationship to viability after transfer. *Reprod Biomed Online* 2001;3:124–32

93. Van den Bergh M, Devreker F, Emiliani S, Englert Y. Glycolytic activity: a possible tool for human blastocyst selection. *Reprod BioMed Online* 2001;3(Suppl 1):8

94. Gardner DK, Lane M, Stevens J, Schoolcraft WB. Noninvasive assessment of human embryo nutrient consumption as a measure of developmental potential. *Fertil Steril* 2001;76:1175–80

95. Houghton FD, Hawkhead JA, Humpherson PG, *et al.* Non-invasive amino acid turnover predicts human embryo developmental capacity. *Hum Reprod* 2002;17:999–1005

96. Lane M, Gardner DK. Nonessential amino acids and glutamine decrease the time of the first three cleavage divisions and increase compaction of mouse zygotes *in vitro*. *J Assist Reprod Genet* 1997;14:398–403

97. Gardner DK, Lane M. Development of viable mammalian embryos *in vitro*: evolution of sequential media. In Cibelli J, Lanza RP, Campbell KHS, West MD, eds. *Principles of Cloning*. San Diego: Academic Press, 2002:187–213

98. Lane M, Gardner DK. Regulation of ionic homeostasis by mammalian embryos. *Semin Reprod Med* 2000;18:195–204

99. Gardner DK, Lane M, Schoolcraft WB. Physiology and culture of the human blastocyst. *J Reprod Immunol* 2002;55:85–100

100. Gardner DK, Lane M, Stevens J, Schlenker T, Schoolcraft WB. Blastocyst score affects implantation and pregnancy outcome: towards a single blastocyst transfer. *Fertil Steril* 2000;73:1155–8

101. Gardner DK, Schoolcraft WB. *In-vitro* culture of human blastocysts. In Jansen R, Mortimer D, eds. *Towards Reproductive Certainty: Fertility and Genetics Beyond 1999*. Carnforth, UK: Parthenon Publishing 1999:378–88

102. Gardner DK. Culture of mammalian embryos in the absense of serum and somatic cells. *Cell Biol Int* 1994;18:1163–79

103. Lane M, Gardner DK. Culture of preimplantation mouse embryos in the presence of amino acids increases post implantation development whilst the concomitant production of ammonium induces birth defects. *J Reprod Fertil* 1994;102:305–12

104. Lane M, Gardner DK. Ammonium affects ICM development, metabolism, intracellular pH, and fetal growth rates. *Biol Reprod* 2002;66(Suppl 1):17

105. Gardner DK, Lane M. Embryo culture. In Gardner DK, Weissman A, Howles C, Shoham Z, eds. *Textbook of Assisted Reproductive Techniques*. London: Martin Dunitz, 2001:203–22

106. Gardner DK, Schoolcraft WB, Wagley L, Schlenker T, Stevens J, Hesla J. A prospective randomized trial of blastocyst culture and transfer in *in-vitro* fertilization. *Hum Reprod* 1998;13:3434–40

107. Biggers JD, Racowsky C. The development of fertilized human ova to the blastocyst stage in KSOMAA medium: is a two-step protocol necessary? *Reprod BioMed Online* 2002;5:133–40

108. Bolton VN, Wren ME, Parsons JH. Pregnancies after *in vitro* fertilization and transfer of human blastocysts. *Fertil Steril* 1991;55:830–2

109. Beebe DJ, Moore JS, Yu Q, *et al*. Microfluidic tectonics: a comprehensive construction platform for microfluidic systems. *Proc Natl Acad Sci USA* 2000;97:13488–93

110. Glasgow IK, Zeringue HC, Beebe DJ, *et al*. Handling individual mammalian embryos using microfluidics. *IEEE Trans Biomed Eng* 2001;48:570–8

111. Gardner DK, Rodriegez-Martinez H, Lane M. Fetal development after transfer is increased by replacing protein with the glycosaminoglycan hyaluronan for mouse embryo culture and transfer. *Hum Reprod* 1999;14:2575–80

112. Gardner DK, Maybach JM, Lane M. Hyaluronan and rHSA increase blastocyst cryosurvival. Presented at the *17th World Congress on Fertility and Sterility*, Melbourne, Australia, November 2001:226

113. Stojkovic M, Kolle S, Pein S, *et al*. Effects of high concentrations of hyaluronan in culture medium on development and survival rates of fresh and frozen–thawed bovine embryos produced *in vitro*. *Reproduction* 2002;124:141–53

114. Lane M, Maybach JM, Hooper K, Hasler JF, Gardner DK. Cryo-survival and development of bovine blastocysts are enhanced by culture with recombinant albumin and hyaluronan. *Mol Reprod Dev* 2003;64:70–8

115. Schoolcraft WB, Lane M, Stevens J, Gardner DK. Increased hyaluronan concentration in the embryo transfer medium results in a significant increase in human embryo implantation rate. *Fertil Steril* 2002;76 (Suppl 3):S5

116. Gardner DK, Lane M. Recombinant human serum albumin and hyaluronan can replace blood-derived albumin in embryo culture media. *Fertil Steril* 2000;74 (Suppl 3):S31

117. Bungum M, Humaidan P, Bungum L. Recombinant human albumin as protein source in culture media used for IVF: a prospective randomized study. *Reprod BioMed Online* 2002;4:233–6

118. Bavister BD, Kinsey DL, Lane M, Gardner DK. Recombinant human albumin supports hamster *in vitro* fertilization. *Hum Reprod* 2003;in press

119. Batt PA, Gardner DK, Cameron AW. Oxygen concentration and protein source affect the development of preimplantation goat embryos *in vitro*. *Reprod Fertil Dev* 1991;3:601–7

120. McKiernan SH, Bavister BD. Different lots of bovine serum albumin inhibit or stimulate *in vitro* development of hamster embryos. *In Vitro Cell Dev Biol* 1992;28A:154–6

121. Reed LC, Lane M, Gardner DK. *In vivo* rates of mouse embryo development can be attained *in vitro*. *Theriogenology* 2003;in press

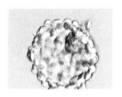

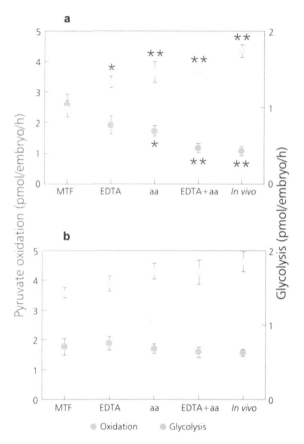

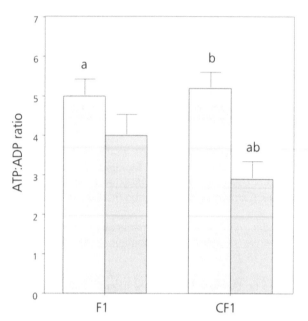

Figure 2.1 Glycolytic activity and pyruvate oxidation of CF1 (a) and F1 (b) 2-cell embryos cultured from the zygote. MTF, mouse tubal fluid medium; aa, amino acids. Significantly different from embryos in MTF: $*p < 0.05$; $**p < 0.01$. Data from reference 13

Figure 2.2 Adenosine nucleotide ratio in CF1 and F1 2-cell embryos cultured from the zygote either under conditions which facilitated development through the 2-cell block (MTF + ethylenediaminetetraacetic acid (EDTA) + amino acids), or under conditions which induced cleavage arrest at the 2-cell stage in CF1 embryos (MTF)[59]. Values are mean ± SEM of ten replicates. Open bars, MTF + EDTA + amino acids; closed bars, MTF. Like pairs are significantly different; a, $p < 0.01$; b, $p < 0.05$. Data from reference 61

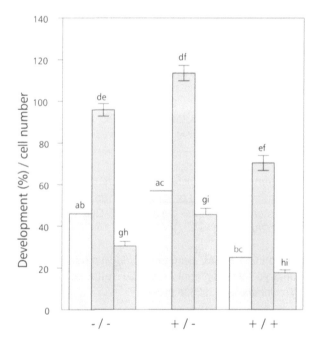

Figure 2.3 Effect of EDTA present in culture medium on the development and differentiation of bovine zygotes to the blastocyst stage: -/- embryos cultured for 72 h in medium SOFaa (synthetic oviduct fluid with amino acids) lacking EDTA followed by culture in medium SOFaa lacking EDTA; +/- embryos cultured for 72 h in medium SOFaa with 100 μmol/l EDTA followed by culture in medium SOFaa lacking EDTA; +/+ embryos cultured for 72 h in medium SOFaa with 100 μmol/l EDTA followed by culture in medium SOFaa with 100 μmol/l EDTA. Open bars represent percentage morula/blastocyst development, dark bars represent total cell number, gray bars represent inner cell mass (ICM) cell number. Like pairs of letters are significantly different: a, h, $p < 0.05$; b, c, d, e, f, g, i, $p < 0.01$. Data from reference 76

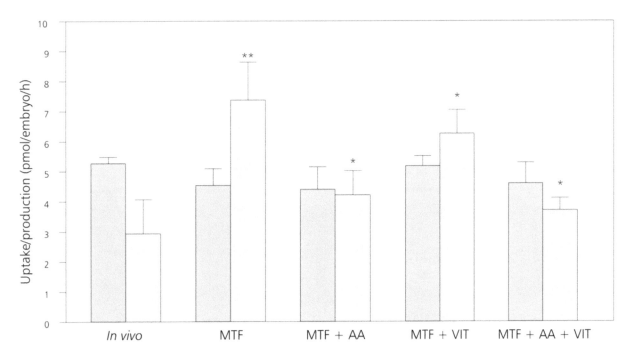

Figure 2.4 Effect of amino acids and vitamins in modified mouse tubal fluid (MTF) medium on glucose uptake and lactate production by mouse blastocysts. MTF + AA: MTF supplemented with 20 amino acids; MTF + VIT: MTF supplemented with vitamins; MTF + AA + VIT: MTF supplemented with Eagle's 20 amino acids and Eagle's vitamins. Open bars represent glucose uptake. Closed bars represent lactate production. Significantly different from *in vivo*-developed blastocysts: *$p < 0.05$; **$p < 0.01$. Data from reference 81

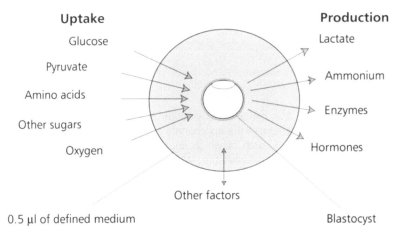

Figure 2.5 Non-invasive assessment of blastocyst nutrient uptake and utilization. Blastocysts are incubated individually in a known volume, e.g. 0.5 μl, of defined medium such as G2[77]. Serial nanoliter samples can then be taken and analyzed for carbohydrates[82], amino acids[83], ammonium[84], oxygen[22] and enzymes[85]. The concomitant measurement of glucose consumption and lactate production can give an indirect measure of glycolytic activity. Glycolytic activity has been shown to be inversely related to both development in culture and subsequent viability. The concomitant measurement of amino acid consumption and ammonium production can give an indirect measure of amino acid utilization. The release of enzymes, such as lactate dehydrogenase, into the surrounding culture medium reflects impairment in membrane integrity, and as such may be useful in assessing freezing damage

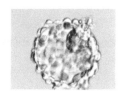

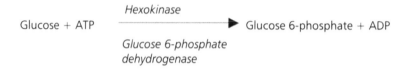

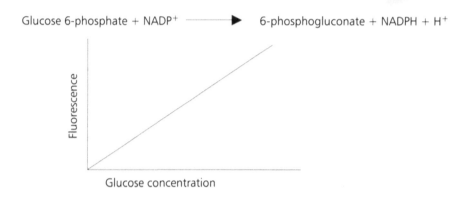

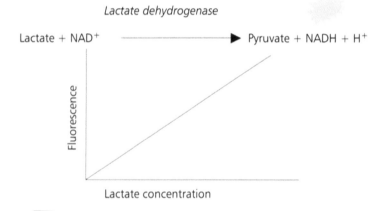

Figure 2.6 Coupling of enzymatic reaction involving the pyridine nucleotides NAD(P)H (reduced nicotinamide–adenine dinucleotide (phosphate)). Under the appropriate conditions, reactions favor the production of either NADH or NADPH, both of which fluoresce when excited by light in the UV range. When these nucleotides are oxidized (i.e. NAD⁺ or NADP⁺), they do not fluoresce. Therefore, in the presence of increasing concentrations of both glucose and lactate, there is a concomitant increase in fluorescence generated by the reaction. The absolute amount of fluorescence can then be calibrated daily by running standards and the concentration of substrates present in the culture medium surrounding the embryo determined. For a more detailed account of substrate assays and the reaction conditions required, see reference 82

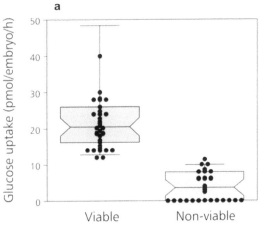

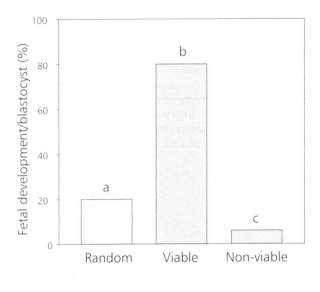

Figure 2.7 Box plots of glucose uptake (a) and lactate production (b) by individual bovine blastocysts after thawing. Blastocysts were classified retrospectively as either 'viable' or 'non-viable' based upon their ability, or otherwise, to re-expand within 14 h post-thaw. The lines across the boxes represent the median, notches representing the interquartile range, therefore including 50% of the data. Whiskers represent 5 and 95% quartiles. After reference 89

Figure 2.8 Fetal development of mouse blastocysts selected prospectively for transfer using glycolytic activity as a metabolic marker of development. 'Viable' blastocysts were those classified with a glycolytic activity close to that of *in vivo*-developed blastocysts, while 'non-viable' blastocysts were those with a highly elevated glycolytic rate. On each day of experiment, a selection of blastocysts were transferred at random. a, b, c: different letters indicate significantly different populations ($p < 0.01$). Data from reference 90

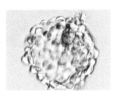

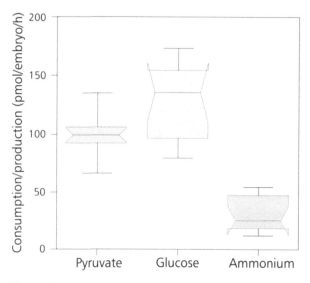

Figure 2.9 Nutrient uptake and ammonium production by individual human blastocysts from the same patients. Data are in the form of a notched box plot where the notches represent the interquartile range, therefore including 50% of the data points. Whiskers represent 5 and 95% quartiles. The line across the box represents the median. Pyruvate (solid box), glucose (open box), ammonium (hatched box). After reference 94

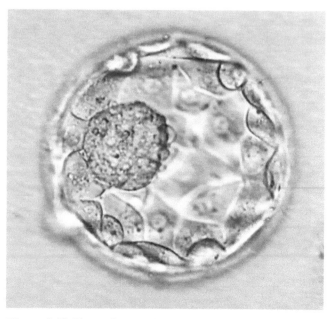

Figure 2.10 Photomicrograph of a human blastocyst cultured in sequential media. Note the development of the ICM and formation of a cohesive epithelium by the trophectoderm cells. Such a blastocyst has an implantation potential (fetal heart rate) of 70%[100]. The scoring of human blastocysts is strongly related to implantation and pregnancy outcome[100,101]

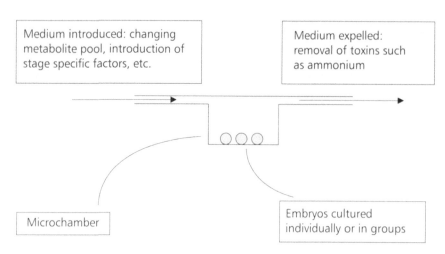

Medium introduced: changing metabolite pool, introduction of stage specific factors, etc.

Medium expelled: removal of toxins such as ammonium

Microchamber

Embryos cultured individually or in groups

Figure 2.11 Schematic diagram of an embryo perfusion culture system. Culture media are continuously passed over the embryo(s). The composition of the culture media can be changed according to the specific requirements of each stage of embryonic development. Toxins such as ammonium are not able to build up and impair embryo development, while more labile components of the culture system are not denatured. Modified from reference 102

3 Human morulae *in vitro*

The mammalian morula

The word *morula* derives from the root morus, the Latin word for 'mulberry'. It was so named in the early days of embryological investigation because of its berry-like shape and appearance, especially notable in amphibians[1]. The human preembryo is said to have become a morula at approximately the 8-cell stage of development, when the process of compaction commences[2]. In the human, up to 16 discrete blastomeres may be observed in growing preembryos, but the existence of such high cell numbers without evidence of compaction is now recognized as detrimental to further development (Figure 3.1). Normal compaction results in the formation of an outer layer of cells that become the trophectoderm of the blastocyst, while inner cells give rise to the inner cell mass (inside–outside theory) (Figure 3.2). The embryonic genome becomes functionally active during, or just before, the morula stage.

Compaction

Compaction is a process that involves the formation of intercellular tight junctions between blastomeres, which become closely apposed and flatten out as the areas of cell contact increase (Figure 3.3). As a result, a cleaving preembryo changes then from a collection of individual cells into a relatively smooth mass with indistinguishable cell outlines (Figure 3.4), the surface of the compacting human morula being characterized by densely distributed microvilli[3]. Contacts and junctions between mammalian blastomeres are dynamic, and change to accommodate the loss of coupling during mitosis[4]. It appears that such coupling is mandatory for further

development, as demonstrated by the observation that inhibited compaction in mice is lethal for the morula[5]. The first evidence of compaction is reflected in a polarization of peripheral blastomeres and a reorganization of cytoplasmic components[2]. Blastomeres or fragments that are unable to form contacts or to communicate appropriately with other blastomeres are generally excluded from the compacting preembryo, often remaining inside the zona pellucida after blastocyst hatching (Figure 3.5). As compaction occurs, cells lose their totipotency as a result of their interactions with one another, and it is believed that this marks the beginning of embryonic DNA transcription.

The time of the onset of compaction varies among species: mouse and rat at the 8-cell stage[6], bovine and rhesus monkey at the 16–32-cell stage[7,8], rabbit at 32–64 cells[8], and pig shortly before blastocyst formation[9]. Human compaction begins after the third mitotic division (8-cell stage) on day 3 and is generally completed by day 4, earlier than in other primate species[3]. What triggers compaction is unknown, but a developmental 'clock' is suggested as being responsible. The process of compaction does not appear to require a strict number of cell divisions, and has been observed to begin before completion of the third cleavage *in vitro*, particularly in slowly developing preembryos (Figure 3.6). In the mouse, inhibition of protein synthesis results in premature compaction[10]. Similarly, removal of cytoplasm from 1-cell mouse embryos results in accelerated compaction, cavitation and blastocyst formation, possibly by reducing some inhibitory factor[11]. Conversely, adding cytoplasm from 1-cell zygotes to cleaved embryos slows subsequent development[12]. These observations suggest that, at least in the mouse, altering

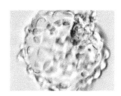

nuclear/cytoplasmic ratios by adding or removing cytoplasm may ultimately impact on developmental rates.

During compaction, a variety of junctions are formed between cells, in sequential order: *gap junctions, adherens junctions, tight junctions* and *desmosomes* (Figures 3.7 and 3.8). Each type plays a fundamental role in cellular communication, adhesion and differentiation[13].

Gap junctions are composed of a membrane protein named connexin. A group of six connexins form *connexson*, which in turn forms an intracellular channel: a gap junction is basically a group of intracellular channels[14]. These transmembrane pores/channels serve as communicators between neighboring cells for transport of metabolites and molecules that regulate cell division, differentiation and apoptosis. Gap junction formation first occurs at the 8-cell stage in the mouse[15], while, in the human, the onset and function of these junctions vary from the 4-cell stage to the early blastocyst stage[16,17]. Electron microscopic studies performed on human morulae show small gap junctions (2–3 nm) within the tight, junctional regions. However, it is unclear whether those of human pre-blastocyst stages are yet functional, since fluorescent dyes do not pass between cells before the blastocyst stage[18]. In one of the few studies specific to intracellular junctions in human preembryos, Hardy and colleagues demonstrated expression of the connexin proteins Cx43, Cx32 and Cx26 in 4-cell to hatched blastocyst stages[17]. Expression of Cx43 was enhanced with increasing development, peaking at the blastocyst stage. Cells of the trophectoderm were noted to be connected by frequent gap junctions, while inner cell masses showed fewer punctate junctions. Abnormal gap junction formation was theorized by these authors to be correlated with reduced conceptus viability. In earlier work involving the microinjection of antibodies against connexin into mouse embryos, the formation of gap junctions was inhibited, causing blastomeres to be extruded[19]. Such uncoupling has also been observed after induction of low intracellular pH, inhibiting gap junction formation[20]. Similar factors may be responsible for 'partial or incomplete' compaction, frequently observed in human preembryos cultured *in vitro* (Figure 3.9).

Adherens junctions include the E (epithelial)-cadherin (uvomorulin) system that is calcium-dependent[21]. In the mouse, E-cadherin is expressed in oocytes and preimplantation embryos during cleavage. Cytoplasmic localization of E-cadherin switches to the membrane regions of adjacent blastomeres in 8-cell specimens, where they mediate early stages of compaction[22]. At the blastocyst stage, E-cadherin is expressed within trophectoderm and inner cell mass, and operates via the E-cadherin connection to the actin cytoskeleton[23]. Antibodies against E-cadherin inhibit compaction; however, they do not inhibit gap junction communication[24]. Furthermore, mouse preimplantation embryos lacking E-cadherin fail to compact, and are rendered non-viable due to an undeveloped trophectoderm[25], possibly as a result of disrupted blastomere polarization during the process of trophectoderm differentiation. In the human, E-cadherin has been described as being expressed in oocytes and cleavage stage preembryos, but limited to the cell surface[26,27]. Other investigators demonstrated cytoplasmic expression of E-cadherin in early preimplantation stages, with trophectoderm localization in the blastocyst[28]. It will be important to investigate possible relationships between failure of compaction and/or blastocyst formation *in vitro* and disturbance in E-cadherin expression in the human.

Tight junctions join adjacent plasma membranes by way of interlinked rows of integral membrane proteins, creating a seal impermeable to the intercellular passage of molecules. They may also result in limited membrane fusion between cells, a situation essential for blastocoel formation (*see* 'Cavitation,' below). Tight junctions interact cytoplasmically with the actin cytoskeleton. The *membrane* proteins responsible for the tight junctions that form a permanent seal between cells include occludin and claudin; the *cytoplasmic* proteins include ZO-1, ZO-2 and cingulin[29]. In addition to forming a seal between cells, tight junctions help to maintain cell polarity, necessary for blastocyst formation and differentiation[30]. In the mouse, tight junctions begin to develop at the late 8-cell stage after compaction, and require previous establishment of the E-cadherin system. The association between tight junctions and E-cadherin was confirmed by experiments using anti-E-cadherin antibody, where tight junction formation was disrupted[29]. Tight junction assembly is regulated in stages during the compaction process[31]. The first stage involves *cytoplasmic* tight junction proteins, particularly the ZO-1α[-] variant, which is regulated by E-cadherin and may be responsible for maintaining cell membrane polarity[29]. In the next stage, cingulin assembles in the apicolateral region of the blastomeres. The final stage of membrane assembly involves the ZO-1α[+] variant and the membrane protein, occludin.

Formation of ZO-1α[+] is thought to be a critical final step in creation of the permeable seal, a prerequisite for cavitation and blastocoel development[13,18]. Interestingly, delayed expression of ZO-1α[+] may prevent occludin transformation, and this delay is possibly involved in developmental arrest of the preembryo. Primitive tight junctions have been observed ultrastructurally in 6–8-cell human preembryos[16,32]. Other studies have shown that tight junctions are well assembled by the morula stage, and are localized to trophectoderm in the developing human blastocyst[18] (Figure 3.10). The expression of ZO-1 proteins in human cleaved preembryos and blastocysts was identified in all stages in the cytoplasm, and localized in trophectoderm junctions in the blastocyst[28].

Desmosomes are small disk-shaped junctions that connect epithelial cells[33]. As with tight junctions, key genes regulate the timing of desmosome expression. It appears that desmosomes help to maintain trophectoderm integrity and stability during blastocyst expansion. Premature desmosome development may interfere with differentiation of the trophectoderm and development of the inner cell mass[13]. In the mouse, desmosomes can be observed between blastomeres and trophectoderm cells[34]. The same is found in human investigations, where single desmosomes have been identified at the 16-cell stage, with extensive desmosome formation occurring between developing trophectoderm cells during cavitation. In the blastocyst, desmosomes are located between trophectoderm cells but are not found between cells of the inner cell mass or between trophectoderm cells that contact the inner cell mass[17] (*see* Figure 3.8).

Ca^{2+} and Mg^{2+} ions are also essential for compaction. Compacting human morulae can be decompacted easily by incubation in Ca^{2+}- and Mg^{2+}-free medium for only a few minutes (Figure 3.11). This method facilitates blastomere biopsy on day 3, involving 6–8-cell stage preembryos that have begun to show cell–cell contact and compaction.

Other factors that may be involved in the process of compaction include carbohydrate antigens, especially the stage-specific embryonic antigen-1 (SSEA-1). This antigen is expressed on the cell surface of mouse embryos after the third cleavage, and is related to the onset of compaction[35]. To investigate the possible role of SSEA-1 during the compaction process, specific oligosaccharides were purified from human milk and added to fully compacted mouse morulae. It was found that blastomeres lost cell–cell contacts and became decompacted after 6–8 h[36]. One possible means of explaining how carbohydrate antigens regulate compaction is to study the Ca^{2+}- and Mg^{2+}-dependent carbohydrate–carbohydrate interaction between cells[37]. At Cornell, we demonstrated expression of the SSEA-1 antigen on both mature human oocytes and cleaved preembryos up to the blastocyst stage of development. The role of SSEA antigens during human embryogenesis and differential expression between mouse and human are discussed in Chapter 4. The presence of specific adhesion molecules and various junctional complexes in human preembryos indicates the complicated nature of the compaction process.

Cavitation

After compaction, and as the preembryo expands, it begins to form a cavity. Cavitation is an essential developmental stage whereby cells differentiate into trophectoderm and inner cell mass. As the extent of cell–cell surface contact increases during compaction, the group of cells located on the outside polarize to form the trophectoderm. The smaller group of cells inside develop into the inner cell mass (*see* Chapter 4). Cavitation involves the accumulation of blastocoelic fluid transported by trophectoderm cells. To accomplish this, trophectoderm cells first depend on complete cellular polarization and then the formation of permeable seals provided by tight junctions which form a belt-like circular line between developing trophectoderm cells[38].

The polarity of blastomeres is regulated by the extent of their contact and location within the preembryo. Cell polarization involves cell surface microvilli and leptin modifications[3,39], irregular allocation of the membrane proteins between apical and basal cell membranes[40] and basal mitochondrial accumulation[41].

The apical membranes of the outer blastomeres of mouse preimplantation embryos possess transport channels that regulate Na$^+$ passage[42], while tight junction proteins, gap junctions and E-cadherin are associated with basal membranes[31,43,44]. In human preembryos, gap junctions are associated with basal and lateral membranes of adjacent blastomeres, while trophectoderm cells of the blastocyst show gap junction formation across their entire surfaces[17]. The irregular

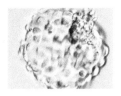

contact between adjacent cells maintains the cell polarity necessary for polarized ion transportation: ions flow in through apical membranes and out through basal membranes into the blastocoel[45].

Accumulation of fluid into the blastocoel is a result of Na^+ transport through the epithelial-like cells of the trophectoderm, and is energy dependent[46] (Figure 3.12). Sodium ions diffuse into the trophectoderm through multiple apical channels[42]. Na/K-adenosine triphosphatase (ATPase), located basolaterally, actively pumps intracellular Na^+ into the blastocoel, and tight junctions moderate containment[47]. Alpha-1 and β-1 subunits of Na/K-ATPase are expressed during mouse preimplantation development, β subunits being essential for the onset of cavitation[48,49]. Consequently, blastocyst expansion is inhibited in the presence of ouabain (an inhibitor of Na/K-ATPase)[50]. Furthermore, ouabain promotes the exchange of intracellular K^+ for extracellular Na^+, indicating that Na/K-ATPase operates in trophectoderm cells in a manner similar to that in, for example, kidney cells[51,52].

It is unknown precisely how intracellular Na^+ levels are regulated in the trophectoderm, but it is likely that other ions are involved, e.g. Cl^-. Apparently, the osmotic gradient resulting from increased Na^+ initiates passive water movement into the blastocoel. This is achieved through 'water channels' that depend on aquaporins, inherent membrane proteins that allow water to pass in the direction of the osmotic gradient[53]. Aquaporins are known to be expressed in mouse preimplantation embryos and blastocysts[54,55]. Intracellular calcium may also play a role in cavitation, since agents such as ethanol and ionomycin that increase intracellular Ca^{2+} also speed the process of cavitation[56,57].

Blastocoelic fluid serves as a culture medium during the crucial development of the inner cell mass[58,59]. Cavitation is clearly an energy-dependent process, and glucose serves as a principal energy source in mammalian preembryos after the 8-cell stage. Cavitation and blastocyst formation in vitro can be greatly influenced by medium composition. Amino acids and other metabolites directly influence normal compaction, cavitation and blastocyst development (see Chapter 2).

In the mouse, cavities are formed to one side of the morula, at the so-called abembryonic pole (Figure 3.13). In the human, cavities appear to develop more centrally (Figure 3.14).

Morphology of the morula

The human morula has generated renewed interest with the routine application of extended culture within clinical in vitro fertilization (IVF) laboratories. Until recently, reports of transferring preembryos on day 4 were limited to cases that involved preimplantation genetic diagnosis (PGD), necessitating a delay of transfer until diagnostic results were obtained. A recent publication contends that this stage of development has been neglected as a transfer option for intrauterine transfer following assisted reproductive technology[60]. The authors demonstrated increased clinical pregnancy rates following the replacement of compacted morulae, and proposed a grading system for day-4 preembryos. On day 4, compacted morulae were assessed for *early compaction* (identified by blastomeres that had begun to form a clustered cell mass, each individual cell being identifiable, but not distinct), *full compaction* (blastomeres were completely adherent, cell boundaries might not be visible, but nuclei could be identified) and *late compaction/early blastocyst* (cell boundaries were visible again, and cell number was significantly increased). Preembryos not showing any evidence of compaction on day 4 were considered slow-growing and not evaluated in the study. Compacted morulae were further assessed for:

(1) The proportion of blastomeres undergoing compaction;

(2) The morphology of compaction;

(3) Previous morphology on days 2 and 3 of development;

(4) The percentage of fragmentation.

The authors then examined subsequent clinical pregnancy rates based on whether or not high-scoring morulae were replaced. When no high-scoring morulae were available, clinical pregnancy was 28.9% and implantation was 15.7%. Ongoing pregnancy was 22.2%. When at least one 'good' morula was transferred, pregnancy, ongoing pregnancy and implantation rates were 50.9%, 37.5% and 25.2%, respectively. When two or more 'good' morulae were transferred, rates were 70.0%, 44.9% and 44.4%, respectively. From these data, the authors concluded that day-4 morulae represent a developmental stage with good selection value for intrauterine replacement.

Under the light microscope, imminent compaction is evidenced by increased *cell–cell contact* between blastomeres. Individual blastomeres become closely apposed but still remain separate (Figures 3.15–3.17).

As the conceptus begins actively *compacting*, individual blastomeres become extremely difficult to distinguish as cells begin to flatten and become closely adherent to one another (Figures 3.18–3.20).

The fully *compacted* morula may appear as a single unit exhibiting multiple nuclei. Sometimes individual blastomeres are excluded from the process; often, cytoplasmic fragments are left behind (Figures 3.21–3.23).

Early cavitation is observed when a sickle-cell-shaped hollowed area or cleft begins to form between fully-adherent blastomeres. As the conceptus continues its development, a true cavity is formed and begins enlarging. For definition purposes, a cavitating morula is said to possess a cavity constituting less than 50% of its total surface area (Figures 3.24–3.26).

Morulae have been seen to *vacuolate* (rather than cavitate) *in vitro*, roughly approximating the appearance of a poorly developing blastocyst, but these soon arrest in their development, secrete no human chorionic gonadotropin (hCG) and have fewer nuclei[61] (Figures 3.27–3.29).

Human morulae can be observed as early as 65 h post-insemination, but are generally noted some hours after that, between days 3 and 4 of development.

References

1. O'Rahilly R, Mèuller F, Streeter GL. *Developmental stages in Human Embryos: Including a Revision of Streeter's 'Horizons' and a Survey of the Carnegie Collection.* Washington, DC: Carnegie Institution of Washington, 1987

2. Hartshorne GM, Edwards RG. Early embryo development. In Adashi EY, Rock JA, Rosenwaks Z, eds. *Reproductive Endocrinology, Surgery, and Technology.* Philadelphia: Lippincott-Raven, 1996:435–50

3. Nikas G, Ao A, Winston RM, Handyside AH. Compaction and surface polarity in the human embryo *in vitro. Biol Reprod* 1996;55:32–7

4. Goodall H, Maro B. Major loss of junctional coupling during mitosis in early mouse embryos. *J Cell Biol* 1986;102:568–75

5. Cheng SS, Costantini F. Morula decompaction (mdn), a preimplantation recessive lethal defect in a transgenic mouse line. *Dev Biol* 1993;156:265–77

6. Reeve WJ. Cytoplasmic polarity develops at compaction in rat and mouse embryos. *J Embryol Exp Morphol* 1981;62:351–67

7. Enders AC, Lantz KC, Schlafke S. The morula–blastocyst transition in two Old World primates: the baboon and rhesus monkey. *J Med Primatol* 1990;19:725–47

8. Koyama H, Suzuki H, Yang X, Jiang S, Foote RH. Analysis of polarity of bovine and rabbit embryos by scanning electron microscopy. *Biol Reprod* 1994;50:163–70

9. Reima I, Lehtonen E, Virtanen I, Flechon JE. The cytoskeleton and associated proteins during cleavage, compaction and blastocyst differentiation in the pig. *Differentiation* 1993;54:35–45

10. Levy JB, Johnson MH, Goodall H, Maro B. The timing of compaction: control of a major developmental transition in mouse early embryogenesis. *J Embryol Exp Morphol* 1986;95:213–37

11. Feng YL, Gordon JW. Removal of cytoplasm from one-celled mouse embryos induces early blastocyst formation. *J Exp Zool* 1997;277:345–52

12. Lee DR, Lee JE, Yoon HS, Roh SI, Kim MK. Compaction in preimplantation mouse embryos is regulated by a cytoplasmic regulatory factor that alters between 1- and 2-cell stages in a concentration-dependent manner. *J Exp Zool* 2001;290:61–71

13. Fleming TP, Ghassemifar MR, Sheth B. Junctional complexes in the early mammalian embryo. *Semin Reprod Med* 2000;18:185–93

14. Kidder GM, Winterhager E. Intercellular communication in preimplantation development: the role of gap junctions. *Front Biosci* 2001;6:D731–6

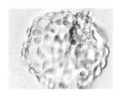

15. Lo CW, Gilula NB. Gap junctional communication in the preimplantation mouse embryo. *Cell* 1979;18:399–409

16. Dale B, Gualtieri R, Talevi R, Tosti E, Santella L, Elder K. Intercellular communication in the early human embryo. *Mol Reprod Dev* 1991;29:22–8

17. Hardy K, Warner A, Winston RM, Becker DL. Expression of intercellular junctions during preimplantation development of the human embryo. *Mol Hum Reprod* 1996;2:621–32

18. Gualtieri R, Santella L, Dale B. Tight junctions and cavitation in the human preembryo. *Mol Reprod Dev* 1992;32:81–7

19. Lee S, Gilula NB, Warner AE. Gap junctional communication and compaction during preimplantation stages of mouse development. *Cell* 1987;51:851–60

20. Leclerc C, Becker D, Buehr M, Warner A. Low intracellular pH is involved in the early embryonic death of DDK mouse eggs fertilized by alien sperm. *Dev Dyn* 1994;200:257–67

21. Takeichi M. Cadherin cell adhesion receptors as a morphogenetic regulator. *Science* 1991;251:1451–5

22. Clayton L, Stinchcombe SV, Johnson MH. Cell surface localisation and stability of uvomorulin during early mouse development. *Zygote* 1993;1:333–44

23. Aberle H, Schwartz H, Kemler R. Cadherin–catenin complex: protein interactions and their implications for cadherin function. *J Cell Biochem* 1996;61:514–23

24. Johnson MH, Maro B, Takeichi M. The role of cell adhesion in the synchronization and orientation of polarization in 8-cell mouse blastomeres. *J Embryol Exp Morphol* 1986;93:239–55

25. Riethmacher D, Brinkmann V, Birchmeier C. A targeted mutation in the mouse E-cadherin gene results in defective preimplantation development. *Proc Natl Acad Sci USA* 1995;92:855–9

26. Campbell S, Swann HR, Seif MW, Kimber SJ, Aplin JD. Cell adhesion molecules on the oocyte and preimplantation human embryo. *Hum Reprod* 1995;10:1571–8

27. Rufas O, Fisch B, Ziv S, Shalgi R. Expression of cadherin adhesion molecules on human gametes. *Mol Hum Reprod* 2000;6:163–9

28. Bloor DJ, Metcalfe AD, Rutherford A, Brison DR, Kimber SJ. Expression of cell adhesion molecules during human preimplantation embryo development. *Mol Hum Reprod* 2002;8:237–45

29. Fleming TP, McConnell J, Johnson MH, Stevenson BR. Development of tight junctions de novo in the mouse early embryo: control of assembly of the tight junction-specific protein, ZO-1. *J Cell Biol* 1989;108:1407–18

30. Stevenson BR, Keon BH. The tight junction: morphology to molecules. *Annu Rev Cell Dev Biol* 1998;14:89–109

31. Fleming TP, Sheth B, Fesenko I. Cell adhesion in the preimplantation mammalian embryo and its role in trophectoderm differentiation and blastocyst morphogenesis. *Front Biosci* 2001;6:D1000–7

32. Tesarik J. Involvement of oocyte-coded message in cell differentiation control of early human embryos. *Development* 1989;105:317–22

33. Garrod D, Chidgey M, North A. Desmosomes: differentiation, development, dynamics and disease. *Curr Opin Cell Biol* 1996;8:670–8

34. Fleming TP, Garrod DR, Elsmore AJ. Desmosome biogenesis in the mouse preimplantation embryo. *Development* 1991;112:527–39

35. Eggens I, Fenderson B, Toyokuni T, Dean B, Stroud M, Hakomori S. Specific interaction between Lex and Lex determinants. A possible basis for cell recognition in preimplantation embryos and in embryonal carcinoma cells. *J Biol Chem* 1989;264:9476–84

36. Fenderson BA, Eddy EM, Hakomori S. Glycoconjugate expression during embryogenesis and its biological significance. *Bioessays* 1990;12:173–9

37. Solter D, Knowles BB. Monoclonal antibody defining a stage-specific mouse embryonic antigen (SSEA-1). *Proc Natl Acad Sci USA* 1978;75:5565–9

38. Watson AJ, Barcroft LC. Regulation of blastocyst formation. *Front Biosci* 2001;6:D708–30

39. Antczak M, Van Blerkom J. Oocyte influences on early development: the regulatory proteins leptin and STAT3 are polarized in mouse and human oocytes and differentially distributed within the cells of the preimplantation stage embryo. *Mol Hum Reprod* 1997;3:1067–86

40. Watson AJ. The cell biology of blastocyst development. *Mol Reprod Dev* 1992;33:492–504

41. Wiley LM. Cavitation in the mouse preimplantation embryo: Na/K-ATPase and the origin of nascent blastocoele fluid. *Dev Biol* 1984;105:330–42

42. Manejwala FM, Cragoe EJ Jr, Schultz RM. Blastocoel expansion in the preimplantation mouse embryo: role of

extracellular sodium and chloride and possible apical routes of their entry. *Dev Biol* 1989;133:210–20

43. Kemler R. From cadherins to catenins: cytoplasmic protein interactions and regulation of cell adhesion. *Trends Genet* 1993;9:317–21

44. Vestweber D, Gossler A, Boller K, Kemler R. Expression and distribution of cell adhesion molecule uvomorulin in mouse preimplantation embryos. *Dev Biol* 1987;124:451–6

45. Nuccitelli R, Wiley LM. Polarity of isolated blastomeres from mouse morulae: detection of transcellular ion currents. *Dev Biol* 1985;109:452–63

46. Biggers JD, Bell JE, Benos DJ. Mammalian blastocyst: transport functions in a developing epithelium. *Am J Physiol* 1988;255:C419–32

47. Watson AJ, Kidder GM. Immunofluorescence assessment of the timing of appearance and cellular distribution of Na/K-ATPase during mouse embryogenesis. *Dev Biol* 1988;126:80–90

48. Watson AJ, Pape C, Emanuel JR, Levenson R, Kidder GM. Expression of Na,K-ATPase α and β subunit genes during preimplantation development of the mouse. *Dev Genet* 1990;11:41–8

49. Gardiner CS, Williams JS, Menino AR Jr. Sodium/potassium adenosine triphosphatase α- and β-subunit and a-subunit mRNA levels during mouse embryo development *in vitro*. *Biol Reprod* 1990;43:788–94

50. DiZio SM, Tasca RJ. Sodium-dependent amino acid transport in preimplantation mouse embryos. III. Na^+–K^+-ATPase-linked mechanism in blastocysts. *Dev Biol* 1977;59:198–205

51. Baltz JM, Smith SS, Biggers JD, Lechene C. Intracellular ion concentrations and their maintenance by Na^+/K^+-ATPase in preimplantation mouse embryos. *Zygote* 1997;5:1–9

52. Watson AJ, Damsky CH, Kidder GM. Differentiation of an epithelium: factors affecting the polarized distribution of Na^+,K^+-ATPase in mouse trophectoderm. *Dev Biol* 1990;141:104–14

53. Deen PM, van Os CH. Epithelial aquaporins. *Curr Opin Cell Biol* 1998;10:435–42

54. Edashige K, Sakamoto M, Kasai M. Expression of mRNAs of the aquaporin family in mouse oocytes and embryos. *Cryobiology* 2000;40:171–5

55. Offenberg H, Barcroft LC, Caveney A, Viuff D, Thomsen PD, Watson AJ. mRNAs encoding aquaporins are present during murine preimplantation development. *Mol Reprod Dev* 2000;57:323–30

56. Stachecki JJ, Armant DR. Regulation of blastocoele formation by intracellular calcium release is mediated through a phospholipase C-dependent pathway in mice. *Biol Reprod* 1996;55:1292–8

57. Stachecki JJ, Armant DR. Transient release of calcium from inositol 1,4,5-trisphosphate-specific stores regulates mouse preimplantation development. *Development* 1996;122:2485–96

58. Dardik A, Schultz RM. Protein secretion by the mouse blastocyst: differences in the polypeptide composition secreted into the blastocoel and medium. *Biol Reprod* 1991;45:328–33

59. Dardik A, Doherty AS, Schultz RM. Protein secretion by the mouse blastocyst: stimulatory effect on secretion into the blastocoel by transforming growth factor-α. *Mol Reprod Dev* 1993;34:396–401

60. Tao J, Tamis R, Fink K. Pregnancies achieved after transferring frozen morula/compact stage embryos. *Fertil Steril* 2001;75:629–31

61. Dokras A, Sargent IL, Barlow DH. Human blastocyst grading: an indicator of developmental potential? *Hum Reprod* 1993;8:2119–27

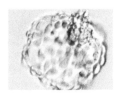

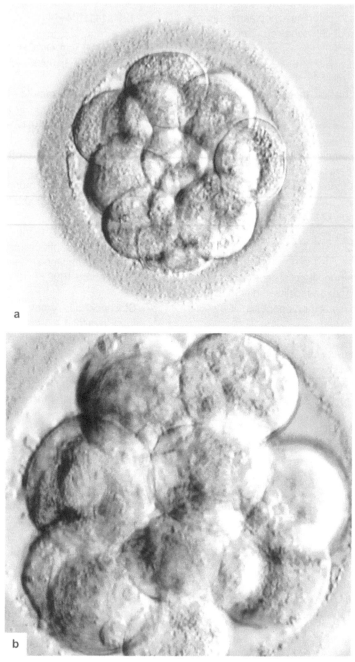

Figure 3.1 Day-3 preembryos that fail to begin compaction by the 8-cell stage of development. (a) Human preembryo on day 3 with 16 blastomeres, displaying no evidence of compaction. Neither compaction nor blastocyst development occurred over the following 3 days; (b) day-3 human preembryo with 14–16 blastomeres, shown here immediately before transfer, that failed to implant after intrauterine transfer

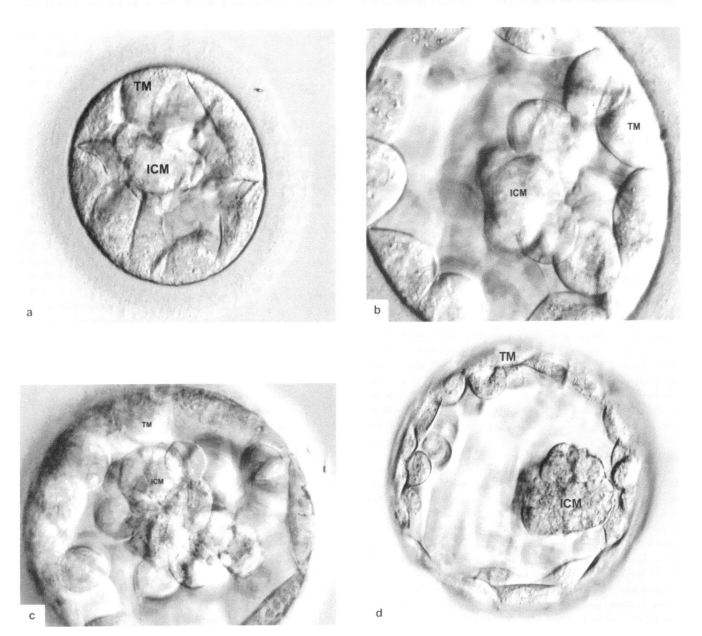

Figure 3.2 Differentiation of inner cell mass (ICM) and trophectoderm (TM) following compaction. (a) Separation of cell types and early cavitation; central inner cell mass and peripheral trophectoderm. The blastocoele can be seen forming between the ICM and TM, occupying nearly 50% of the surface area; (b) morula at more advanced stage of cavitation. Clear formation of the ICM, its migration from a central to more polar position, and a peripheral TM. ICM cells are rounded while TM cells are elliptical and polarized. Blastocoele encompasses approximately 50% of the surface area; (c) centrally-developing ICM shows dispersed cells beginning to join together; (d) fully expanded blastocyst with compacted ICM and cohesive, multicellular TM

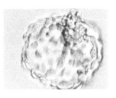

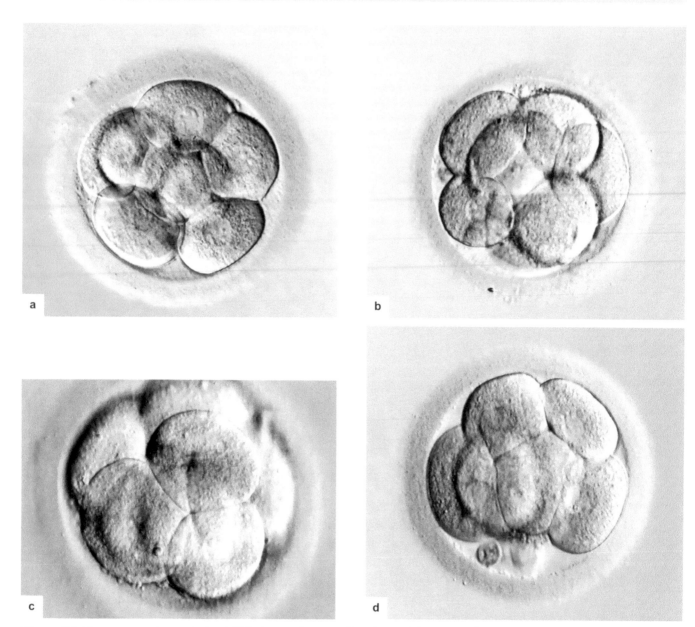

Figure 3.3 Human preembryos during initial stages of compaction, termed the stage of cell–cell contact. Blastomeres become closely apposed to one another and cell junctions begin to form between them. (a)–(d) Early cell–cell contact when blastomeres may still be counted easily

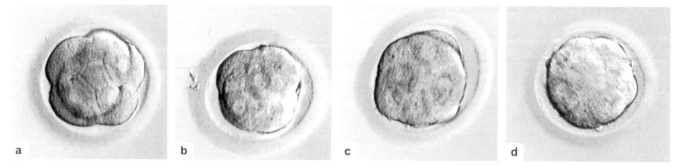

Figure 3.4 Human preembryos exhibiting increased cell–cell contact. As the areas of cell contact increase, individual cell membranes are less defined. (a) Blastomeres are closely apposed but can still be counted; (b) with increased contact, blastomeres cannot be counted easily; (c) and (d) fully compacted morula; cell membranes cannot be distinguished but nuclei can be counted

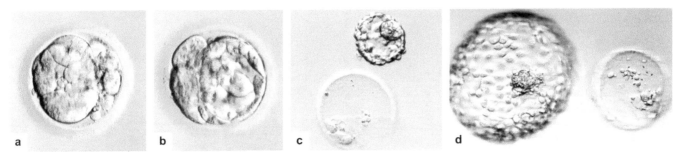

Figure 3.5 Blastomeres and fragments unable to form appropriate contacts are generally excluded from the compaction process. (a) Compacted morula at the onset of cavitation. Fragments and/or blastomeres not participating in the process are shown to the right; (b) two to three large, vacuolating blastomeres to the left are excluded from compaction and cavitation; (c) and (d) cells and/or fragments excluded from the blastocyst remain in the zona pellucida after hatching

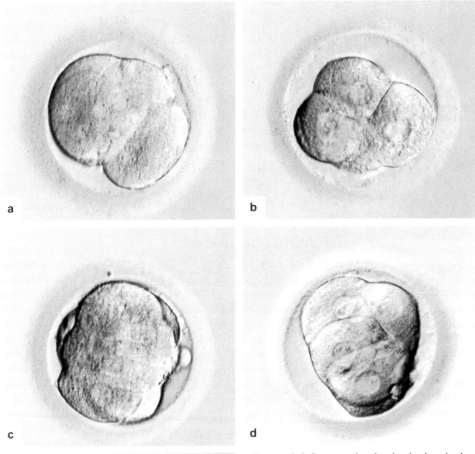

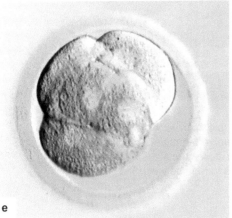

Figure 3.6 Compaction in slowly developing preembryos before the 8-cell stage. (a)–(e) The fact that compaction occurs in slowly developing human preembryos (4–7-cell stages) on day 4 supports the idea of a developmental clock regulating the process. These preembryos usually do not form viable blastocysts

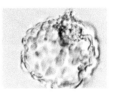

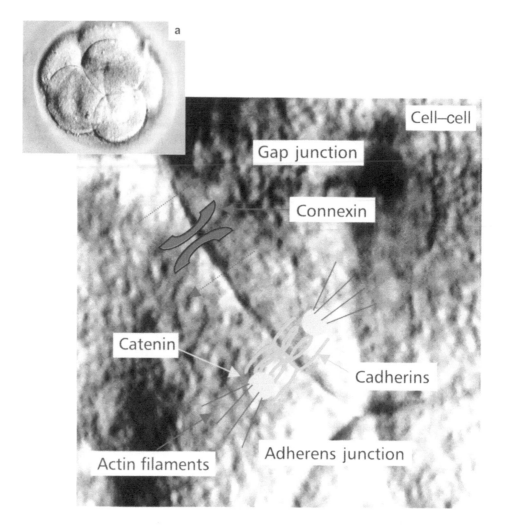

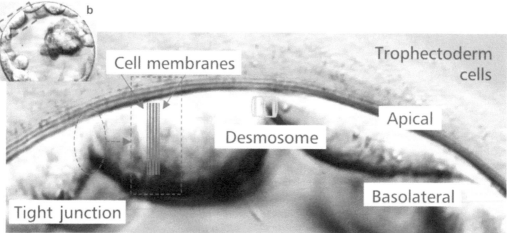

Figure 3.7 Schematic presentation of cell junctions. (a) Gap junctions are comprised of connexins that form gaps between blastomere membranes. Adherens junctions involve the cadherin system connected to actin filaments via catenins; (b) tight junctions are extremely close connections formed between membranes of TM cells. Desmosomes are disk-shaped junctions formed between TM cells

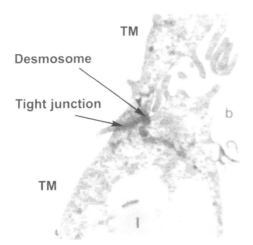

Figure 3.8 Transmission electron micrograph of human blastocyst showing cell junctions between two trophectoderm cells, i.e. tight junction and desmosome (arrows). Photograph courtesy of Henry A. Sathananthan

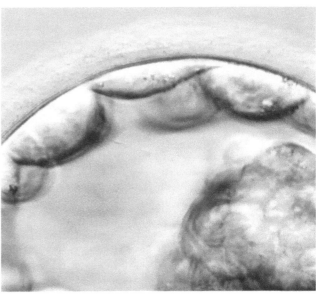

Figure 3.10 High-power magnification of the trophectoderm cells of a human blastocyst. TM cells are elongated, elliptical in shape, and have polarized membranes. Tight junctions mediate connections between these cells

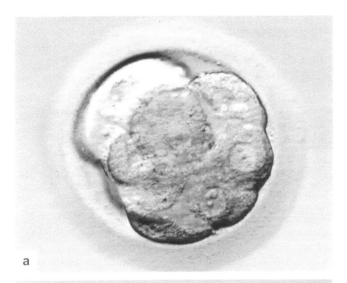

Figure 3.9 Partial/incomplete compaction. (a) Partial compaction frequently seen in human preembryos cultured *in vitro*. One or more blastomeres of the preembryo will not participate in the compaction process; (b) exclusion of one large, vacuolated blastomere does not impede compaction of the remainder of the conceptus

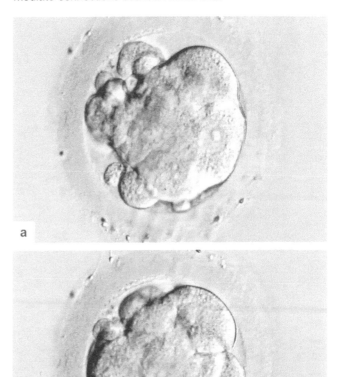

Figure 3.11 Human morula exposed briefly to Ca^{2+}- and Mg^{2+}-free medium. (a) Compacted morula exhibiting some excluded cells before treatment; (b) morula after treatment showing decompaction as evidenced by the loss of blastomere coupling

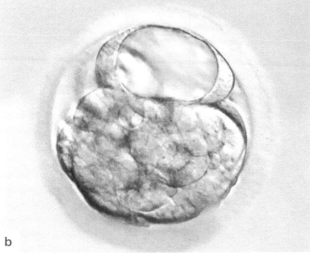

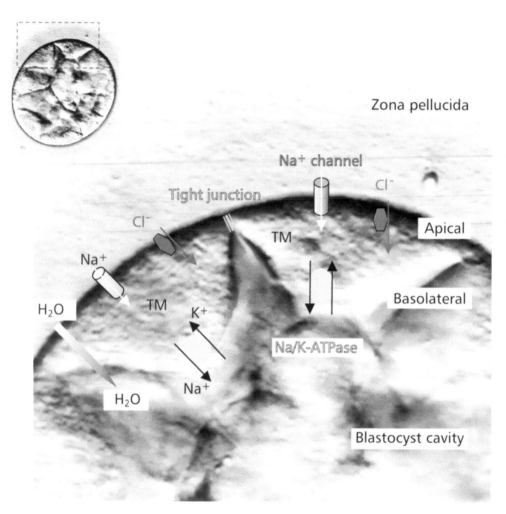

Zona pellucida

Na+ channel

Cl⁻

Tight junction

Cl⁻

Apical

Na+

TM

Na+

TM

K+

Basolateral

H₂O

Na/K-ATPase

H₂O

Na+

Blastocyst cavity

Figure 3.12 Schematic representation of the cavitation process. TM cells are polarized apically, facing the zona pellucida; basal membranes face the blastocoele. Tight junctions between TM cells form permeable seals necessary for fluid accumulation. Sodium ions diffuse through TM cells via sodium channels. NA/K-ATPase, located basolaterally, is responsible for the active pumping of intracellular sodium into the blastocoele. The resulting osmotic gradient initiates passive water movement into the blastocoele. Tight junctions moderate containment

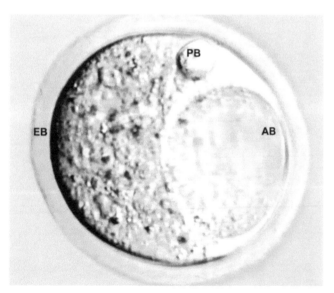

Figure 3.13 Exocentric cavitation of the mouse morula. The cavity forms at the abembryonic (AB) pole, while the ICM forms at the embryonic (EB) pole. The AB/EB orientation depends upon polar body (PB) position

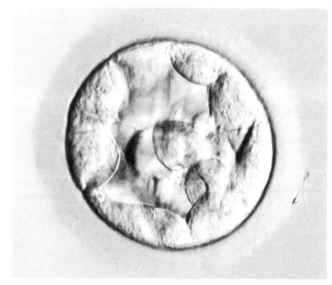

Figure 3.14 Central cavitation of the human morula. The cavity forms centrally, surrounding ICM cells as they separate from the developing TM. There are notable differences between mouse (Figure 3.13) and human cavitation

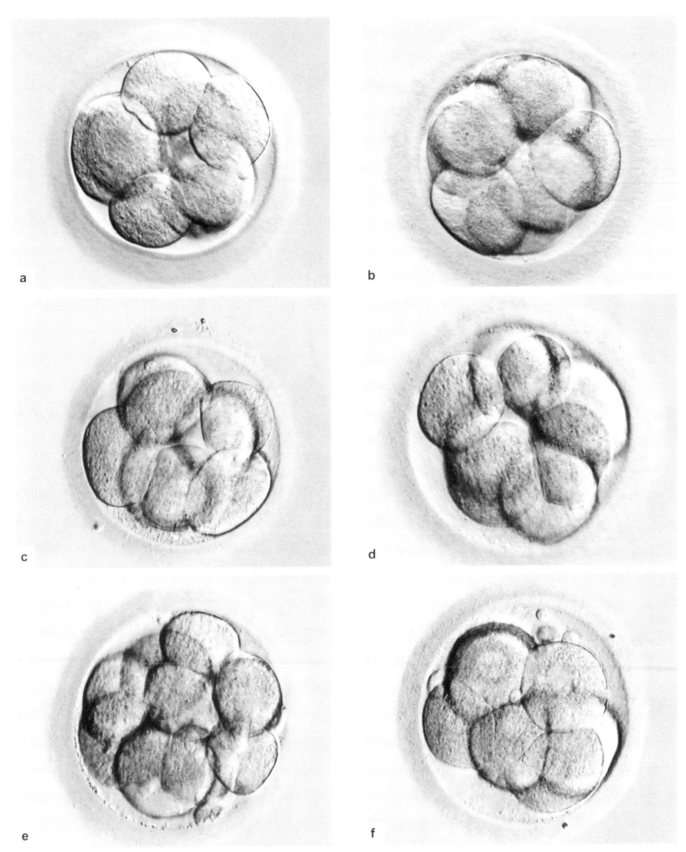

Figure 3.15 (a)–(f) Human preembryos on day 3 (8–10 blastomeres) exhibiting minimal cell–cell contact. Blastomeres are counted easily

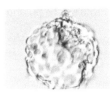

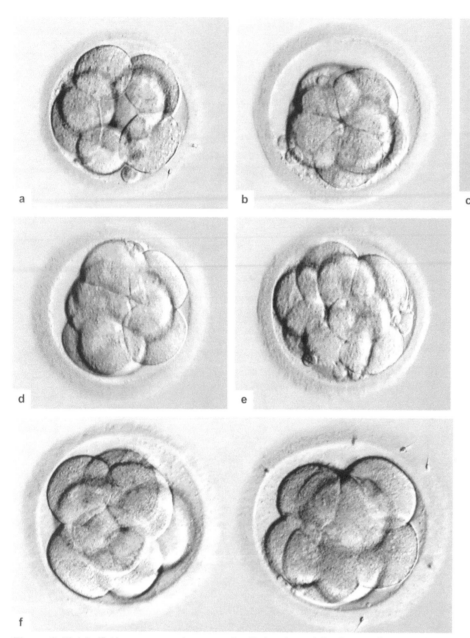

Figure 3.16 (a)–(f) Human preembryos on day 3 showing minimal to moderate cell–cell contact. Membranes of blastomeres can still be seen clearly

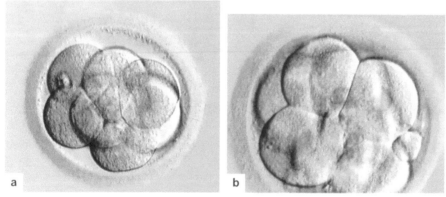

Figure 3.17 (a) and (b) Moderate cell–cell contact between blastomeres

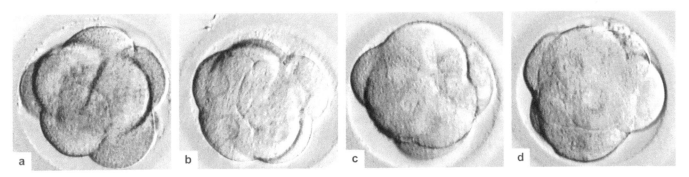

Figure 3.18 (a)–(d) Full cell–cell contact between blastomeres (compaction). Individual blastomere membranes are becoming difficult to recognize

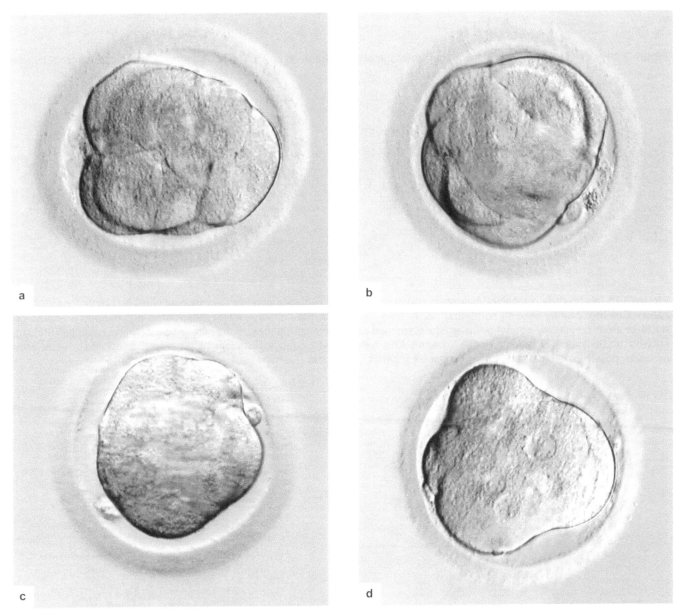

Figure 3.19 (a)–(d) Compacting human morulae on day 4. Tightly compacted cells are observed. Compacted human morulae on day 4 showing multiple nuclei of different sizes and shapes, indicating possible multinucleation

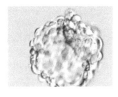

77

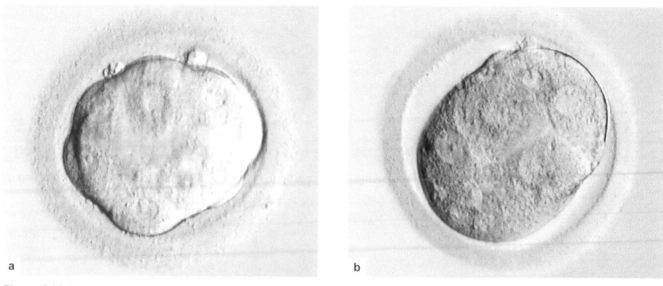

Figure 3.20 (a) and (b) Human morulae at the final stage of compaction on day 4. Individual cell membranes are no longer visible

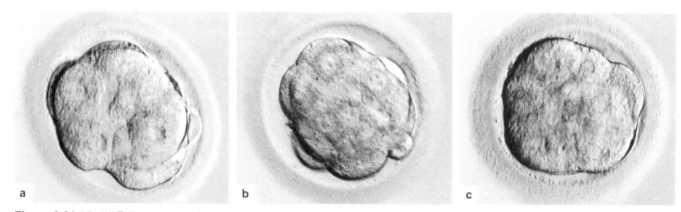

Figure 3.21 (a)–(c) Fully compacted human morulae on day 4; first evidence of minor decompaction just before the onset of cavitation. Cell membranes become somewhat visible once again. One may observe either cytoplasmic accumulations around cell nuclei or areas completely clear of cytoplasm (at presumed blastomere peripheries). If the latter areas increase, cavitation and subsequent blastocyst development may be impaired. This may indicate intracytoplasmic, instead of extracytoplasmic, water accumulation, possibly stemming from an abnormal early cavitation process (Na/K-ATPase)

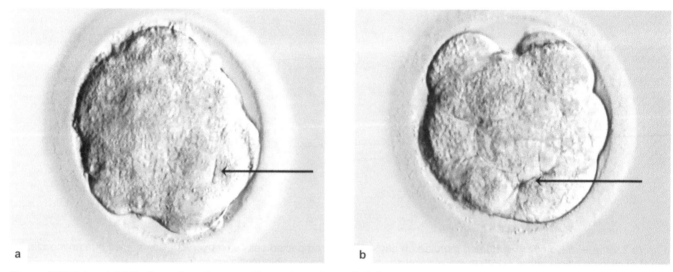

Figure 3.22 (a) and (b) Further minor decompaction; extremely small clefts are appearing between cells, indicating the very beginning of cavitation

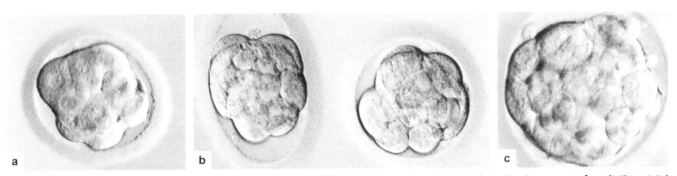

Figure 3.23 Compaction → decompaction → cavitation. (a) Slight decompaction; small clefts indicating onset of cavitation; total cell number is increasing; (b) two decompacting, early cavitating morulae. Some decompaction is taking place and cell number is increasing just before the onset of cavitation; (c) human morula showing increased cell division (thus, an increase in cell number) and minor decompaction and clefting just before cavitation

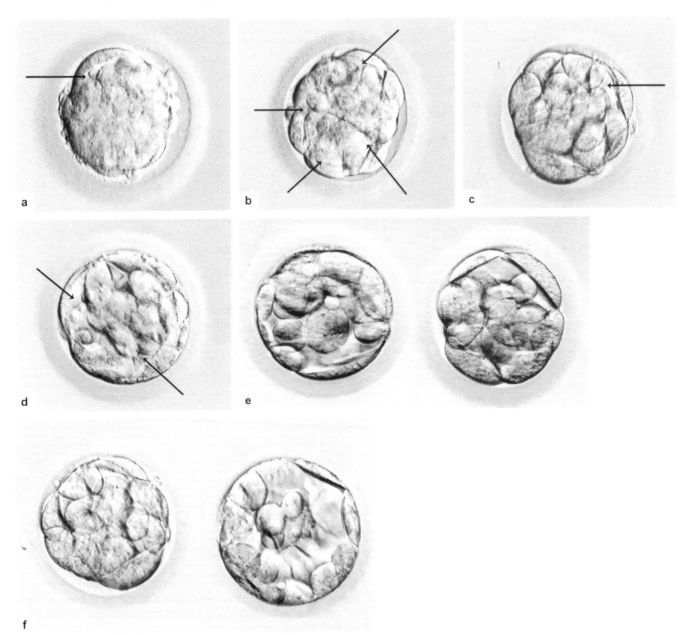

Figure 3.24 (a)–(f) Beginning of cavitation. Small fluid-filled areas are formed between adjacent cells of the morula. In time, these areas will enlarge to form a single cavity, the blastocoele. Cells differ in size and shape. No clear ICM can yet be discerned

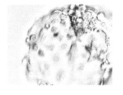

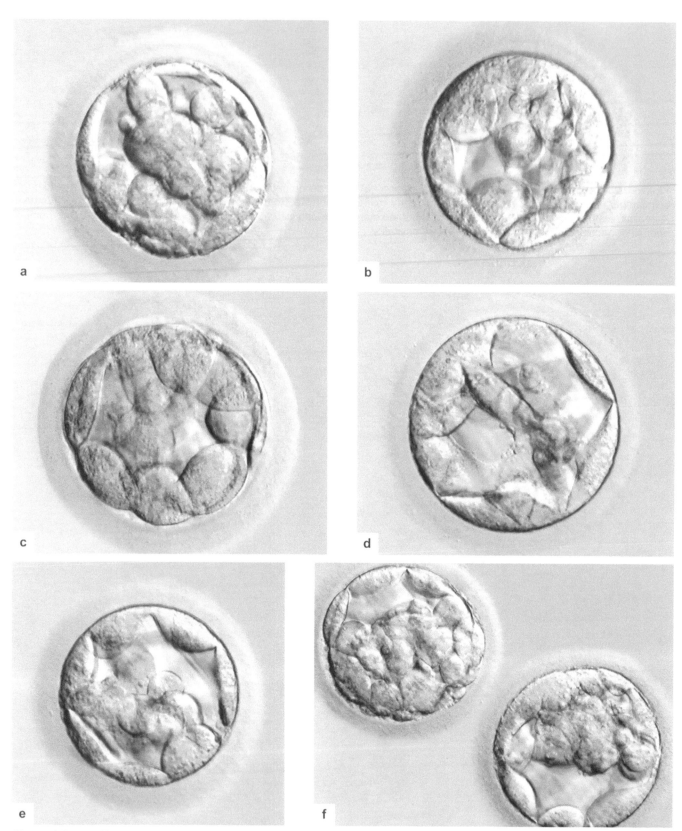

Figure 3.25 (a)–(f) Advancing cavitation in human morulae. Increased accumulation of blastocyst fluid can be observed. Early morphological differences between the rounded cells of the inner cell mass and elliptical cells of the trophectoderm are apparent. The blastocoele still occupies less than 50% of the blastocyst surface area

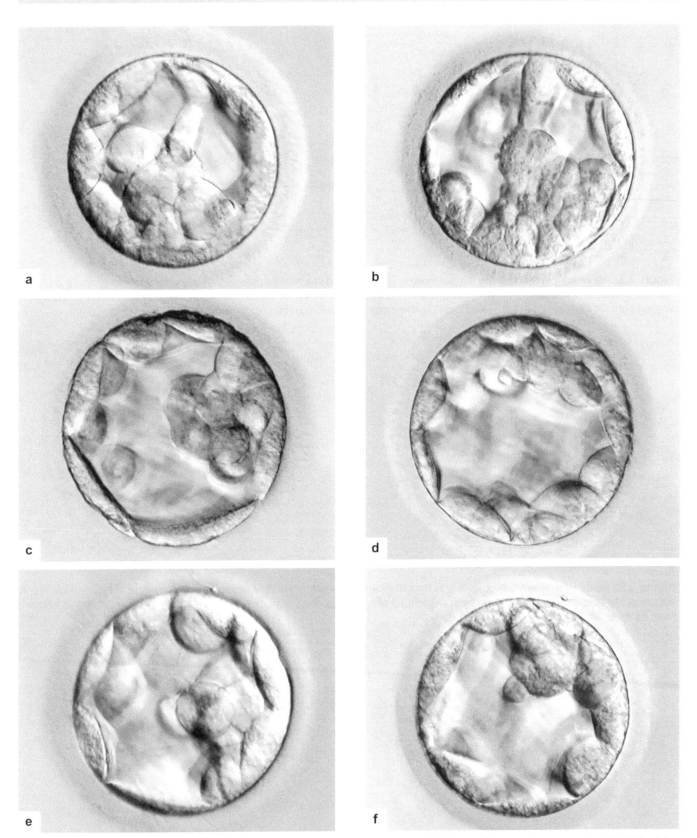

Figure 3.26 (a)–(f) Final stage of cavitation in the human morula (Cornell criteria). The cavity occupies approximately 50% of the morula surface area. Although no increase in overall size has yet occurred (no overall expansion), these conceptuses may be called early blastocysts by others, since cells have clearly separated to inner cell mass and trophectoderm components

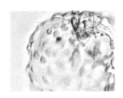

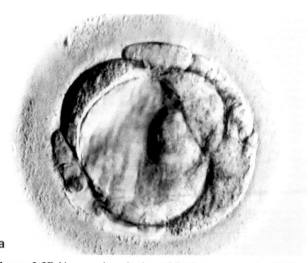
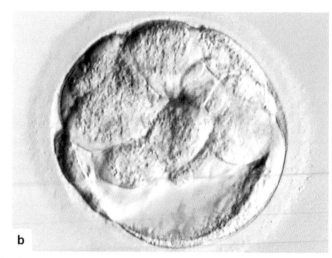

a

b

Figure 3.27 Abnormal cavitation of the human morula. (a) Cavitation in a morula made up of few blastomeres. Typically, a low cell number is observed in this type of abnormal morula before compaction. While the mechanisms contributing to cavity formation are active (if only in few cells), the future blastocyst is compromised; (b) exocentric, single-sided cavitation, or vacuolization

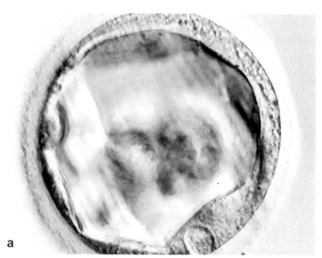
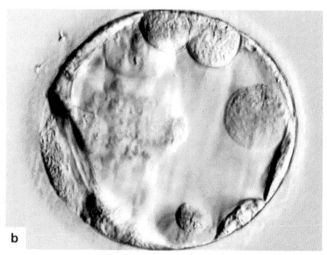

a

b

Figure 3.28 (a) and (b) Typical vacuolization in human morulae. Single, unhealthy appearing cells are pushed to the side due to accumulating fluid. Some individual cells are associated with the fluid-filled area, but overall morphology is quite poor. Specimens such as these always arrest at this stage

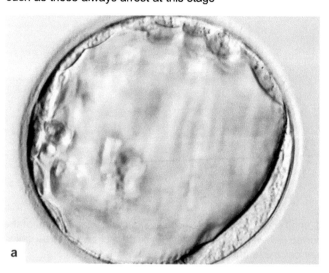
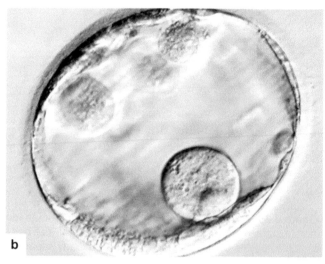

a

b

Figure 3.29 (a) and (b) Vacuolated morulae on day 5. These are completely filled with fluid, although no ICM or TM has formed. There is, however, a notable increase in overall size and the zona pellucida thins under fluid pressures. These conceptuses always arrest and never hatch

4 Cell allocation and differentiation

During blastocyst development, two distinguishable cell types are formed, those of the inner cell mass and those of the trophectoderm. Trophectoderm represents the first truly differentiated cell line to be established in the newly formed conceptus, differences between these cells and those of the inner cell mass becoming apparent as the trophectoderm and inner cell mass separate and migrate to their new positions during cavitation (Figure 4.1).

During blastocyst formation, trophectoderm cells become elliptical and exhibit polarization, whereas cells of the inner cell mass remain rounded and morphologically undifferentiated (Figure 4.2). Trophectoderm cells connect to one another over small surface areas, while cells of the inner cell mass become tightly compacted and closely apposed. The position and development of the trophectoderm and inner cell mass are not random, but are dependent on genetic, morphological and developmental mechanisms. Regulated at the start of the fertilization process, or even earlier in some mammals, this involves a distinct polarization. In most mammals, including the human, polarization and formation of the embryonic axes are fundamental to mammalian pre- and post-implantation development[1].

Mammalian oocytes express a polarized organization in which specific maternal proteins, *leptin* and *STAT3*, are expressed at the 'animal' (anterior) pole of growing oocytes and on trophectoderm cells of blastocysts[2]. The second polar body position marks the anterior pole, the posterior pole being opposite, and the polar axis marks the position of the first cleavage plane (Figure 4.3). It was suggested by Piotrowska and Zernicka-Goetz, and later questioned by Davies and Gardner, that the mouse oocyte may be polarized in regard to sperm entry; thus, the site of sperm entry is believed to predict the first cleavage plane, and may also predict embryonic and abembryonic regions of the future blastocyst[3,4]. The human oocyte, in contrast, is not polarized in this manner, and the observation that fragments from human oocytes (cytoplasts) can form a pronucleus after incubation with spermatozoa provides evidence that there is no specific sperm entry site[5,6].

During fertilization, polarized nucleoli are apparent within the pronuclei, and mitochondria become aggregated around pronuclei[7,8]. The first cleavage plane in mouse and human zygotes is established by the position of the second polar body, which serves as a marker of the polar axis from zygote to blastocyst stages (Figures 4.4 and 4.5). The anterior–posterior axes and dorsal–ventral axes determine anterior–posterior and embryonic–abembryonic poles (Figures 4.6 and 4.7). These axes are well established in the mouse, but less clear in the human[7].

In a lineage-tracing study performed in the mouse, totipotent 2-cell stage blastomeres were reported to contribute equally to inner cell mass and trophectoderm cell lines[9]. The validity of this conclusion has been questioned subsequently, however, since a growing body of evidence suggests that polarity plays a major role in murine development[10]. In the mouse at least, blastomeres of the 2-cell stage can develop into either embryonic or abembryonic components. It has been demonstrated further that one blastomere at the 2-cell stage cleaves earlier than the other and preferentially contributes to the embryonic part of the developing

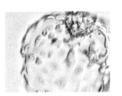

blastocyst[11]. Recall here that the onset of embryonic gene expression in the mouse begins at the 2-cell stage, as opposed to the 4–8-cell stages in humans.

Experiments on human preembryos, in which a tracing dye was injected into a single blastomere at the 2–8-cell stage, showed later random distribution of dye between inner cell mass and trophectoderm cells[12]. Future studies must investigate the fate of single blastomere development within the concept of preembryo polarization, possibly by using cell-permeable dyes, since the intracellular injection technique might have been responsible for delaying cell division and altering developmental outcome[13]. In the human, blastomeres of the 8-cell stage have been thought to be genetically equal, a prerequisite for preimplantation genetic diagnosis (PGD). However, if developmental differences between blastomeres do exist before the third cleavage, then genetic analyses of individual blastomeres at the 8-cell stage will evaluate only one of the future developmental lineages, either inner cell mass or trophectoderm. This concern is supported by studies using Oct4 and β-human chorionic gonadotropin (β-hCG) (markers of the inner cell mass and trophectoderm, respectively), where neither was expressed uniformly within blastomeres of cleavage stage preembryos[14,15].

Mouse blastomeres at the first cleavage are clearly totipotent, since the two can each develop into a normal blastocyst when separated[16]. This totipotency appears to become limited soon thereafter, because isolated 4–8-cell blastomeres are often observed to develop abnormally, primarily as trophectoderm[17]. In humans, however, it is clear from the experience of PGD that removal of one or two blastomeres at the 8-cell stage does not necessarily compromise subsequent development[18]. Conversely, removal of one blastomere at the 4-cell stage or earlier impairs further development, and results in a reduction in the total number of cells of the inner cell mass[19].

Various models for the basis of mammalian cell allocation and differentiation have been proposed over the years. These include: the inside–outside hypothesis, the polarization hypothesis and the cleavage-driven hypothesis[20] (Figure 4.8).

Tarkowski and Wroblewska proposed the inside–outside hypothesis, wherein the fate of blastomeres is described as being a consequence of their differing locations within the preembryo[17]. These investigators detailed a situation where inner blastomeres of the 8-cell stage preembryo are destined to form the inner cell mass and those outside to form the trophectoderm. In accord with this, isolated blastomeres from 4–8-cell mouse and 8-cell human preembryos, no longer totipotent (see Glossary), are capable of developing only into trophectoderm-like vesiculated structures, and subsequently fail to form inner cell masses and normal trophectoderm, probably owing to a reduction in cellular mass[21].

The polarization hypothesis proposes that, during the fourth cleavage to 16 cells, polarized surfaces and a cytoskeleton develop in an outside to inside direction[22]. Subsequent cleavage generates daughter cells with different developmental fates.

The newer cleavage-driven hypothesis includes elements of the previous two hypotheses and incorporates the idea of blastomeres becoming predisposed at the first cleavage to contribute to embryonic portions of the blastocyst[20]. According to this theory, blastocyst polarity arises from early asymmetric cleavage of the preembryo.

Each of these hypotheses will require scientific verification in a human model, since the only analyses to date relate to the morphology of early development[7]. From such investigations carried out in our laboratory, it appears that the human preembryo enters compaction at the 8-cell stage and that further cleavage is inhibited until the compaction process is completed (Figures 4.9 and 4.10). Following compaction, some blastomeres are immediately allocated to the outside, where they begin to proliferate rapidly to form the trophectoderm. This separation of cells is clearly evident during cavitation and subsequent blastocyst formation (Figures 4.11 and 4.12). A few cells remaining inside the morula ultimately form the inner cell mass.

Connections between blastomeres, their polarization, and cellular orientation within the preembryo regulate embryonic differentiation (see Chapter 3). The ratio of cells contributing to each cell type is tightly controlled. The blastocyst is polarized, with the inner cell mass localized at the embryonic pole[7]. The inner cell mass represents a group of cells that are tightly connected and pluripotent (see Glossary), while trophectoderm cells have smaller areas of their surfaces connected, serve as protectors of the inner cell mass and are differentiated for this function. If trophectoderm cells are removed, the morphology of the inner cell mass changes rapidly and pluripotency is lost (Figure 4.13). In the mouse, the inner cell mass regulates trophectoderm development and its distribution within the blastocyst. Fibroblast growth factor-4 has been shown to be involved in this process[23]. It is unclear just how cells of the inner cell mass direct trophectoderm differentiation and distribution, since daughter cells on the outside of the morula usually form the trophectoderm[24]. Interestingly, parthenogenic mouse conceptuses develop into blastocysts with lower total cell numbers and lower inner cell mass/trophectoderm cell ratios, implicating gene imprinting as an important factor even during preimplantation development[25].

Blastocyst cell number

For successful development and implantation, the total number of cells in the blastocyst and the inner cell mass/trophectoderm cell ratio are genetically and developmentally regulated[26]. The average cell cycle in mouse trophectoderm requires 17.5 h, while that of the inner cell mass is 24 h. Thus, the trophectoderm proliferates more rapidly as compared to the inner cell mass, averaging one extra full cell division per 24 h[24,27].

In the human also, the trophectoderm proliferates more rapidly as compared to the inner cell mass. Trophectoderm cell numbers double from the onset of cavitation on day 4 to the formation of the blastocyst on day 5, while the numbers in the inner cell mass double between days 5 and 6. During blastocyst expansion, cells of the trophectoderm divide at a rate of one-half a division per 24 h more rapidly than cells of the inner cell mass[28]. Still, quantitative studies of the human blastocyst demonstrate great variability in total cell number. Generally, total cell numbers in normal human blastocysts should exceed 60 cells. The human blastocyst has approximately 60 cells on day 5, up to 160 cells on day 6 and over 200 cells after hatching on day 7[28-30]. In the mouse, the inner cell mass/trophectoderm ratio changes during blastocyst development from 40 : 60 to 25 : 75; in the human, approximately 40% of the final cell number is made up of inner mass cells[28]. The exact mechanisms that control cell number in the human and primate blastocyst are unknown. These mechanisms are conserved during early cleavage stages, as evidenced by the fact that rhesus monkey blastocysts developing after separation of the blastomeres (after artificial twinning) contain half the number of total cells while maintaining the same inner cell mass/trophectoderm ratios[31] (*see* Chapter 12). Apoptotic processes may be one of the possible systems involved in regulating blastocyst cell number[32].

Quantitative analysis of the total blastocyst cell number can be performed by using various techniques that visualize individual cell nuclei. As an example, the total cell number in living specimens can be evaluated easily using cell permeable fluorescence nuclear dyes, e.g. Hoechst (Figure 4.14). Other methods include fixation and staining with nuclear dyes (propidium iodide, Giemsa® or 4',6-diamidino-2-phenylindole). To quantify and compare the numbers of cells in the inner cell mass and trophectoderm, differential staining techniques were developed[33]. Techniques include differential staining of whole specimens, or isolation and staining of the inner cell mass alone[34]. These techniques are based on the high permeability of the trophectoderm and the relatively poor permeability of the tightly connected inner cell mass.

Immunological techniques include the use of a species-specific antiserum followed by complement, with propidium iodide used to stain the nuclei of lysed trophectoderm cells; cells of the inner cell mass are then stained with permeable dyes[27]. A modification of this technique involves using trinitrobenzenesulfonic acid (TNMS) instead of antiserum[28].

Differential staining through chemical permeabilization techniques can be achieved using Ca^{2+} ionophore A23187 in combination with nuclear fluorochromes; however, lysing of trophectoderm cells is a necessary preliminary, based on an osmotic response that causes membrane vesiculation[35]. Modifications of this technique include the labeling of trophectoderm with fluorescent-labeled lectins, e.g. wheat-germ agglutinin[36], or using the detergent Triton X-100® to permeabilize trophectoderm cells[37].

Blastocyst quality can be evaluated by both non-invasive and invasive techniques. Non-invasive techniques include evaluating the timing of blastocyst expansion, trophectoderm morphology and inner cell mass characteristics. Other non-invasive techniques include the metabolic evaluation of nutrient uptake and/or production. Recently, it was shown that depletion of leucine and formation of alanine are positively correlated with normal blastocyst formation and implantation in the human[38].

Invasive techniques generally result in a loss of viability. They include, among others, karyotyping, fluorescence *in situ* hybridization (FISH) for analysis of chromosome structure or number (aneuploidy, mosaicism) and analysis of mitotic or apoptotic indices.

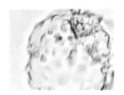

Gene expression and regulation

The genes involved in blastocyst formation are largely unknown, but are probably induced or regulated by activation of some preembryonic genes at the 4–8-cell stage in the human. Known genes include those for sodium/potassium adenosine triphosphatase and ZO-1α[+39,40] (*see* Chapter 3).

The preimplantation embryo development gene (*Ped* gene) is located in the Q region of the major histocompatibility complex in mice, and has fast- and slow-cleaving forms. In more rapidly growing preembryos, this gene induces faster cleavage and a higher total cell number in the subsequent blastocyst[41]. It has been suggested that human leukocyte antigen-G (HLA-G), expressed in human blastocysts, is homologous to the *Ped* gene in mice[42].

As might be expected, gene expression differs between the inner cell mass and the trophectoderm. These differences probably reflect the loss of totipotency and formation of differentiated trophectoderm cells. One well-known marker of totipotency is *Oct4*. This transcription factor is crucial for maintaining totipotency in early cleaving preembryos, is responsible for maintaining pluripotency in the inner cell mass and is later restricted to germ cells during embryogenesis[43]. In the absence of *Oct4*, early lethality occurs due to the differentiation as trophectoderm of those cells that would normally give rise to the inner cell mass[44]. Another important role for *Oct4* is the maintenance of embryonic stem cells in an undifferentiated state, it being down-regulated before cells are triggered to differentiate[45].

Oct4 is differentially expressed in various species including the human[46]. In humans, *Oct4* is expressed on the oocyte and throughout development to the blastocyst stage[47,48]. The distribution of *Oct4* varies between blastomeres of human preembryos, suggesting a possible directive mechanism towards inner cell mass (*Oct4*-positive) or trophectoderm (*Oct4*-negative) lineages[14]. In the human blastocyst, *Oct4* is expressed primarily in the inner cell mass, where mRNA expression is approximately 31 times higher than in the trophectoderm[49] (Figure 4.15). Elevated *Oct4* expression is maintained in undifferentiated embryonic stem cells as they develop from the inner cell mass. Recently, poor results with somatic cell cloning were associated with abnormal and/or failed expression of *Oct4* in cloned mouse embryos and blastocysts[50].

Trophectoderm-associated genes regulate membrane polarity during the compaction and cavitation stages necessary for normal trophectoderm formation (*see* Chapter 3). One might be the helix-loop-helix transcription factor (*Hxt*), a gene that is increasingly expressed in mouse morulae, trophectoderm and placenta[51]. In addition, transforming growth factor type β2 (TGF-β 2) is expressed in outer cells of the morula and in trophectoderm, while the inner cell mass is unstained[52]. Also, the β subunit of human chorionic gonadotropin (β-hCG), a trophectoderm marker, is expressed in human cleavage-stage preembryos, and hCG is later secreted from the trophectoderm cells of the blastocyst[15,53,54].

Carbohydrates are further elements that play a role in preimplantation development. Glycans, which are glycoprotein-rich carbohydrates, are characteristic of early embryonic cells that carry a number of carbohydrate markers. As in other cell systems, surface carbohydrates play a critical role in the cell–cell interactions of mammalian preembryos[55,56]. Stage-specific embryonic antigens (SSEAs) are surface glycoconjugates associated with glycolipids, glycoproteins and proteoglycans, and are developmentally regulated[57].

In the mouse, SSEA-3 and SSEA-4 are glycolipid antigens evident during oogenesis, which are expressed in oocytes and cleavage stage preembryos but which disappear by the blastocyst stage[58]. In contrast, SSEA-1 is expressed from the 8-cell stage, participates in the process of compaction[59], is later expressed mainly in the inner cell mass, and in embryonic stem cells serves as a marker of non-differentiation[60,61].

In the human, SSEA-3 and -4 antigens are markers of undifferentiated stem cells, while the presence of SSEA-1 indicates a differentiated state. These species-specific differences have been confirmed by our own studies with human and mouse oocytes and preembryos (Figures 4.16–4.18)[62]. SSEA-3 and -4 expression becomes restricted to the inner blastomeres of the compacting human morula (support for the inside–outside theory), indicating that human cell differentiation begins by this stage and continues throughout the process of cell allocation. Subsequently, the inner cell mass expresses SSEA-3 and -4, while cells of the trophectoderm do not.

Mature human oocytes express SSEA-1 while immature oocytes appear not to; preembryos and blastocysts

Table 4.1   Expression of stage-specific embryonic antigen SSEA: mouse and human

	SSEA-1	SSEA-3	SSEA-4
Mouse oocyte	–	+	+
Human oocyte	+mature/–immature	+	+
Mouse embryo	– < 8-cell/ + ≥ 8-cell	+	+
Human preembryo	+	+	+
Mouse blastocyst	+	–	–
inner cell mass	+	–	–
trophectoderm	+	–	–
Human blastocyst	+	+/–	+/–
inner cell mass	+	+	+
trophectoderm	+	–	–
Mouse embryonic stem cell	+	–	–
Human embryonic stem cell	–	+	+

express it consistently. A comparison of SSEA expression in both human and mouse is presented in Table 4.1.

Henderson and colleagues recently confirmed most of our results of SSEA expression in human blastocysts[63]. The differences that they found before the 8-cell stage may be technical in nature. We stained live specimens, as did Solter and Knowles in their original experiments[60], while Henderson used fixed material in which we had earlier noted only faint or no staining.

The techniques involving SSEA staining in living specimens will allow selection of SSEA-3- and -4-positive inner cell masses for future embryonic stem cell culture, and undifferentiated stem cells for manipulation.

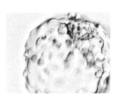

References

1. Edwards RG, Beard HK. Oocyte polarity and cell determination in early mammalian embryos. *Mol Hum Reprod* 1997;3:863–905

2. Antczak M, Van Blerkom J. Oocyte influences on early development: the regulatory proteins leptin and STAT3 are polarized in mouse and human oocytes and differentially distributed within the cells of the preimplantation stage embryo. *Mol Hum Reprod* 1997;3:1067–86

3. Piotrowska K, Zernicka-Goetz M. Role for sperm in spatial patterning of the early mouse embryo. *Nature (London)* 2001;409:517–21

4. Davies TJ, Gardner RL. The plane of first cleavage is not related to the distribution of sperm components in the mouse. *Hum Reprod* 2002;17:2368–79

5. Santella L, Alikani M, Talansky BE, Cohen J, Dale B. Is the human oocyte plasma membrane polarized? *Hum Reprod* 1992;7:999–1003

6. Levron J, Willadsen S, Munne S, Cohen J. Formation of male pronuclei in partitioned human oocytes. *Biol Reprod* 1995;53:209–13

7. Scott LA. Oocyte and embryo polarity. *Semin Reprod Med* 2000;18:171–83

8. Van Blerkom J, Davis P, Alexander S. Differential mito-chondrial distribution in human pronuclear embryos leads to disproportionate inheritance between blastomeres: relationship to microtubular organization, ATP content and competence. *Hum Reprod* 2000;15:2621–33

9. Balakier H, Pedersen RA. Allocation of cells to inner cell mass and trophectoderm lineages in preimplantation mouse embryos. *Dev Biol* 1982;90:352–62

10. Gardner RL. Specification of embryonic axes begins before cleavage in normal mouse development. *Development* 2001;128:839–47

11. Piotrowska K, Wianny F, Pedersen RA, Zernicka-Goetz M. Blastomeres arising from the first cleavage division have distinguishable fates in normal mouse development. *Development* 2001;128:3739–48

12. Mottla GL, Adelman MR, Hall JL, Gindoff PR, Stillman RJ, Johnson KE. Lineage tracing demonstrates that blastomeres of early cleavage-stage human preembryos contribute to both trophectoderm and inner cell mass. *Hum Reprod* 1995;10:384–91

13. Dyce J, George M, Goodall H, Fleming TP. Do trophectoderm and inner cell mass cells in the mouse blastocyst maintain discrete lineages? *Development* 1987;100:685–98

14. Hansis C, Tang YX, Grifo JA, Krey LC. Analysis of *Oct-4* expression and ploidy in individual human blastomeres. *Mol Hum Reprod* 2001;7:155–61

15. Hansis C, Grifo JA, Tang YX, Krey LC. Assessment of β-HCG, β-LH mRNA and ploidy in individual human blastomeres. *Reprod BioMed Online* 2002;5:156–61

16. Tarkowski AK. Experiments on the development of isolated blastomeres of mouse eggs. *Nature (London)* 1959;184:1286–7

17. Tarkowski AK, Wroblewska J. Development of blastomeres of mouse eggs isolated at the 4- and 8-cell stage. *J Embryol Exp Morphol* 1967;18:155–80

18. Hardy K, Martin KL, Leese HJ, Winston RM, Handyside AH. Human preimplantation development in vitro is not adversely affected by biopsy at the 8-cell stage. *Hum Reprod* 1990;5:708–14

19. Tarin JJ, Conaghan J, Winston RM, Handyside AH. Human embryo biopsy on the 2nd day after insemination for preimplantation diagnosis: removal of a quarter of embryo retards cleavage. *Fertil Steril* 1992;58:970–6

20. Zernicka-Goetz M. Patterning of the embryo: the first spatial decisions in the life of a mouse. *Development* 2002;129:815–29

21. Geber S, Winston RM, Handyside AH. Proliferation of blastomeres from biopsied cleavage stage human embryos *in vitro*: an alternative to blastocyst biopsy for preimplantation diagnosis. *Hum Reprod* 1995;10:1492–6

22. Johnson MH, Ziomek CA. The foundation of two distinct cell lineages within the mouse morula. *Cell* 1981;24:71–80

23. Leunda-Casi A, de Hertogh R, Pampfer S. Control of trophectoderm differentiation by inner cell mass-derived fibroblast growth factor-4 in mouse blastocysts and corrective effect of FGF-4 on high glucose-induced trophoblast disruption. *Mol Reprod Dev* 2001;60:38–46

24. Fleming TP. A quantitative analysis of cell allocation to trophectoderm and inner cell mass in the mouse blastocyst. *Dev Biol* 1987;119:520–31

25. Mognetti B, Sakkas D. Defects in the allocation of cells to the inner cell mass and trophectoderm of parthenogenetic mouse blastocysts. *Reprod Fertil Dev* 1996;8:1193–7

26. Winston NJ, Braude PR, Pickering SJ, *et al.* The incidence of abnormal morphology and nucleocytoplasmic ratios in 2-, 3- and 5-day human pre-embryos. *Hum Reprod* 1991;6:17–24

27. Handyside AH, Hunter S. A rapid procedure for visualising the inner cell mass and trophectoderm nuclei of mouse blastocysts *in situ* using polynucleotide-specific fluorochromes. *J Exp Zool* 1984;231:429–34

28. Hardy K, Handyside AH, Winston RM. The human blastocyst: cell number, death and allocation during late preimplantation development *in vitro*. *Development* 1989;107:597–604

29. Steptoe PC, Edwards RG, Purdy JM. Human blastocysts grown in culture. *Nature (London)* 1971;229:132–3

30. Fong CY, Bongso A. Comparison of human blastulation rates and total cell number in sequential culture media with and without co-culture. *Hum Reprod* 1999;14:774–81

31. Mitalipov SM, Yeoman RR, Kuo HC, Wolf DP. Monozygotic twinning in rhesus monkeys by manipulation of *in vitro*-derived embryos. *Biol Reprod* 2002;66:1449–55

32. Hardy K. Apoptosis in the human embryo. *Rev Reprod* 1999;4:125–34

33. Van Soom A, Vanroose G, de Kruif A. Blastocyst evaluation by means of differential staining: a practical approach. *Reprod Domest Anim* 2001;36:29–35

34. Solter D, Knowles BB. Immunosurgery of mouse blastocyst. *Proc Natl Acad Sci USA* 1975;72:5099–102

35. de la Fuente R, King WA. Use of a chemically defined system for the direct comparison of inner cell mass and trophectoderm distribution in murine, porcine and bovine embryos. *Zygote* 1997;5:309–20

36. de la Fuente R, King WA. Developmental consequences of karyokinesis without cytokinesis during the first mitotic cell cycle of bovine parthenotes. *Biol Reprod* 1998;58:952–62

37. Thouas GA, Korfiatis NA, French AJ, Jones GM, Trounson AO. Simplified techniques for differential staining of inner cell mass and trophectoderm cells of mouse and bovine blastocysts. *Reprod BioMed Online* 2001;3:25–9

38. Houghton FD, Hawkhead JA, Humpherson PG, *et al.* Non-invasive amino acid turnover predicts human embryo developmental capacity. *Hum Reprod* 2002;17:999–1005

39. Watson AJ, Westhusin ME, De Sousa PA, Betts DH, Barcroft LC. Gene expression regulating blastocyst formation. *Theriogenology* 1999;51:117–33

40. Sheth B, Fesenko I, Collins JE, *et al.* Tight junction assembly during mouse blastocyst formation is regulated by late expression of ZO-1 α+ isoform. *Development* 1997;124:2027–37

41. McElhinny AS, Kadow N, Warner CM. The expression pattern of the Qa-2 antigen in mouse preimplantation embryos and its correlation with the *Ped* gene phenotype. *Mol Hum Reprod* 1998;4:966–71

42. Jurisicova A, Casper RF, MacLusky NJ, Mills GB, Librach CL. HLA-G expression during preimplantation human embryo development. *Proc Natl Acad Sci USA* 1996;93:161–5

43. Pesce M, Anastassiadis K, Scholer HR. *Oct-4*: lessons of totipotency from embryonic stem cells. *Cells Tissues Organs* 1999;165:144–52

44. Pesce M, Scholer HR. *Oct-4*: control of totipotency and germline determination. *Mol Reprod Dev* 2000;55:452–7

45. Pesce M, Scholer HR. *Oct-4*: gatekeeper in the beginnings of mammalian development. *Stem Cells* 2001;19:271–8

46. Kirchhof N, Carnwath JW, Lemme E, Anastassiadis K, Scholer H, Niemann H. Expression pattern of *Oct-4* in preimplantation embryos of different species. *Biol Reprod* 2000;63:1698–705

47. Abdel-Rahman B, Fiddler M, Rappolee D, Pergament E. Expression of transcription regulating genes in human preimplantation embryos. *Hum Reprod* 1995;10:2787–92

48. Verlinsky Y, Morozov G, Verlinsky O, *et al.* Isolation of cDNA libraries from individual human preimplantation embryos. *Mol Hum Reprod* 1998;4:571–5

49. Hansis C, Grifo JA, Krey LC. *Oct-4* expression in inner cell mass and trophectoderm of human blastocysts. *Mol Hum Reprod* 2000;6:999–1004

50. Boiani M, Eckardt S, Scholer HR, McLaughlin KJ. *Oct4* distribution and level in mouse clones: consequences for pluripotency. *Genes Dev* 2002;16:1209–19

51. Cross JC, Flannery ML, Blanar MA, *et al.* Hxt encodes a basic helix-loop-helix transcription factor that regulates trophoblast cell development. *Development* 1995;121:2513–23

52. Slager HG, Lawson KA, van den Eijnden-van Raaij AJ, de Laat SW, Mummery CL. Differential localization of TGF-β2 in mouse preimplantation and early postimplantation development. *Dev Biol* 1991;145:205–18

53. Bonduelle ML, Dodd R, Liebaers I, Van Steirteghem A, Williamson R, Akhurst R. Chorionic gonadotrophin-β

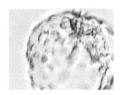

mRNA, a trophoblast marker, is expressed in human 8-cell embryos derived from tripronucleate zygotes. *Hum Reprod* 1988;3:909–14

54. Fishel SB, Edwards RG, Evans CJ. Human chorionic gonadotropin secreted by preimplantation embryos cultured *in vitro*. *Science* 1984;223:816–18

55. Poirier F, Kimber S. Cell surface carbohydrates and lectins in early development. *Mol Hum Reprod* 1997;3:907–18

56. Muramatsu T. Developmentally regulated expression of cell surface carbohydrates during mouse embryogenesis. *J Cell Biochem* 1988;36:1–14

57. Fenderson BA, Eddy EM, Hakomori S. Glycoconjugate expression during embryogenesis and its biological significance. *Bioessays* 1990;12:173–9

58. Shevinsky LH, Knowles BB, Damjanov I, Solter D. Monoclonal antibody to murine embryos defines a stage-specific embryonic antigen expressed on mouse embryos and human teratocarcinoma cells. *Cell* 1982;30:697–705

59. Fenderson BA, Zehavi U, Hakomori S. A multivalent lacto-*N*-fucopentaose III-lysyllysine conjugate decompacts preimplantation mouse embryos, while the free oligosaccharide is ineffective. *J Exp Med* 1984;160:1591–6

60. Solter D, Knowles BB. Monoclonal antibody defining a stage-specific mouse embryonic antigen (SSEA-1). *Proc Natl Acad Sci USA* 1978;75:5565–9

61. Smith AG, Heath JK, Donaldson DD, *et al*. Inhibition of pluripotential embryonic stem cell differentiation by purified polypeptides. *Nature (London)* 1988;336:688–90

62. Zaninovic N, Veeck LL, Rosenwaks Z. Stage-specific expression of embryonic antigens SSEA-1, SSEA-3, and SSEA-4 on human conceptuses using vital staining. *Fertil Steril* 2001;76:S33–S34

63. Henderson JK, Draper JS, Baillie HS, *et al*. Preimplantation human embryos and embryonic stem cells show comparable expression of stage-specific embryonic antigens. *Stem Cells* 2002;20:329–37

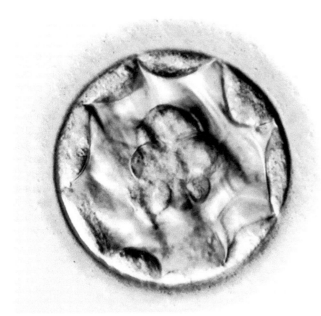

Figure 4.1 Human blastocyst displaying grade 1 expansion; no thinning of the zona pellucida and greater than 50% of the total volume filled with fluid. Clear morphological differences can be observed between the inner cell mass (center) and the trophectoderm (circling the blastocoele)

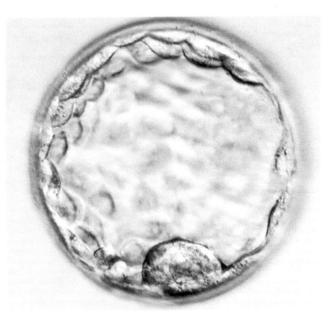

Figure 4.2 Fully expanded human blastocyst (grade 3), with thin zona pellucida and fully filled blastocoele. The rounded/oval inner cell mass (ICM; 6-o'clock) is made up of a group of highly compacted cells. The trophectoderm (TM) is cohesive and comprised of many cells. Cells of the inner cell mass are rounded while trophectoderm cells are elliptical and polarized

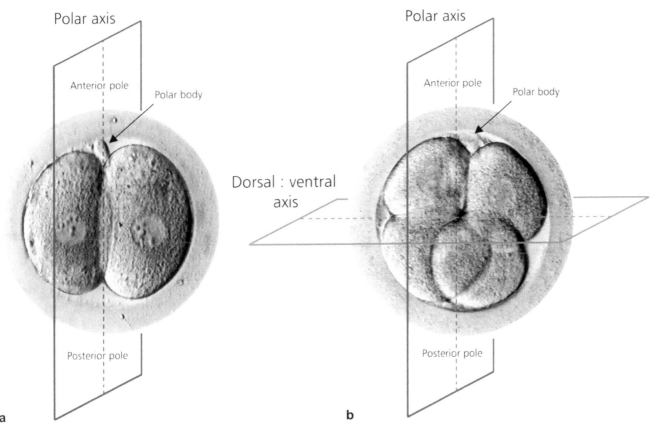

a

b

Figure 4.3 The anterior–posterior (A–P) polar axis and the dorsal–ventral axis in 2-cell and 4-cell human preembryos. (a)The second polar body marks the anterior pole and the orientation of the polar axis which determines the first cleavage plane of the zygote, while the posterior pole is opposite (A–P axis); (b) the second polar body marks the polar axis and first cleavage plane, while the dorsal–ventral axis marks the second cleavage plane. The second cleavage is equatorial and perpendicular to the first cleavage

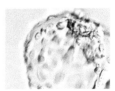

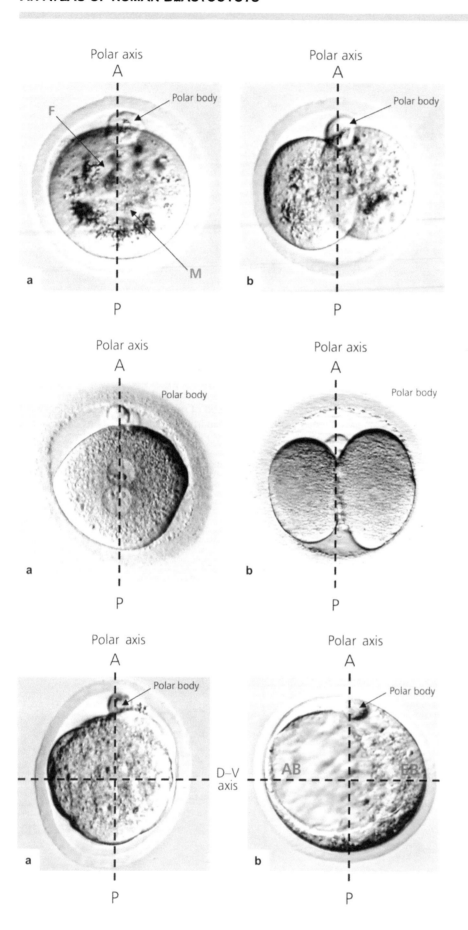

Figure 4.4 The anterior–posterior (A–P) polar axis in the mouse pronuclear oocyte and mouse 2-cell stage embryo. (a) Pronuclear polarity is indicated by pronuclear alignment along the polar axis. F = female pronucleus in close proximity to the polar body; M = male pronucleus; (b) the second polar body marks the polar axis and first cleavage plane of the two-cell mouse embryo

Figure 4.5 The anterior–posterior (A–P) polar axis in the human pronuclear oocyte and human 2-cell stage pre-embryo. (a) Polarized pre-zygote with pronuclear alignment along the polar axis. Pronuclei can rotate and become organized in a polarized formation; (b) the second polar body indicates the first cleavage plane and marks the polar axis throughout development to the blastocyst stage

Figure 4.6 The anterior–posterior axes (A–P) and dorsal–ventral axes (D–V) in the mouse morula and mouse blastocyst. (a) The second polar body (PB) marks the A–P axis (reflects the A–P axis of the zygote). The D–V axis is perpendicular to the A–P axis; (b) the blastocoele occupies the abembryonic (AB) pole while the inner cell mass occupies the embryonic (EB) pole

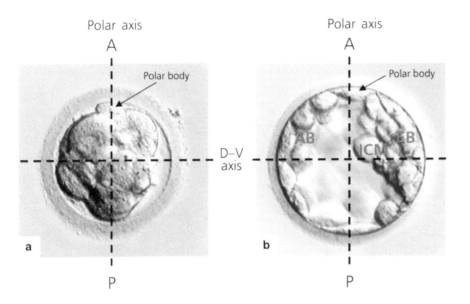

Polar axis

D–V axis

Figure 4.7 The anterior–posterior axes (A–P) and dorsal-ventral axes (D–V) in the human morula and blastocyst. (a) The establishment of axes in the human morula and blastocyst is less clear since one observes central ICM formation and a surrounding blastocoele; (b) in the expanded human blastocyst, the ICM is associated with one pole of the blastocyst, the embryonic pole

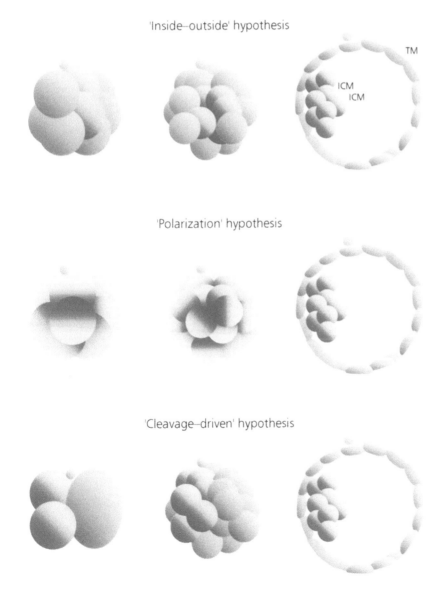

'Inside–outside' hypothesis

'Polarization' hypothesis

'Cleavage–driven' hypothesis

Figure 4.8 Models of cell allocation and differentiation in mammalian blastocyst. The 'Inside–outside' hypothesis is based on the localization of individual blastomeres within cleaved preembryos and the existence of different environments surrounding inner and outer blastomeres. Blastomeres inside the preembryo form the ICM while those outside form trophectoderm.

The 'Polarization' hypothesis is based on the polarization of each individual blastomere, where subsequent divisions generate daughter cells that exhibit different cytoplasmic compositions and different developmental fates.

The 'Cleavage-driven' hypothesis is based on the early asymmetric cleavage of the preembryo. The blastomere that cleaves earlier, at the 2-cell stage, is predisposed to contribute to embryonic (ICM) cells, while slower-cleaving blastomere gives rise to abembryonic (TM) cells

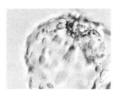

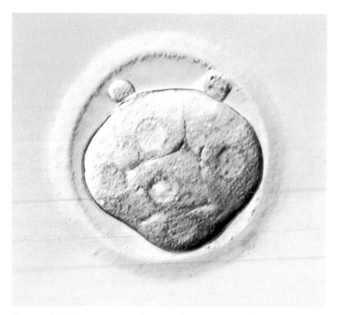

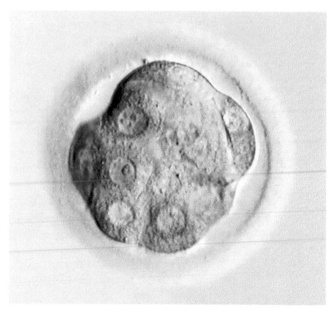

Figure 4.9 Human preembryo at the compacted morula stage on day 4. This preembryo entered compaction at the 6–8-cell stage and further cell divisions were inhibited until compaction was complete. Blastomere membranes are closely apposed; several nuclei and the two polar bodies are identified easily

Figure 4.10 Compacted human morula on day 4. Similar to the example in Figure 4.9, this morula did not complete further cell divisions until after compaction was finished and cavitation had begun. Nine to ten nuclei with a varying number of nucleoli are clearly visible

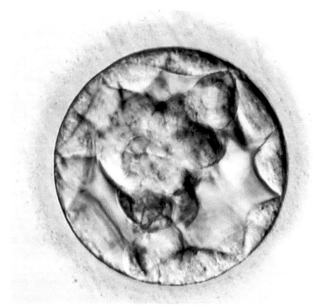

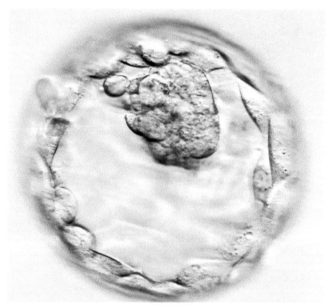

Figure 4.11 Cavitating morula on late day 4. Cells inside are ICM cells, which are round in shape and are loosely aggregated. Cells located peripherally are trophectoderm cells, which show polarized alignment, with one pole facing the zona pellucida while the other faces blastocoele. Cell number begins increasing once again just before the onset of cavitation

Figure 4.12 Blastocyst-stage conceptus with dominant inner cell mass and trophectoderm cells. The ICM has become smaller and extremely compacted, and forms a rounded shape. Trophectoderm cells become smaller in size with each division and take on a more elliptical shape due to increased pressure from the enlarging blastocoele

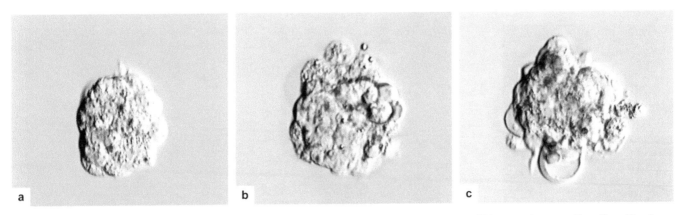

Figure 4.13 Morphology of an inner cell mass isolated from a human day-7 blastocyst. The ICM was subsequently cultured in standard stage II sequential medium. ICM isolation involves removal of the zona pellucida with pronase followed by sequential incubation in both mouse anti-human serum and complement. (a) The isolated ICM shows an intact, compacted structure; (b) the same ICM after 2 hours of culture, showing partial decompaction and initiation of membrane blebbing; (c) 6 hours post-isolation showing membrane blebbing and vesiculation with some cell lysing and possible fragmentation. This ICM likely lost its pluripotency

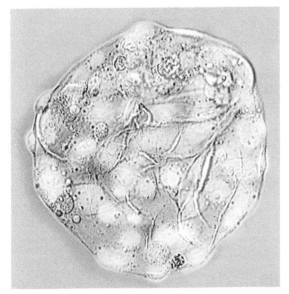

Figure 4.14 Visualization of cell nuclei in a living zona-free human blastocyst stained with Hoechst 33342. Photograph taken under double exposure using differential interference contrast (DIC) for the living image, and under UV light to demonstrate blue-stained nuclei

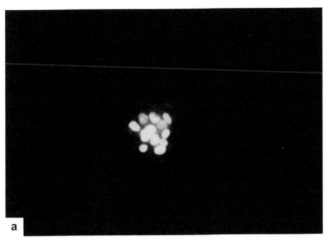
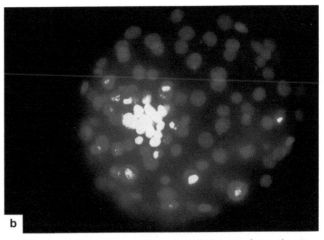

Figure 4.15 *Oct4* expression in an expanded human blastocyst. (a) *Oct4* expression in the nuclei of the ICM (green); trophectoderm is negative; (b) the same blastocyst showing ICM-specific expression of *Oct4* (green) while trophectoderm nuclei stain negatively (blue only), double exposure. Cell nuclei stain blue with Hoechst 33342; *Oct4*+ nuclei stain aqua (overlapping green- and blue-stained nuclei)

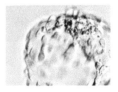

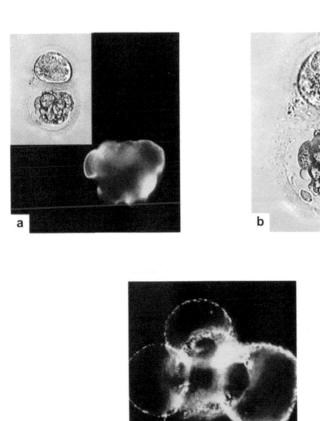
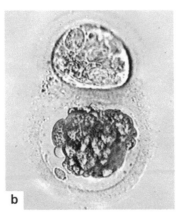
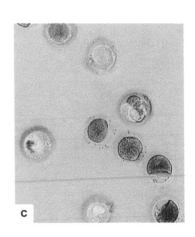

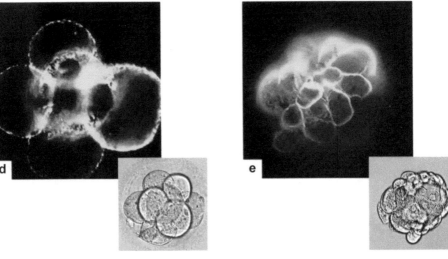

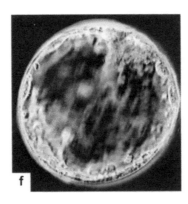

Figure 4.16 Expression of the SSEA-1 in living human oocytes, preembryos, and blastocysts. (a) Binovular oocyte: lower oocyte was at MII of maturation at collection, was fertilized by ICSI, and produced a fragmented preembryo on day 3; upper oocyte was at PI of maturation at collection, and never matured. The lower preembryo membranes stain positively for SSEA-1 (green) by fluorescein isothiocyanate (FITC), while the upper immature oocyte stains negatively; (b) double exposure (DIC/FITC) of the same binovular oocyte. The lower preembryo expresses SSEA-1 (red); (c) SSEA-1 is expressed in mature oocytes (green) while immature oocytes fail to stain; (d) spatial membrane expression of SSEA-1 in a human preembryo (green); (e) SSEA-1 expression in a human morula after zona pellucida removal; (f) uniform expression of SSEA-1 in a human blastocyst; both the ICM and TM stain positively

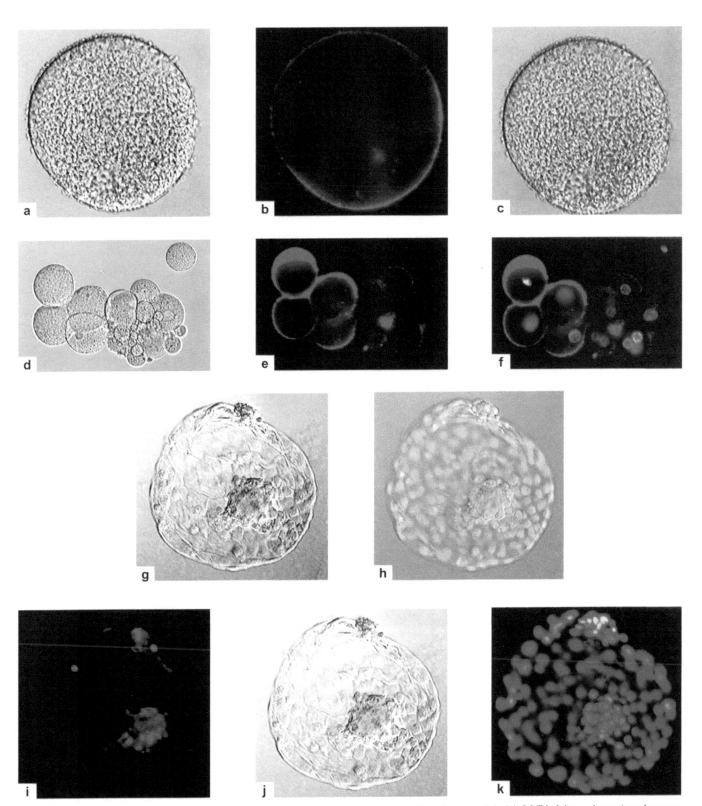

Figure 4.17 Expression of SSEA-3 in living human oocytes, preembryos, and blastocysts. (a)–(c) SSEA-3 in an immature human oocyte; (a) DIC; (b) SSEA-3 antibody marked with phycoerythrin R (PE) (red); (c) DIC/PE; (d)–(f) SSEA-3 in blastomeres of a human cleaved preembryo; (d) DIC; (e) SSEA-3-PE (red); (f) SSEA-3-PE (red) / DAPI (nuclei-blue); (g)–(k) SSEA-3 in a human blastocyst; (g) DIC; (h) DIC/DAPI (nuclei-blue); (i) SSEA-3-PE in ICM cell membranes only (other cells, possibly undifferentiated TM cells or separated ICM cells showed positive staining); (j) DIC/SSEA-3-PE; (k) SSEA-3-PE/DAPI

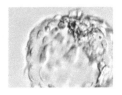

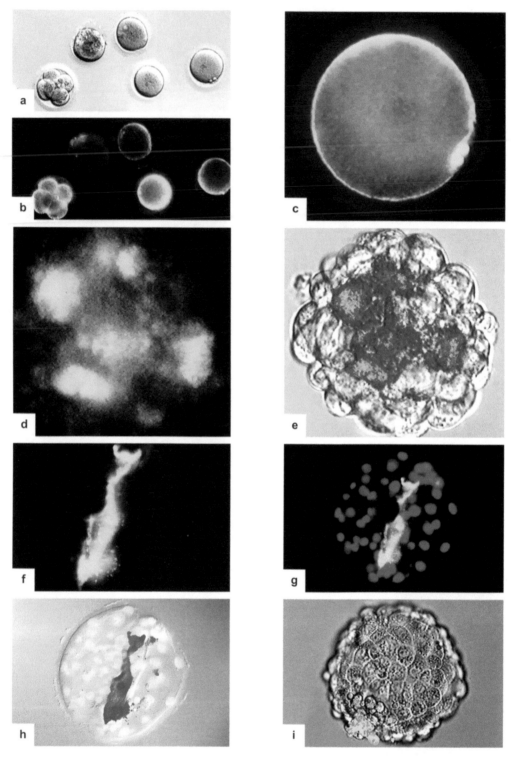

Figure 4.18 Expression of SSEA-4 in living human oocytes, preembryos, and blastocysts. (a) and (b) SSEA-4 in human oocytes and preembryos; (a) DIC; (b) SSEA-4 antibody marked with FITC (green). Mature oocytes and preembryos exhibited positive staining for SSEA-4 while the degenerating immature oocyte showed only faint positive staining; (c) SSEA-4 expression in a mature human oocyte with two polar bodies; (d) and (e) SSEA-4 in a human morula; (d) SSEA-4-FITC expressed in the membranes of the inner cells only (future ICM cells?); (e) SSEA-4-FITC/DIC showing expression in inner cells, which supports the 'Inside-outside' hypothesis of cell allocation for blastocyst development; (f)–(i) SSEA-4 expression in a human blastocyst; (f) SSEA-4-FITC staining of ICM only; (g) SSEA-4-FITC (green)/DAPI (nuclei stained blue); (h) triple staining: SSEA-4-FITC (red due to overlapping colors)/DAPI (blue nuclei)/DIC; (i) SSEA-4-FITC staining (green) of ICM only in human blastocyst

5 Human blastocysts *in vitro*

Approximately 24 h after the morula forms, intercellular spaces begin to enlarge to create a central fluid-filled cavity called the *blastocoel*. The cells of the developing human blastocyst form a spherical shell enclosing the blastocoel, with one pole distinguished by a thicker accumulation of cells that makes up the inner cell mass (Figure 5.1). Although the pluripotent cells of the inner cell mass can form every type of cell found in the human body, they cannot form an entire organism since they are unable to give rise to the placenta and supporting tissues necessary for development in the human uterus.

The outer ring of cells of the blastocyst constitutes the trophectoderm (Figure 5.2). While the inner cell mass gives rise to the actual embryo, the trophectoderm gives rise to the placenta and other supporting structures of pregnancy.

In vivo fertilized blastocysts have been examined after being washed from the uterine cavity. Using uterine lavage performed 5 days after the luteinizing hormone peak, John Buster and his colleagues collected 25 specimens from five fertile donors who had undergone artificial insemination[1,2]. After examination, all recovered preembryos were transferred to recipients and resulted in three intrauterine and one tubal pregnancy. Morphological development of the specimens ranged from degenerating oocytes to mature blastocysts and all intrauterine pregnancies were established with blastocysts. A 12-cell conceptus with degenerating blastomeres was associated with the tubal pregnancy. It is of extreme interest to note that not all oocytes and preembryos collected from these donors were viable, nor were they all morphologically attractive. This perhaps

points to the innate inefficiency of the human reproductive process which results in only one of four exposures to intercourse ending in a viable pregnancy.

Blastocysts are generally observed *in vitro* sometime after 100 h post-insemination. If left in culture for 5 or 6 days after insemination, 26–65% of preembryos will reach this stage, depending on culture methods and medium composition[3-7]. Most *in vitro* fertilization (IVF) programs choose to transfer blastocysts after 5 days of culture, but the occasional clinic opts for transfer on later days, either waiting for further development of slowly growing blastocysts or delaying transfer until hatching occurs[8,9].

Early and late stages in blastocyst development can be recognized by both the thickness of the zona pellucida and the overall size of the blastocyst. In early blastocyst formation, the zona is thick and the diameter of the conceptus has changed little; one observes the blastocoel filling with fluid (Figure 5.3). At late stages, the blastocyst increases in overall size from the accumulated fluid, and a single ring of trophoblastic (trophectoderm) cells surrounds the cavity; the inner cell mass is clearly delineated and the zona has stretched very thin, to a mere outline (Figure 5.4). It may exist in this expanded state for 24 h or more before *hatching* from the zona pellucida[10] (*see* Chapter 7). In culture, the human blastocyst can be seen to expand, collapse, and re-expand during late stages. Once the blastocyst has shed its glycoprotein layer, it is free to implant in the uterine wall.

Of interest is that the blastocyst appears to have a built-in time clock. It has been observed that a cavity will often begin coalescing in the day-4 or -5 preembryo

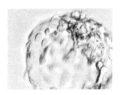

regardless of the number of cells present, or even after one-quarter of its cells have been removed at an earlier stage for biopsy purposes. It has been debated whether this time clock is related to chronological age, associated with the number of nuclear divisions that have taken place, or both. Cleaving preembryos have been treated experimentally with chemical agents that interrupt the cell cycle by disrupting microtubules and microfilaments. Although cell division stops under these conditions, nuclear division continues. Once exposure to the drug is discontinued, compaction and blastocyst formation occur, although fewer cells than normal are present and many of these are multinucleated[11]. In related experiments, 4-cell mouse preembryos were treated with cytochalasin-D to inhibit cytokinesis. When cytochalasin-D was removed, preembryos were capable of forming 'blastocysts' at the same time as controls, but contained only four polyploid cells. Although they possessed the ability to hatch and implant after intrauterine transfer, none were instrumental in producing living young[12]. It is now generally accepted, and may well be true, that the speed of cleavage is less important than the number of cells that eventually make up the blastocyst.

In 1954, Hertig and colleagues recorded counts of 158 and 107 cells in two blastocysts collected at the time of hysterectomy[13]. In 1972, Croxatto and associates estimated 186 cells in a blastocyst obtained after uterine flushing[14]. Today, either we can speculate that multinucleated cells accounted for some excessive distortion of cell number in these earlier reports, or we are forced to recognize that the culturing systems used for early in vitro investigations did not produce the same cell numbers that actually occur in vivo. In 1989, nuclear fluorescent staining was used to obtain an average cell count in nine in vitro-derived blastocysts. In this study, only 58 ± 8.1 cells were counted, with a wide range of 24–90[15]. Similarly, based on the results of examining 57 human specimens, Winston and colleagues estimated that two-thirds of cavitated preembryos on day 5 possessed fewer than 32 cells, and that these were multinucleated at high rates[16]. These last authors speculated that the majority of preembryos developing in vitro fail to complete sufficient cell cycles to produce blastocysts with cell numbers adequate to allow for normal differentiation of an inner cell mass. In the mouse, there is indeed some evidence to suggest that more rapidly dividing blastomeres contribute preferentially to the inner cell mass of the blastocyst[17] (see Chapter 4). Clearly, history has demonstrated the need to improve culturing systems and further define accurate measurements to determine viability in the conceptuses we so carefully nurture in our laboratories.

Coculture techniques were once believed to be necessary for encouraging preembryos to reach blastocyst stages of development. Whether coculture cells themselves impart factors favorable to support growth, or whether they utilize unnecessary medium components and/or absorb toxins, is not clearly defined. Perhaps the cells are helpful for each of these reasons, especially under conditions where culture media or environmental factors are suboptimal. In the 1990s, an occasional study showed no differences in results obtained after coculture versus conventional culture[18], but most publications demonstrated enhanced rates of development after placing preembryos on various cell-type monolayers, most notably Vero® cells (African green monkey kidney cells), autologous endometrial cells, autologous granulosa and cumulus cells, or bovine oviductal cells[19-26]. However, in the past few years, some of the original proponents of coculture techniques have openly declared the better suitability of sequential medium systems for extended culture[27].

As we will see emerging throughout this discussion, a true need exists for a marker of preembryo viability, one that will serve to guide embryologists in determining precisely what should be replaced to enhance pregnancy without exposing the patient to high-order multiple gestation. It has been proposed that one approach might involve the transfer of a single, or at most two, healthy blastocysts[28]. Reviewing the literature, one finds that there are reports of blastocyst implantation rates that do not surpass[29], marginally surpass[23] and greatly surpass[30] the implantation rates of day-2 and -3 transferred conceptuses (for more detail, see Chapter 6). In the article by Gardner and colleagues[30], blastocysts implanted in utero at rates in excess of 46% in a defined patient population (mean age 34.5 years, mean basal follicle stimulating hormone (FSH) 6.9 IU/l, normal uterus, no contraindication to pregnancy), representing a two-fold increase over rates in matched controls (eight patients in study group; 15 patients in control group). The culturing condition, specifically the sequential culture medium used in this study, appears to play a large role in encouraging the continued growth of viable conceptuses to advanced stages (see Chapter 2). Indeed, high rates of blastocyst development have been attained after exposing preembryos to tailored culture medium components according to the precise stage of development[31].

The prospect of using non-invasive techniques to select appropriate preembryos and blastocysts for transfer is a relatively new and intriguing area of investigation. It has been suggested that, in the near future, human blastocysts may be studied using ultramicrofluorescence techniques to select those with the greatest potential for implantation. In the mouse, excellent correlation was found between blastocysts with a high glucose uptake/low lactate production (as an estimate of glycolytic activity) and fetal development[32]. Even more recently, the concept of non-invasive amino acid profiling has caught the attention of the scientific community, since the procedure has the exciting potential to select developmentally competent single human preembryos for transfer[33]. The application of these and other new methods may revolutionize laboratory techniques in the future.

Influence of maternal age on successful outcome after blastocyst transfer

In one study of 300 women between the ages of 18 and 45 years undergoing blastocyst transfer, the impact of maternal age was studied[34]. Fertilized oocytes were cultured for up to 144 h, and subsequently transferred when at least one attained an expanded blastocyst stage. The rate of cycle cancellation before oocyte retrieval increased significantly with age, and the average number of oocytes per retrieval and the proportion of cycles with expanded blastocysts declined significantly. While pregnancy rates per stimulation declined with age, pregnancy rates per transfer were approximately 50% across the entire age range. In this study, the decline in female fertility with age was concluded to be the result of reduced numbers of oocytes and the inability of fertilized oocytes to develop to the blastocyst stage. Implantation and pregnancy rates appeared to be unaffected by advancing age when blastocysts actually formed, a finding also observed by other investigators[35]. Other authors have surmised that biological ovarian age, rather than chronological age, determines blastocyst development potential and subsequent pregnancy rates[28].

At Cornell, we have observed a similar trend towards higher clinical pregnancy rates in selected patients suitable for day-5 transfer over the age of 40. Nonetheless, the miscarriage rate, as reflected by a lower ongoing pregnancy rate in these women, is still higher than in younger women undergoing blastocyst transfer (Tables 5.1 and 5.2).

Similarly, Pantos and colleagues[36] found that blastocyst development rates, clinical pregnancy rates and implantation rates were reduced across the board in women over age 40 receiving blastocysts for transfer on day 5 or 6 (22.2%, 21.1% and 8.9%, respectively vs. 40.5%, 44.6% and 19.9% in younger controls). In addition, clinical miscarriage rates were significantly higher in the older age group (25% vs. 13% in younger controls).

Monozygotic twinning and blastocyst transfer

Monozygotic (MZ) twinning results from the division of a single fertilized oocyte into two genetically identical preembryos, and is thought to occur in 0.42% of all deliveries[37]. Several studies have shown an increased risk for MZ twinning following day-5 transfer. Rates per clinical pregnancy range from 0%[38] to 12.5%[39]. Most reports are intermediate to these numbers, Behr and associates reporting an incidence of 5.0% per day-5 pregnancy[40] and da Costa and associates reporting an incidence of 3.9%[41]. The Cornell program has experienced an MZ twinning rate per clinical pregnancy of 0.49% for day-3 transfer (not significantly different from natural conception) and 3.4% per day-5 transfer (significantly higher than natural conception).

While MZ twins are thought to result from the division of a single fertilized oocyte to form two genetically identical preembryos, the precise mechanism(s) responsible for this division are not known. However, several observations have yielded theoretical explanations of the process. For example, the occurrence of inner cell mass 'splitting' might cause duplication of the preembryo at an early developmental stage (Figures 5.5 and 5.6)[42,43]. This splitting hypothesis was supported by animal studies showing that mechanical cleavage of mammalian preembryos *in vitro* could produce identical twins[44,45]. While these microsurgical approaches proved effective in the laboratory, the *de novo* fission apparently required for spontaneous MZ twinning has never been directly observed. It was very recently proposed that increased levels of glucose in culture media may predispose the inner cell mass to apoptotic changes, and if apoptotic cells are polarized in a linear fashion, cells of the inner cell mass may separate during hatching[46].

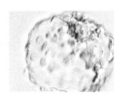

Table 5.1   Results from all day-5 transfers, with and without actual blastocysts transferred

Age (years)	Number of patients	Blastocysts transferred/transfer (n)	Clinical pregnancy/transfer (%)	Ongoing pregnancy/transfer (%)	Multiple pregnancy/transfer (%)	Sacs/blastocyst transferred (%)
< 30	67	1.99 ± 0.12	72	69	37	59
30–33	104	2.04 ± 0.27	81	74	46	65
34–36	75	2.04 ± 0.26	68	57	32	53
37–39	53	2.11 ± 0.46	59	49	28	45
≥ 40	29	2.62 ± 0.67	66	41	17	37
Total	328	2.09 ± 0.38	71	62	36	55

Table 5.2   Results from all transfer cycles involving at least one true blastocyst

Age (years)	Number of patients	Blastocysts transferred/transfer (n)	Clinical pregnancy/transfer (%)	Ongoing pregnancy/transfer (%)	Multiple pregnancy/transfer (%)	Sacs/blastocyst transferred (%)
< 30	64	1.98 ± 0.12	75	72	38	61
30–33	91	2.00 ± 0.21	86	78	52	71
34–36	71	2.03 ± 0.24	70	61	34	56
37–39	47	2.09 ± 0.40	62	51	30	48
≥ 40	26	2.65 ± 0.62	69	46	19	39
Total	299	2.07 ± 0.35	75	66	38	58

The timing of twinning can be inferred from the structure of the placenta, membranes and yolk sac(s). The earlier is the twinning event, the greater is the degree to which each embryo is provided with adequate extraembryonic structures. Twin embryos that are formed early are therefore more autonomous and physiologically independent than those resulting from later twinning events[47].

Talansky and Gordon proposed that zona drilling experiments facilitated twinning by inducing a conformational change in some mouse blastocysts[48]. Specifically, some blastocoels associated with micromanipulation assumed a 'figure of eight' shape as the cells attempted to squeeze through the artificially created hole in the zona pellucida. Other investigators found murine blastocoel expansion unimpeded after natural hatching in most cases[42], but observed trapping 5 days post-manipulation in others that received zona drilling (59/132, or 45%). One human blastocyst experimentally treated with partial zona dissection in this study hatched partially on day 8 and was noted to 'fold double and split', resulting in two distinctly separate but grossly unequal blastocoels. However, this connection between assisted hatching and MZ twinning remains highly speculative, as blastocoels and inner cell masses have never been observed to divide evenly and completely after passing through an artificial zona opening, either in humans or in any animal model. A review of six cases of MZ twins either with naturally thin zonae or where zona micromanipulation was performed suggested that zona architecture plays an important role in the development of MZ twins[49]. Other investigators reported five cases of MZ twins after assisted hatching from 142 pregnancies, and concluded that monoamniotic multiple gestations were increased in zona-manipulated cycles[50]. Recently, Schachter and co-workers reported an overall increase in MZ twinning with assisted reproductive treatment, but concluded that this increase is irrespective of treatment modality or micromanipulative techniques[51].

The relevance of MZ twinning in view of assisted conception outcomes is based on the markedly increased hazards attendant to pregnancies of this type. Twin–twin transfusion syndrome[52,53] and fetal entanglement/umbilical cord accidents[54], and other developmental anomalies[55], are much more common among MZ twin gestations than in singleton pregnancies[56].

The subjects of MZ twinning and infertility treatments converged soon after the realization that IVF could be associated with an increased frequency of MZ twinning[57]. This observation was refined by a study of more than 2500 multiple births[58], which postulated that ovulation induction itself, not culture conditions, was responsible for the markedly higher rate of MZ twinning following infertility treatments. Increased numbers of monoamniotic multiple gestations following zona-manipulated cycles have been reported[50], but this was based on self-reported, anonymous data supplied by 42 IVF centers in the USA. More recently, a 12-fold increase in MZ twins (chorionicity not specified) was identified in a series of more than 600 patients who received single preembryo transfer[59].

An analysis of factors affecting zona characteristics is appropriate, since the zona pellucida is central to several theories regarding MZ twinning. A synthesis of findings from earlier studies[49,57,58] suggests that at least three factors are influential in MZ twinning among patients receiving infertility treatments: ovulation induction, certain IVF culture conditions and zona architecture/micromanipulation. With these three variables occurring together so often in modern clinical infertility practice, multiple regression analysis to determine the specific contribution of each intervention has proved difficult to perform. If the natural rate of MZ twinning (0.42%) may be considered valid in settings of spontaneous conception and single implantation, then the increase in the observed MZ twinning rate after blastocyst transfer may be partially explained by the increased number of implantations. Importantly, the clinical rarity of MZ twinning challenges the study of this phenomenon in the context of IVF, as relevant investigations require large samples (> 10 000 cases) to detect meaningful differences with suitable statistical power[60].

Figures 5.7–5.10 depict day-5 blastocysts, which, after transfer to the uterine cavity, generated MZ twins. Outcomes are noted.

Male/female sex ratios and birth weight after blastocyst transfer

It has been postulated by several researchers that Y-bearing preembryos (males) develop at faster rates than X-bearing ones (females). If this theory is proved accurate, one might expect a skew in sex ratios after day-5 transfer, as the most advanced blastocysts are almost always replaced preferentially. In one very interesting study, the number of cells and metabolic activity of male and female human preembryos were examined to determine whether male preembryos were more advanced than female ones following *in vitro* fertilization[61]. The metabolic activity of normally fertilized preembryos was assessed daily by non-invasive measurements of pyruvate and glucose uptake and lactate production between days 2 and 6 after insemination. On day 6, the numbers of nuclei from the trophectoderm and inner cell masses of blastocysts were counted by differential labeling and fluorescence microscopy. Nuclei were then recovered, and the sex of the preembryos identified using nested primers to amplify the amelogenin gene and pseudogene sequences on the X and Y chromosomes, respectively. Development of male and female preembryos were then compared. From 69 of 178 (39%) preembryos that developed to the blastocyst stage, the sex of 57 was determined: 21 (37%) were male and 36 (63%) female. The number of cells in male preembryos was significantly greater on day 2 ($p < 0.005$), and this difference was maintained through the blastocyst stage (in both the trophectoderm and the inner cell mass). Pyruvate uptake was significantly higher by male preembryos between days 2 and 5 ($p < 0.05$). Glucose uptake and lactate production were significantly higher in male preembryos on days 4–5 ($p < 0.05$). Extrapolation from differences in the number of cells indicated that female preembryos were approximately 4.5 h delayed in their development from day 2 onwards, compared to male preembryos.

Although many thousands of children must be born before the statistical relevance of this finding can be proved, it is interesting to examine smaller numbers. In

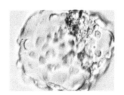

1999, Menezo and colleagues[62] reported that blastocysts transferred on day 5 after development in either coculture or sequential media systems gave rise to the birth of more male offspring, namely 225 males versus 158 females (59% vs. 41%). Contrary to this finding, replacement of thawed blastocysts did not demonstrate more males, perhaps consistent with the fact that those which were frozen actually developed more slowly to the blastocyst stage as compared to ones transferred fresh. In a report from Australia, no statistically significant shift in the male/female birth ratio was observed after blastocyst replacement, but the numbers were small and a trend towards more males was similarly observed (92 males versus 71 females or 56% vs. 44%)[8]. In this last study, transfers involved blastocysts which were also transferred on days 6 and 7, possibly diluting the impact of rapid cleavage.

The male/female live birth ratio for the USA and the world is 1.05, or 51% males versus 49% females *(UN Population Division; http:/esa.un.org/unpp [panel 2])*. In our program, day-3 transfer has resulted in an expected male/female ratio of 51 : 49. The male/female ratio for day-5 transfer in our program is 56 : 44, an intriguing 'mini-skew' that will be followed closely as numbers of children born after blastocyst transfer continue to grow.

No differences have been observed in the birth weights of live-born infants conceived through blastocyst transfer[8,62], a finding dissimilar to that reported for domestic animals[63].

Grading systems used for blastocysts

Different grading systems have been proposed for scoring human blastocysts. One of the most popular was developed by David Gardner and his colleagues in the late 1990s[64]. With this system, blastocysts are given a numerical score from 1 to 6 on the basis of their degree of expansion and hatching status as follows: 1, an early blastocyst with a blastocoel that is less than half of the volume of the embryo; 2, a blastocyst with a blastocoel that is half of or greater than half of the volume of the embryo; 3, a full blastocyst with a blastocoel completely filling the embryo; 4, an expanded blastocyst with a blastocoel volume larger than that of the early embryo, with a thinning zona; 5, a hatching blastocyst with the trophectoderm starting to herniate though the zona; and 6, a hatched blastocyst, in which the blastocyst has completely escaped from the zona. For blastocysts graded as 3–6 (i.e. full blastocysts onwards), the

development of the inner cell mass is assessed as follows: A, tightly packed, many cells; B, loosely grouped, several cells; or C, very few cells. The trophectoderm is also assessed as follows: A, many cells forming a cohesive epithelium; B, few cells forming a loose epithelium; or C, very few large cells. Using this scheme, it was shown clearly that clinical pregnancy rates in excess of 60% could be attained by the transfer of at least one high-scoring blastocyst greater than or equal to 3AA[38].

In early 2000, we modified Gardner's three-part grading system to fit the needs of the Cornell program. A blastocyst is defined as having a blastocoel filling greater than half the volume of the conceptus, and early stages must possess cells that suggest the formation of an inner cell mass; cavitating morulae possess smaller blastocoels, and developing inner cell masses are unidentifiable. Our current system is detailed in Figures 5.11a and 5.11b. Briefly, blastocysts are similarly given a numerical score from 1 to 6 on the basis of their degree of expansion and hatching status, but with slight modifications to Gardner's methods: 1, an early blastocyst (blastocoel filling greater than half of the volume of the conceptus), but without overall increase in size as compared to earlier stages; 2, a true blastocyst (blastocoel filling greater than half of the volume of the conceptus) with slight expansion in overall size and some thinning of the zona pellucida; 3, a full blastocyst (blastocoel filling greater than half of the volume of the conceptus) with overall size fully enlarged and a very thin zona pellucida; 4, a hatching blastocyst (no biopsy, assisted hatching, or other major zona-manipulation); 5, a fully hatched blastocyst, completely removed from the zona pellucida (no biopsy, assisted hatching or other major zona-manipulation); and 6, a hatching or hatched blastocyst resulting from manipulations that have created a substantial hole in the zona pellucida. For blastocysts graded as 1–6 (i.e. any defined blastocyst), the development of the inner cell mass is assessed as follows: A, tightly packed, compacted cells; B, larger, loosely grouped cells or formation of a cellular bridge; C, no inner cell mass distinguishable; or D, cells of the inner cell mass appear degenerative. The trophectoderm is assessed as follows: A, many healthy cells forming a cohesive epithelium; B, few, but healthy cells, large in size, forming a loose epithelium; C, unhealthy, very large or unevenly distributed cells, may appear as few cells squeezed to the side; or D, cells appear degenerative.

Using this system, transfers with at least one 1BD blastocyst (any real blastocyst by definition; 91% of cycles undergoing extended culture) result in a 75% clinical pregnancy rate and a 59% implantation rate. Transfers with at least one 3AA, 3AB or 3BA blastocyst result in a 78% clinical pregnancy rate and 63% implantation rate. The fact that there is so little difference between cycles with 'early' and 'late' blastocysts indicate that *any* blastocyst on day 5 will lead to good pregnancy and implantation results. Only cycles without defined blastocysts on day 5 demonstrate significantly lower potential, although pregnancy and implantation are by no means negated (31% clinical pregnancy and 17% implantation).

Individual grading parameters

Little attention has been given to individual grading parameters (blastocyst expansion, inner cell mass quality or trophectoderm quality) as separate and individual parameters. At Cornell, we analyzed blastocysts from 156 patients on day 5[65]. Non-hatching blastocysts were assessed for blastocoel expansion, inner cell mass morphology and trophectoderm morphology, as described above. Only blastocysts with known implantation results were included in the study.

In general, there was positive correlation between overall blastocyst quality and implantation rate (for example, transfer of a 3AA blastocyst approached a 70% implantation rate). Examining individual parameters, there were no significant differences between degree of blastocyst expansion and implantation rate (3 = 67%, 2 = 58% and 1 = 53%, a slight trend) or inner cell mass compaction and implantation rate (A = 68%, B = 62% and C = 61%, a slight trend). In contrast, significantly higher implantation rates were achieved by transferring blastocysts with grade A trophectoderm (76%) compared to B (56%; $p < 0.05$) or C (50%; $p < 0.05$). While the morphology of the blastocyst measured with a three-part grading system impacted upon overall implantation, the quality (number and size of cells) of the trophectoderm influenced implantation to the greatest degree as a single parameter; expansion and inner cell mass morphology appeared to impact upon implantation to a lesser degree. The trophectoderm is probably the most important individual factor for implantation, as it plays a crucial role in blastocyst attachment, trophoblast development and subsequent uterine invasion. Following implantation, a good quality inner cell mass will direct embryo development.

Optimal inner cell mass size and shape

In contrast, a recent publication discredits the previously described grading systems as being vague and poorly defined[66]. The authors state that the observed differences using such systems simply reflect differences in developmental timing events rather than differences in actual quality. They further contend that combining multiple assessment factors into a single grading system without first demonstrating the importance of each factor independently is counterproductive and potentially misleading. They go on to propose alternative markers of blastocyst quality, namely the quantitative measurement of inner cell mass (ICM) size and shape, quantitative measurement of blastocyst expansion and quantitative analysis of trophectoderm cell number, first assessing the predictive value of each measure independently, then combining features with significant predictive value to form a unified grading system. What they discovered was quite interesting: the ICMs of implanting blastocysts were significantly larger than of those failing to implant (5023 μm^2 vs. 4312 μm^2, $p = 0.008$). Logistic regression analysis revealed an approximately linear positive relationship between ICM size and implantation ($p = 0.01$). Implantation rates ranged from approximately 20% for 2000-μm^2 ICMs to nearly 50% for ICMs of 6000 μm^2. A continuous model such as this is likely to reflect an accurate description of the relationship between ICM size and implantation potential. However, for simplification, they subsequently divided blastocysts into 'large' and 'small' ICM categories using a break-point that maximized the difference between the two groups. Implantation was significantly higher among blastocysts with ICM measurements > 4500 μm^2 compared with those having smaller ICMs (45% vs. 23%, $p = 0.006$). Optimal ICM size was therefore defined as 'large', measuring > 4500 μm^2. Inner cell masses measuring < 3800 μm^2 were associated with particularly low implantation rates (18%, $p = 0.0028$ vs. large ICMs). Blastocysts with ICMs falling between these large and small size ranges implanted at an intermediate rate of 32%, which was statistically indistinguishable from the rates for either smaller or larger ICMs. The authors failed to detect any statistically significant difference in ICM shape between implanting and non-implanting preembryos, but noted that implantation rates were highest for blastocysts with slightly oval-shaped ICMs. Blastocysts were then grouped according to whether their ICMs fell within the optimal size and/or shape ranges. 'Top-quality' blastocysts with ICMs within both optimal size and

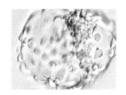

optimal shape ranges implanted at a rate of 60% (Figure 5.12). Implantation rates were much lower for those with ICMs that were optimally sized only (29%), optimally shaped only (32%) or suboptimally sized and shaped (19%).

The implantation rate for unexpanded blastocysts (10%) was significantly lower than that of high-scoring blastocysts, but no differences were seen in the mean diameter of implanting and non-implanting blastocysts that were expanded at the time of transfer (195 µm vs. 194 µm, $p = 0.81$). The number of trophectoderm cells observed in a cross-sectional circumference plane was also nearly identical between implanting and non-implanting conceptuses (11.0 vs. 10.8, $p = 0.64$).

From this study, it was concluded that quantitative measurements of the inner cell mass are highly indicative of implantation potential, and that these measurements provide more predictive value for implantation when compared to the qualitative assessment of developmental timing events. Whether or not this conclusion is accurate will be determined only after other investigators apply these methods, replicate the published results and determine the basis for the correlative findings.

Blastocyst development and intracytoplasmic sperm injection

It was suggested in 1994 that blastocyst development rates may be reduced when oocytes are fertilized by sperm derived from suboptimal semen samples[67]. Since that time, other investigators have reported lower blastocyst formation rates associated with intracytoplasmic sperm injection (ICSI) procedures using suboptimal sperm when compared to non-ICSI treatment[68–71]. Possible hypotheses for impaired blastocyst formation after ICSI have ranged from defective sperm DNA and delayed male pronucleus formation to abnormal male centrosome control through the first cleavages and inappropriate or delayed genomic activation.

Extended culture has even been proposed as a means of weeding out chromosomal abnormalities contributed by defective spermatozoa. This idea has resulted from the concern that the use of ICSI may contribute to increased numbers of abnormal offspring[72,73]. The relationship between poor preembryo quality and the existence of low morphological 'normalcy' of a semen sample has certainly been suggested[74]. It has been proposed that, by using a selection process such as extended culture to identify preembryos most likely to develop normally, chances of an errant paternal genome being inherited by ICSI might be reduced[75]. While an interesting speculation, recent studies suggest that the phenotypic manifestation of paternal genomic abnormalities probably does not occur before implantation and, therefore, blastocyst transfer may not diminish the likelihood of inheriting genetic defects involving 'male factor' loci[76].

Experience in the Cornell program indicates that blastocyst development is not impaired after ICSI procedures are carried out. Although slightly poorer development after ICSI initially occurred in our first year of day-5 transfer trials, rates of clinical pregnancy and implantation have since evened out for conventional insemination and ICSI groups, both being in the region of 71% and 55%, respectively, for all preembryos transferred, actual blastocysts or not.

Enzymatic removal of the zona pellucida before blastocyst transfer

It is theorized that the zona pellucida is required during early preembryonic development, at the 2-cell to 8-cell stages, but may not be necessary after compaction occurs. The first report of an ongoing human pregnancy following the intrauterine transfer of day-6 zona-free blastocysts was presented in early 1997[77]. In this case report, a patient had undergone eight previous transfers without success; preembryos were cocultured on Vero® cells until blastocyst stages, and their zonae removed with 0.5% pronase. Clinical pregnancy was established after the transfer of two zona-free blastocysts, and led to an ongoing singleton gestation. In a follow-up report by the same authors published in 1998, 19 additional women (mean age 32.6 years, and 2.1 previous failed attempts) had zona-free blastocysts transferred[78]. Clinical pregnancy and implantation rates were 53% and 33%, respectively. The multiple pregnancy rate was 40%. Based on these studies, it appears that zona-manipulated blastocysts implant relatively well. The authors suggest that enzymatic treatment of the zona may allow better anchorage and dialog of the blastocyst with the endometrium. Other investigators have reported similar outcomes after the transfer of zona-free blastocysts[79].

Blastocyst development after manipulation of the zona pellucida

Artificially created holes, cuts or flaps are sometimes made purposefully in the zonae pellucidae of selected preembryos. This occurs routinely during biopsy, assisted hatching and ICSI procedures. These breeches, if large enough, may affect subsequent blastocyst expansion and hatching events (*see* Chapter 7). Blastocyst development after biopsy for preimplantation genetic diagnosis differs considerably from what is routinely observed in non-manipulated conceptuses. Because a relatively large hole is created in the zona pellucida during the biopsy procedure, either with chemical agents or 'burned' with a laser, premature hatching often occurs without coincident expansion of the blastocyst or gradual thinning of the zona pellucida. Cavitating morulae and early non-expanded blastocysts are often observed to herniate through the artificially made holes in the zona pellucida (Figures 5.13–5.15). Preembryos subjected to assisted hatching procedures follow much the same course after blastocysts form if chemical agents are used to breech the zona (Figures 5.16 and 5.17), whereas assisted hatching techniques utilizing a mechanical tearing action are associated with slits or flaps rather than actual holes, and have been implicated in blastocyst entrapment during expansion and hatching. Small punctures made with an ICSI pipette during assisted fertilization procedures are likely to either reseal or be too tiny to permit easy escape of the expanding blastocyst.

Uterine receptivity and blastocyst transfer

In the rabbit, preembryos have been shown to implant at greater rates as the interval between ovulation and transfer increases. This finding has been attributed to the transfer being carried out concurrent to higher circulating progesterone levels in the mother. It has been put forth that this state tends to inhibit uterine contractions[80]. It was subsequently determined that uterine junctional zone contractions progressively decrease as the cycle moves into the luteal phase, and that fewer contractions are associated with improved pregnancy rates[81]. It has additionally been demonstrated that day 5 is favorable for the human in terms of decreased uterine contractility[82].

Time line for optimal blastocyst development

Based on studies performed at Cornell, examining a timely first cleavage and the importance of observing growth to the 8-cell stage by the morning of day 3[83], we worked out a model for optimal blastocyst development (Table 5.3). Other factors could certainly be incorporated into the time line such as standards for pronuclear size and alignment, morphological features felt to be of importance during cleavage stages or inner cell/trophectoderm characteristics, but these would require that preembryos be 'perfect' rather than simply 'timely'. Briefly, the time line covers the two major points listed above and sets up minimal growth parameters for assessing adequate blastocyst development by the time of intrauterine transfer (Figure 5.18).

Figures 5.19–5.23 depict groups of preembryos that were serially photographed on days 3, 4 and 5 of development (preembryo/morula/blastocyst stage). Some closely follow the proposed time line, others do not. Outcomes are noted.

Figure 5.24 depicts sequential photographs of mouse preembryos developing to the hatching blastocyst stage.

Blastocysts known to implant

Figures 5.25–5.35 present blastocysts on day 5 of culture that are known to have implanted after transfer to the uterine cavity. Each led to a fetal heartbeat by ultrasound, and most often produced a living, healthy child. Where this is not the case, the obstetrical outcome is indicated in the legend.

Favorable blastocysts that failed to implant

Figure 5.36 shows highly graded blastocysts that failed to implant after intrauterine transfer.

Unfavorable development on day 5 with implantation

Figure 5.37 demonstrates poorly graded day 5 conceptuses that led to ongoing pregnancies after transfer.

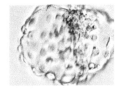

Table 5.3 Time line for optimal blastocyst development

Time line	Actual time	Minimal expected observation
Hour 0	15.00, day 0	insemination or ICSI
Before hour 24 (ICSI)	15.00, day 1	cleavage to the 2-cell stage, ≤ 10% fragments
Before hour 26 (insemination)	17.00, day 1	cleavage to the 2-cell stage, ≤ 10% fragments
Before hour 42	09.00, day 2	cleavage to the 4-cell stage, ≤ 10% fragments
Before hour 66	09.00, day 3	cleavage to the 8-cell stage, ≤ 10% fragments
Before hour 72	15.00, day 3	evidence of increased cell–cell contact
Before hour 90	09.00, day 4	evidence of uniform compaction
Before hour 100	19.00, day 4	evidence of central cavitation
Before hour 114	09.00, day 5	grade 2 blastocyst expansion
Before hour 120	15.00, day 5	transfer; grade 3 blastocyst expansion
Before hour 144	15.00, day 6	if not transferred, evidence of hatching or already hatched

ICSI, intracytoplasmic sperm injection

Abnormal blastocyst development

Blastocysts can form despite possessing discernable inner cell masses (Figure 5.38), with very small inner cell masses (Figure 5.39) or with abnormally developed inner cell masses (Figure 5.40). They may also form despite having exhibited extensive vacuolization during development fig. 5.41). Cells constituting the trophectoderm may also display abnormal features (Figure 5.42).

Recall that, although the pluripotent cells of the inner cell mass can form every type of cell found in the human body, they cannot form an entire organism since they are unable to give rise to the placenta and supporting tissues necessary for development in the human uterus. While the inner cell mass gives rise to the actual embryo, the trophectoderm gives rise to the placenta and other supporting structures of pregnancy. It has been observed that some blastocysts possess non-viable trophectoderm cells despite exhibiting healthy-appearing inner cell masses. In such specimens, the trophectoderm eventually degenerates, while the inner cell mass proliferates and enlarges (Figure 5.43). It has been proposed that because these specimens are incapable of establishing a viable pregnancy, their inner cell masses might be useful, without ethical objection, for potentially life-saving therapies resulting from appropriately designed stem cell research.

References

1. Buster JE, Bustillo M, Rodi IA, *et al*. Biologic and morphologic development of donated human ova recovered by nonsurgical uterine lavage. *Am J Obstet Gynecol* 1985;153:211–17

2. Buster JE. Embryo donation by uterine flushing and embryo transfer. *Clin Obstet Gynaecol* 1985;12:815–24

3. Alves da Motta EL, Alegretti JR, Baracat EC, Olive D, Serafini PC. High implantation and pregnancy rates with transfer of human blastocysts developed in preimplantation stage one and blastocyst media. *Fertil Steril* 1998;70:659–63

4. Behr B, Pool TB, Milki AA, Moore D, Gebhardt J, Dasig D. Preliminary clinical experience with human blastocyst development *in vitro* without co-culture. *Hum Reprod* 1999;14:454–7

5. Dokras A, Sargent IL, Barlow DH. Human blastocyst grading: an indicator of developmental potential? *Hum Reprod* 1993;8:2119–27

6. Gardner DK, Lane M, Kouridakis K, Schoolcraft WB. Complex physiologically based serum-free culture media increase mammalian embryo development. In Gomel V, Leung PCK, eds. *In Vitro Fertilization and Assisted Reproduction, Proceedings of the Tenth World Congress*, Monduzzi Editoire, Bologna, 1997:187–91

7. Schoolcraft WB, Gardner DK, Lane M, Schlenker T, Hamilton F, Meldrum DR. Blastocyst culture and transfer: analysis of results and parameters affecting outcome in two *in vitro* fertilization programs. *Fertil Steril* 1999;72:604–9

8. Kausche A, Jones GM, Trounson AO, Figueiredo F, MacLachlan V, Lolatgis N. Sex ratio and birth weights of infants born as a result of blastocyst transfers compared with early cleavage stage embryo transfers. *Fertil Steril* 2001;76:688–93

9. Sagoskin AW, Han T, Graham JR, Levy MJ, Stillman RJ, Tucker MJ. Healthy twin delivery after day 7 blastocyst transfer coupled with assisted hatching. *Fertil Steril* 2002;77:615–17

10. Cohen J, Simons RF, Edwards RG, Fehilly CB, Fishel SB. Pregnancies following the frozen storage of expanding human blastocysts. *J In Vitro Fertil Embryo Transf* 1985;2:59–64

11. Surani MA, Barton SC, Burling A. Differentiation of 2-cell and 8-cell mouse embryos arrested by cytoskeletal inhibitors. *Exp Cell Res* 1980;125:275–86

12. Pratt HP, Chakraborty J, Surani MA. Molecular and morphological differentiation of the mouse blastocyst after manipulations of compaction with cytochalasin D. *Cell* 1981;26:279–92

13. Hertig AT, Rock J, Adams EC, Mulligan WJ. On the preimplantation stages of the human ovum: a description of four normal specimens ranging from the second to fifth day of development. *Contrib Embryol* 1954;35:199

14. Croxatto HB, Diaz S, Fuentealba B, Croxatto HD, Carrillo D, Fabres C. Studies on the duration of egg transport in the human oviduct. I. The time interval between ovulation and egg recovery from the uterus in normal women. *Fertil Steril* 1972;23:447–58

15. Hardy K, Handyside AH, Winston RM. The human blastocyst: cell number, death and allocation during late preimplantation development *in vitro*. *Development* 1989;107:597–604

16. Winston NJ, Braude PR, Pickering SJ, *et al*. The incidence of abnormal morphology and nucleocytoplasmic ratios in 2-, 3- and 5-day human preembryos. *Hum Reprod* 1991;6:17–24

17. Pedersen RA. Early mammalian embryogenesis. In Knobil E, Neill JD, eds. *The Physiology of Reproduction*. New York: Raven Press, 1988:187

18. Van Blerkom J. Development of human embryos to the hatched blastocyst stage in the presence or absence of a monolayer of Vero® cells. *Hum Reprod* 1993;8:1525–39

19. Barmat LI, Liu HC, Spandorfer SD, *et al*. Autologous endometrial co-culture in patients with repeated failures of implantation after *in vitro* fertilization–embryo transfer. *J Assist Reprod Genet* 1999;16:121–7

20. Desai NN, Kennard EA, Kniss DA, Friedman CI. Novel human endometrial cell line promotes blastocyst development. *Fertil Steril* 1994;61:760–6

21. Freeman MR, Whitworth CM, Hill GA. Granulosa cell co-culture enhances human embryo development and pregnancy rate following *in-vitro* fertilization. *Hum Reprod* 1995;10:408–14

22. Mansour RT, Aboulghar MA, Serour GI, Abbass AM. Co-culture of human pronucleate oocytes with their cumulus cells. *Hum Reprod* 1994;9:1727–9

23. Menezo YJ, Sakkas D, Janny L. Co-culture of the early human embryo: factors affecting human blastocyst formation *in vitro*. *Microsc Res Tech* 1995;32:50–6

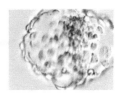

24. Nieto FS, Watkins WB, Lopata A, Baker HW, Edgar DH. The effects of coculture with autologous cryopreserved endometrial cells on human *in vitro* fertilization and early embryo morphology: a randomized study. *J Assist Reprod Genet* 1996;13:386–9

25. Quinn P, Margalit R. Beneficial effects of coculture with cumulus cells on blastocyst formation in a prospective trial with supernumerary human embryos. *J Assist Reprod Genet* 1996;13:9–14

26. Wiemer KE, Hoffman DI, Maxson WS, *et al*. Embryonic morphology and rate of implantation of human embryos following co-culture on bovine oviductal epithelial cells. *Hum Reprod* 1993;8:97–101

27. Menezo YJ, Hamamah S, Hazout A, Dale B. Time to switch from co-culture to sequential defined media for transfer at the blastocyst stage. *Hum Reprod* 1998;13:2043–4

28. Scholtes MC, Zeilmaker GH. Blastocyst transfer in day-5 embryo transfer depends primarily on the number of oocytes retrieved and not on age. *Fertil Steril* 1998;69:78–83

29. Bolton VN, Wren ME, Parsons JH. Pregnancies after *in vitro* fertilization and transfer of human blastocysts. *Fertil Steril* 1991;55:830–2

30. Gardner DK, Vella P, Lane M, Wagley L, Schlenker T, Schoolcraft WB. Culture and transfer of human blastocysts increases implantation rates and reduces the need for multiple embryo transfers. *Fertil Steril* 1998;69:84–8

31. Gardner DK, Lane M, Calderon I, Leeton J. Environment of the preimplantation human embryo *in vivo*: metabolite analysis of oviduct and uterine fluids and metabolism of cumulus cells. *Fertil Steril* 1996;65:349–53

32. Gardner DK. Routine culture to blastocyst – the solution to high order multiple pregnancy with IVF. Presented at the *Tenth Annual Conference on In Vitro Fertilization and Embryo Transfer*, Santa Barbara, UCLA-sponsored symposium, July, 1997:263

33. Houghton FD, Hawkhead JA, Humpherson PG, *et al*. Non-invasive amino acid turnover predicts human embryo developmental capacity. *Hum Reprod* 2002;17:999–1005

34. Shapiro BS, Richter KS, Harris DC, Daneshmand ST. Influence of patient age on the growth and transfer of blastocyst-stage embryos. *Fertil Steril* 2002;77:700–5

35. Janny L, Menezo YJ. Maternal age effect on early human embryonic development and blastocyst formation. *Mol Reprod Dev* 1996;45:31–7

36. Pantos K, Athanasiou V, Stefanidis K, Stavrou D, Vaxevanoglou T, Chronopoulou M. Influence of advanced age on the blastocyst development rate and pregnancy rate in assisted reproductive technology. *Fertil Steril* 1999;71:1144–6

37. Bulmer MG. *The Biology of Twinning in Man*. Oxford: Clarendon Press, 1970

38. Gardner DK, Lane M, Stevens J, Schlenker T, Schoolcraft WB. Blastocyst score affects implantation and pregnancy outcome: towards a single blastocyst transfer. *Fertil Steril* 2000;73:1155–8

39. Tarlatzis BC, Qublan HS, Sanopoulou T, Zepiridis L, Grimbizis G, Bontis J. Increase in the monozygotic twinning rate after intracytoplasmic sperm injection and blastocyst stage embryo transfer. *Fertil Steril* 2002;77:196–8

40. Behr B, Fisch JD, Racowsky C, Miller K, Pool TB, Milki AA. Blastocyst-ET and monozygotic twinning. *J Assist Reprod Genet* 2000;17:349–51

41. da Costa AA, Abdelmassih S, de Oliveira FG, *et al*. Monozygotic twins and transfer at the blastocyst stage after ICSI. *Hum Reprod* 2001;16:333–6

42. Malter HE, Cohen J. Blastocyst formation and hatching *in vitro* following zona drilling of mouse and human embryos. *Gamete Res* 1989;24:67–80

43. Van Langendonckt A, Wyns C, Godin PA, Toussaint-Demylle D, Donnez J. Atypical hatching of a human blastocyst leading to monozygotic twinning: a case report. *Fertil Steril* 2000;74:1047–50

44. Willadsen SM. A method for culture of micromanipulated sheep embryos and its use to produce monozygotic twins. *Nature (London)* 1979;277:298–300

45. Ozil JP. Production of identical twins by bisection of blastocysts in the cow. *J Reprod Fertil* 1983;69:463–8

46. Menezo YJ, Sakkas D. Monozygotic twinning: is it related to apoptosis in the embryo? *Hum Reprod* 2002;17:247–8

47. Machin GA, Keith LG. *An Atlas of Multiple Pregnancy: Biology and Pathology*. Carnforth, UK: Parthenon Publishing, 1999

48. Talansky BE, Gordon JW. Cleavage characteristics of mouse embryos inseminated and cultured after zona pellucida drilling. *Gamete Res* 1988;21:277–87

49. Alikani M, Noyes N, Cohen J, Rosenwaks Z. Monozygotic twinning in the human is associated with the zona pellucida architecture. *Hum Reprod* 1994;9:1318–21

50. Slotnick RN, Ortega JE. Monoamniotic twinning and zona manipulation: a survey of US IVF centers correlating zona manipulation procedures and high-risk twinning frequency. *J Assist Reprod Genet* 1996;13:381–5

51. Schachter M, Raziel A, Friedler S, Strassburger D, Bern O, Ron-El R. Monozygotic twinning after assisted reproductive techniques: a phenomenon independent of micromanipulation. *Hum Reprod* 2001;16:1264–9

52. Peramo B, Ricciarelli E, Cuadros-Fernandez JM, Huguet E, Hernandez ER. Blastocyst transfer and monozygotic twinning. *Fertil Steril* 1999;72:1116–17

53. Talbert DG, Bajoria R, Sepulveda W, Bower S, Fisk NM. Hydrostatic and osmotic pressure gradients produce manifestations of fetofetal transfusion syndrome in a computerized model of monochorial twin pregnancy. *Am J Obstet Gynecol* 1996;174:598–608

54. Nyberg DA, Filly RA, Golbus MS, Stephens JD. Entangled umbilical cords: a sign of monoamniotic twins. *J Ultrasound Med* 1984;3:29–32

55. Schinzel AA, Smith DW, Miller JR. Monozygotic twinning and structural defects. *J Pediatr* 1979;95:921–30

56. Powers WF. Twin pregnancy, complications and treatment. *Obstet Gynecol* 1973;42:795–808

57. Edwards RG, Mettler L, Walters DE. Identical twins and *in vitro* fertilization. *J In Vitro Fertilization Embryo Transf* 1986;3:114–17

58. Derom C, Vlietinck R, Derom R, Van den Berghe H, Thiery M. Increased monozygotic twinning rate after ovulation induction. *Lancet* 1987;1:1236–8

59. Blickstein I, Verhoeven HC, Keith LG. Zygotic splitting after assisted reproduction. *N Engl J Med* 1999;340:738–9

60. Sills ES, Moomjy M, Zaninovic N, *et al*. Human zona pellucida micromanipulation and monozygotic twinning frequency after IVF. *Hum Reprod* 2000;15:890–5

61. Ray PF, Conaghan J, Winston RM, Handyside AH. Increased number of cells and metabolic activity in male human preimplantation embryos following *in vitro* fertilization. *J Reprod Fertil* 1995;104:165–71

62. Menezo YJ, Chouteau J, Torello J, Girard A, Veiga A. Birth weight and sex ratio after transfer at the blastocyst stage in humans. *Fertil Steril* 1999;72:221–4

63. McEvoy TG, Sinclair KD, Young LE, Wilmut I, Robinson JJ. Large offspring syndrome and other consequences of ruminant embryo culture *in vitro*:

relevance to blastocyst culture in human ART. *Hum Fertil (Camb)* 2000;3:238–46

64. Gardner DK, Schoolcraft WB. *In vitro* culture of the human blastocyst. In Jansen R, Mortimer D, eds. *Towards Reproductive Certainty: Infertility and Genetics Beyond 1999*. Carnforth, UK: Parthenon Publishing, 1999:378–88

65. Zaninovic N, Berrios R, Clarke RN, Bodine R, Ye Z, Veeck LL. Blastocyst expansion, inner cell mass (ICM) formation, and trophectoderm (TM) quality: is one more important for implantation? Presented at the *57th Annual Meeting of the American Society for Reproductive Medicine*, Orlando, FL, October 2001

66. Richter KS, Harris DC, Daneshmand ST, Shapiro BS. Quantitative grading of a human blastocyst: optimal inner cell mass size and shape. *Fertil Steril* 2001;76:1157–67

67. Janny L, Menezo YJ. Evidence for a strong paternal effect on human preimplantation embryo development and blastocyst formation. *Mol Reprod Dev* 1994;38:36–42

68. Jones GM, Trounson AO, Lolatgis N, Wood C. Factors affecting the success of human blastocyst development and pregnancy following in vitro fertilization and embryo transfer. *Fertil Steril* 1998;70:1022–9

69. Miller JE, Smith TT. The effect of intracytoplasmic sperm injection and semen parameters on blastocyst development *in vitro*. *Hum Reprod* 2001;16:918–24

70. Shoukir Y, Chardonnens D, Campana A, Sakkas D. Blastocyst development from supernumerary embryos after intracytoplasmic sperm injection: a paternal influence? *Hum Reprod* 1998;13:1632–7

71. Wun WS, Wun CC, Valdes CT, Dunn RC, Grunert GM. Blastocyst formation is a good indicator for attainment of assisted reproduction. *Chin J Physiol* 1997;40:237–42

72. Bonduelle M, Joris H, Hofmans K, Liebaers I, Van Steirteghem A. Mental development of 201 ICSI children at 2 years of age. *Lancet* 1998;351:1553

73. Bowen JR, Gibson FL, Leslie GI, Saunders DM. Medical and developmental outcome at 1 year for children conceived by intracytoplasmic sperm injection. *Lancet* 1998;351:1529–34

74. Ombelet W, Fourie FL, Vandeput H, *et al*. Teratozoospermia and in-vitro fertilization: a randomized prospective study. *Hum Reprod* 1994;9:1479–84

75. Sakkas D. The use of blastocyst culture to avoid inheritance of an abnormal paternal genome after ICSI. *Hum Reprod* 1999;14:4–5

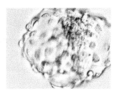

76. Banerjee S, Lamond S, McMahon A, Campbell S, Nargund G. Does blastocyst culture eliminate paternal chromosomal defects and select good embryos?: inheritance of an abnormal paternal genome following ICSI. *Hum Reprod* 2000;15:2455–9

77. Fong CY, Bongso A, Ng SC, Anandakumar C, Trounson A, Ratnam S. Ongoing normal pregnancy after transfer of zona-free blastocysts: implications for embryo transfer in the human. *Hum Reprod* 1997;12:557–60

78. Fong CY, Bongso A, Ng SC, Kumar J, Trounson A, Ratnam S. Blastocyst transfer after enzymatic treatment of the zona pellucida: improving *in-vitro* fertilization and understanding implantation. *Hum Reprod* 1998;13:2926–32

79. Jones GM, Trounson AO, Gardner DK, Kausche A, Lolatgis N, Wood C. Evolution of a culture protocol for successful blastocyst development and pregnancy. *Hum Reprod* 1998;13:169–77

80. Adams CE. Retention and development of eggs transferred to the uterus at various times after ovulation in the rabbit. *J Reprod Fertil* 1980;60:309–15

81. Fanchin R, Righini C, Olivennes F, Taylor S, de Ziegler D, Frydman R. Uterine contractions at the time of embryo transfer alter pregnancy rates after *in-vitro* fertilization. *Hum Reprod* 1998;13:1968–74

82. Fanchin R, Ayoubi JM, Righini C, Olivennes F, Schonauer LM, Frydman R. Uterine contractility decreases at the time of blastocyst transfers. *Hum Reprod* 2001;16:1115–19

83. Zaninovic N, Veeck L, Clarke RN, Rosenwaks Z. Early assessment of human preembryos as an indicator for potential blastocyst development. Presented at the *56th Annual Meeting of the American Society for Reproductive Medicine*, San Diego, CA, October 2000

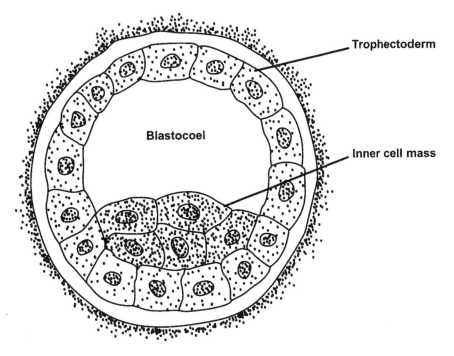

Early blastocyst

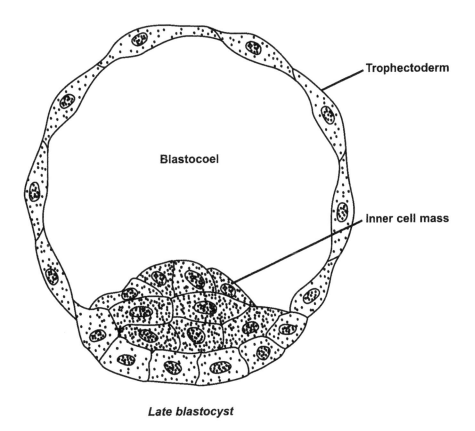

Late blastocyst

Figure 5.1 Schematic: early and late blastocyst stages

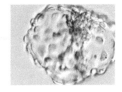

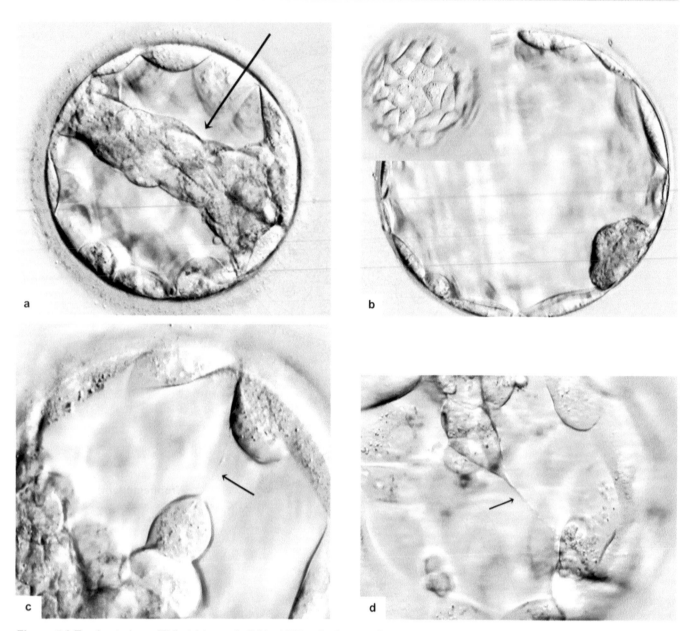

Figure 5.2 Trophectoderm (TM). (a) Large individual TM cells; inner cell mass (ICM) forms a band that spans the blastocoele; (b) smaller individual TM cells as compared to (a) and compacted ICM; insert focuses on TM cells; (c) on high magnification, one observes quite large TM cells that appear pushed to one side; a cytoplasmic 'string' can be seen between separating cells. According-ing to Scott (*Semin Reprod Med* 2000;18:171), the persistence of these processes after full expansion of the blastocyst correlates negatively with subsequent implantation; (d) high magnification of a cytoplasmic 'string' between developing ICM and TM

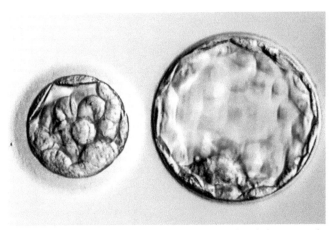

Figure 5.3 Blastocoelic enlargement. To the left, an early cavitating morula; to the right, an expanded blastocyst. Note the enlarging blastocoele and thinning zona pellucida as development advances

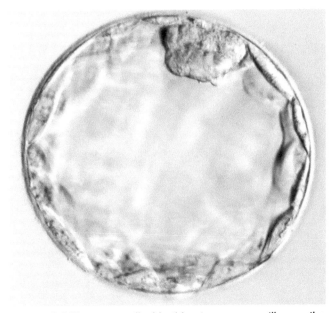

Figure 5.4 The zona pellucida thins to a mere outline as the blastocoele enlarges

Figure 5.5 Inner cell mass trapping as hatching occurs through a small hole. Note part of the ICM inside the zona pellucida and part outside, which could, theoretically, lead to ICM 'splitting'

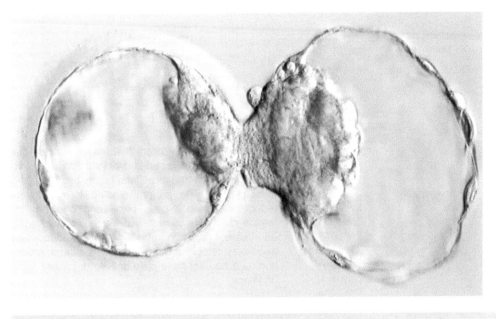

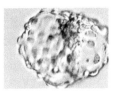

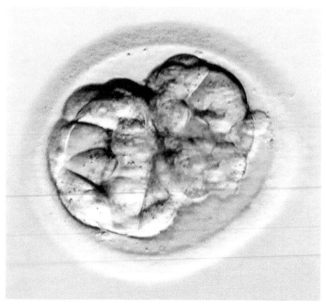

Figure 5.6 Developing blastocyst that appears to possess two separately cavitating segments

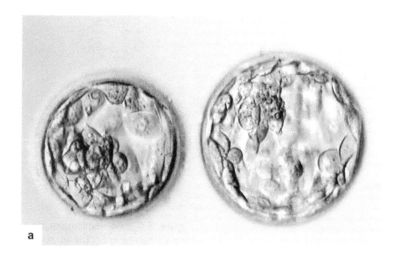

a

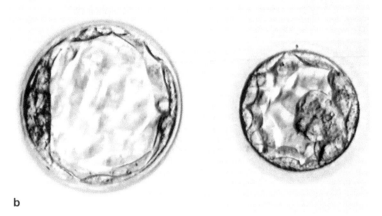

b

Figure 5.7 Day-5 transfers that led to monozygotic twins. (a) Two transferred blastocysts that led to two gestational sacs and three fetal hearts by ultrasound investigation. The patient elected to selectively reduce the monozygotic twins and one healthy female child was ultimately delivered; patient aged 36 years; (b) two blastocysts replaced; two sacs/three fetal hearts by ultrasound; natural reduction; one healthy male child delivered; patient aged 38 years

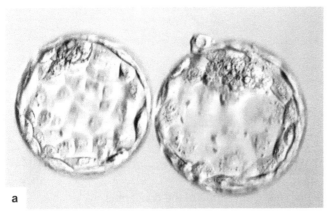
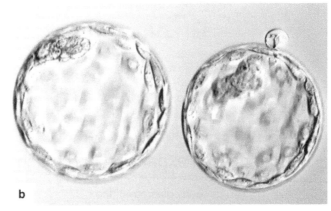

a   b

Figure 5.8 Day-5 transfers that led to monozygotic twins. (a) Two blastocysts replaced; two identical males and one female delivered; patient aged 27 years; (b) two blastocysts replaced; two identical males and third male sibling delivered; patient aged 36 years

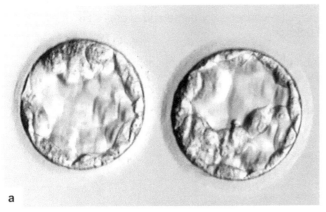
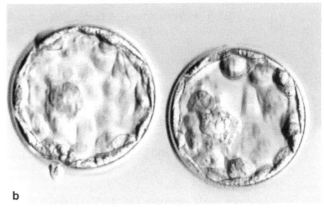

a   b

Figure 5.9 Day-5 transfers that led to monozygotic twins. (a) Two blastocysts replaced; two gestational sacs/three fetal hearts noted by ultrasound investigation. The monozygotic twins were miscarried; one female delivered to this oocyte recipient; patient aged 45 years; (b) two blastocysts replaced; two gestational sacs/three fetal hearts noted by ultrasound investigation. The monozygotic twins were reduced; one female delivered; patient aged 31 years

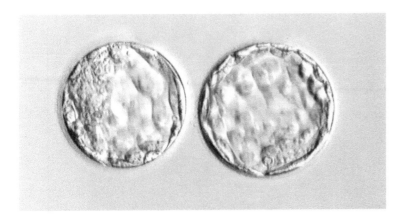

Figure 5.10 Day-5 transfer that led to monozygotic twins. Two blastocysts replaced; two gestational sacs/three fetal hearts noted by ultrasound investigation. The monozygotic twins were reduced; one male delivered; patient aged 42 years

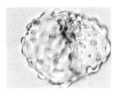

Grading criteria for human blastocysts

Cavitating morula < 50% cavity

Blastocyst ≥ 50% cavity

Degree of expansion and hatching status:

(1) Early blastocyst; the blastocoel filling more than half the volume of the conceptus, but no expansion in overall size as compared to earlier stages

(2) Blastocyst; the blastocoel filling more than half of the volume of the conceptus, with slight expansion in overall size and notable thinning of the zona pellucida

(3) Full blastocyst; a blastocoel more than 50% of the conceptus volume and overall size fully enlarged with a very thin zona pellucida

(4) Hatching blastocyst; non-preimplantation genetic diagnosis. The trophectoderm has started to herniate through the zona

(5) Fully hatched blastocyst; non-preimplantation genetic diagnosis. Free blastocyst fully removed from zona pellucida

(6) Hatching or hatched blastocyst; preimplantation genetic diagnosis

Inner cell mass (ICM) grading:

(A) Tightly packed, compacted cells

(B) Larger, loose cells

(C) No ICM distinguishable

(D) Cells of ICM appear degenerative

Trophectoderm grading:

(A) Many healthy cells forming a cohesive epithelium

(B) Few, but healthy cells, large in size

(C) Poor, very large, or unevenly distributed cells; may appear as few cells squeezed to the side

(D) Cells of the trophectoderm appear degenerative

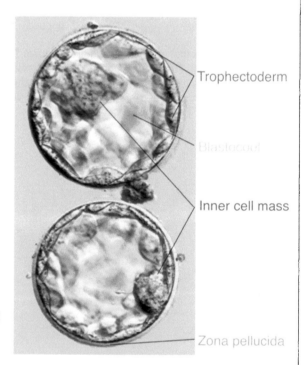

Figure 5.11 Blastocyst grading schemes used by the Cornell program. (a) Grading system detailed in text and photograph; (b) grading system detailed by individual photographs (*see next page*)

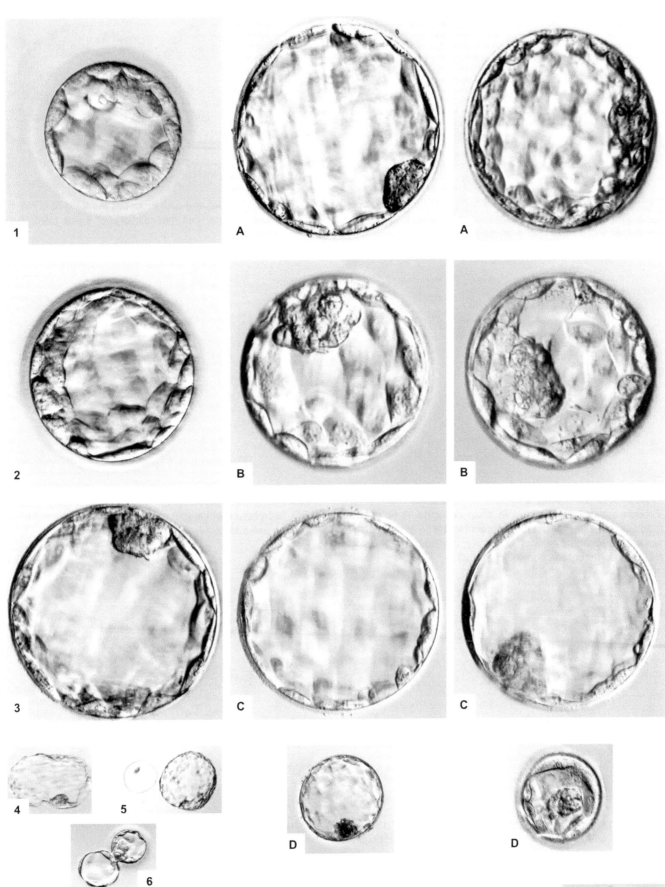

Figure 5.11 Continued

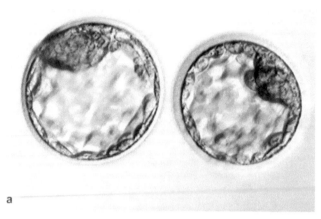
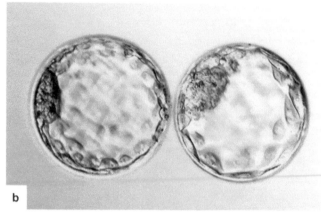

a

b

Figure 5.12 Blastocysts graded for 'top-quality' inner cell masses. (a) Large, compacted, and oval inner cell masses; both blastocysts implanted and two females were delivered; (b) large, compacted, and oval inner cell masses; one of these blastocysts implanted and a male child was delivered

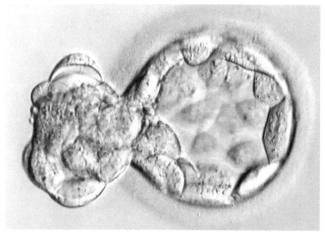
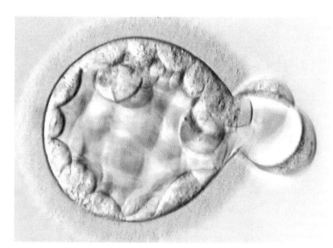

Figure 5.13 Cavitating morula/early blastocyst herniating through artificially-made hole in zona pellucida. A hole was made on day 3 during biopsy for preimplantation genetic diagnosis; the conceptus was ultimately diagnosed as being monosomic for chromosomes 15 and 22

Figure 5.14 Early blastocyst, diagnosed for trisomy 13 after PGD, seen here herniating through the artificially made hole in the zona pellucida

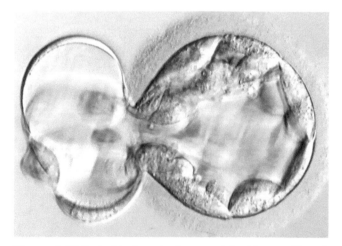
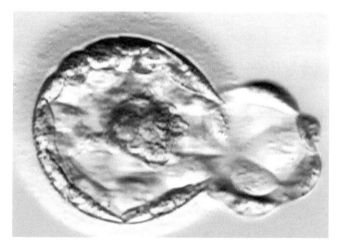

Figure 5.15 Early blastocyst, diagnosed for trisomy 13 and trisomy 21 after PGD, seen here herniating through artificially made hole in zona pellucida

Figure 5.16 Non-expanded blastocyst after PGD, herniating through biopsy site in zona pellucida

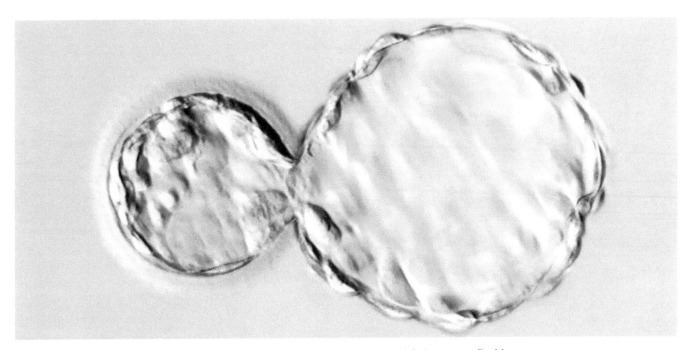

Figure 5.17 Late blastocyst after PGD, herniating through artificially made hole in zona pellucida

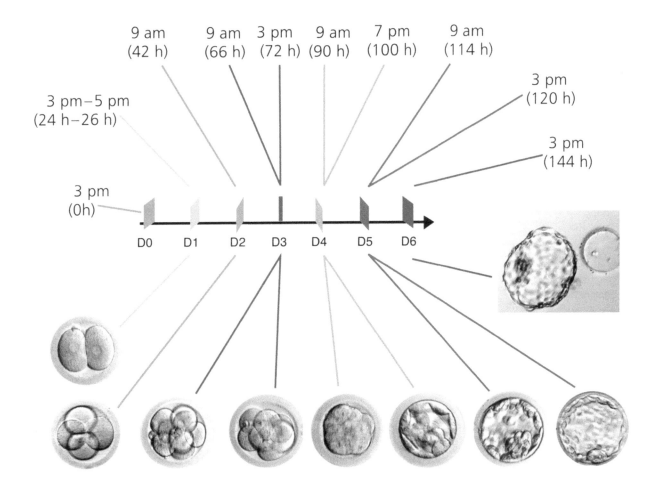

Figure 5.18 Time line for optimal blastocyst development

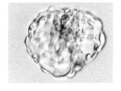

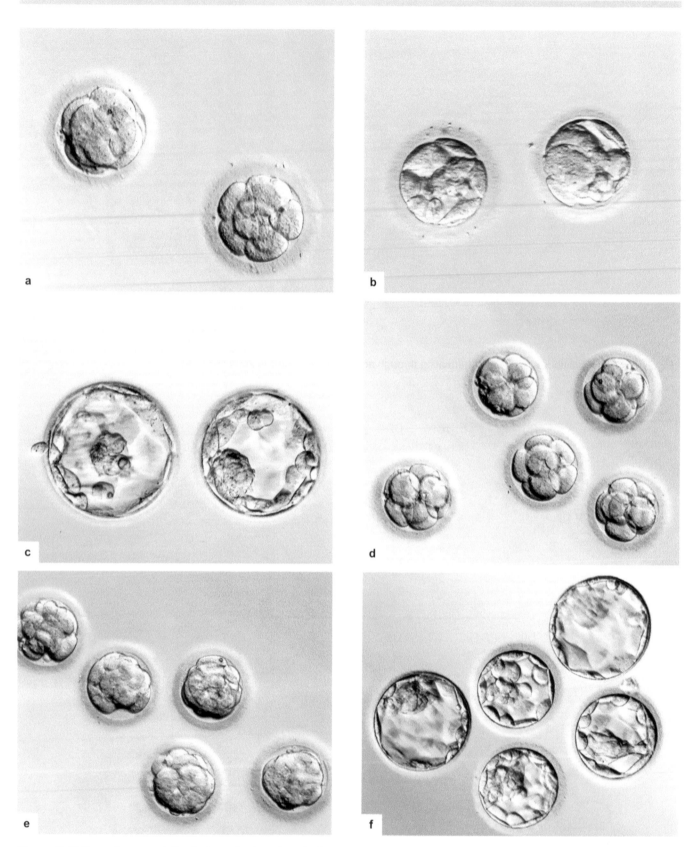

Figure 5.19 Preembryos serially photographed on days 3, 4, and 5 of development (preembryo/morula/blastocyst stages); patient aged 32 years. (a)–(c) Two preembryos photographed over 3 days and transferred on day 5. Neither implanted; (d)–(f) five preembryos from the same patient, photographed over 3 days and cryopreserved on day 5. Because the patient did not become pregnant after fresh transfer, she returned to have these blastocysts thawed. Three were thawed and replaced; an ongoing pregnancy with one fetal heart is currently in progress beyond 20 weeks

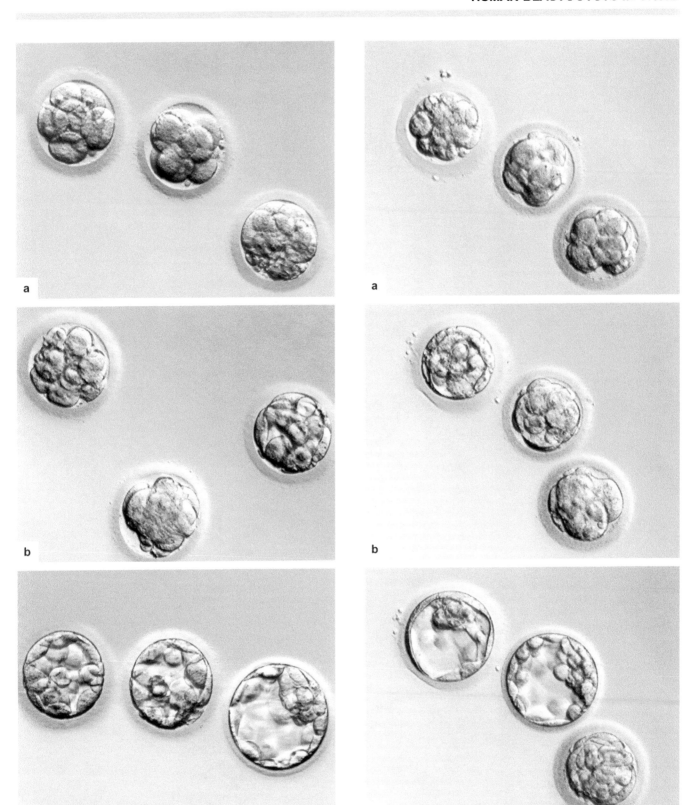

a

b

c

a

b

c

Figure 5.20 Preembryos serially photographed on days 3, 4, and 5 of development (preembryo/morula/blastocyst stages); patient aged 32 years. (a)–(c) Three preembryos photographed over 3 days, two of which were transferred on day 5 (the one on the left and the one on the right in photograph (c). An ongoing pregnancy with one fetal heart is currently in progress beyond 20 weeks

Figure 5.21 Preembryos serially photographed on days 3, 4, and 5 of development (preembryo/morula/blastocyst stages); patient aged 29 years. (a)–(c) Three preembryos photographed over 3 days, one of which was transferred on day 5 (middle blastocyst in photograph (c) along with a second blastocyst not shown. A pregnancy with two fetal hearts was established which is ongoing beyond 20 weeks

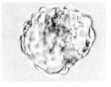

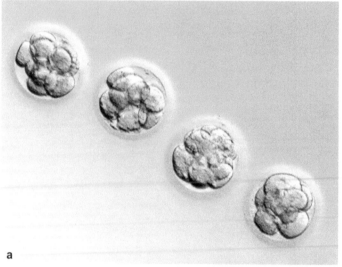

a

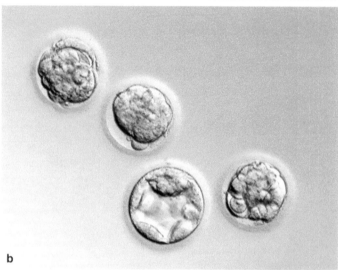

b

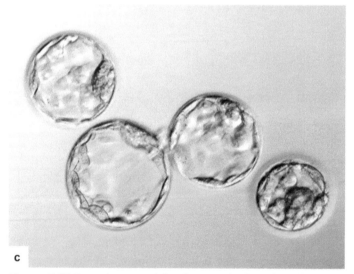

c

Figure 5.22 Preembryos serially photographed on days 3, 4, and 5 of development (preembryo/morula/blastocyst stages); patient aged 29 years. (a)–(c) Four preembryos photographed over 3 days, two of which were transferred on day 5 (the two blastocysts to the left in photograph (c). Both implanted and a twin pregnancy is ongoing beyond 20 weeks

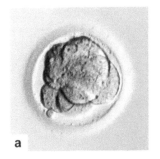
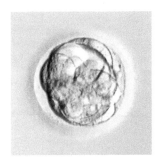
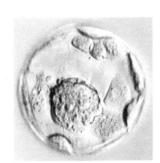

a

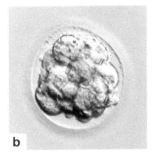
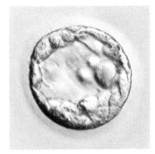
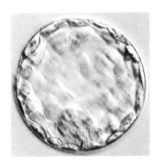

b

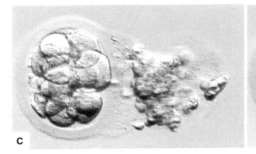
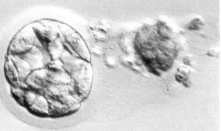

c

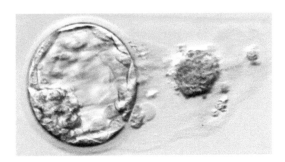

Figure 5.23 Individual preembryos serially photographed on days 3, 4, and 5. (a) On the afternoon of day 3, cell–cell aggregation (earliest evidence of impending compaction) is noted; on day 4, cavitation begins to occur between still large blastomeres; on day 5, the blastocyst possesses a round and compacted inner cell mass despite having a trophectoderm that is made up of few, large cells. This conceptus was frozen for future replacement in an oocyte recipient patient; no thaw has yet been carried out on this 36-year-old woman; (b) on the afternoon of day 3, ten blastomeres are noted; on day 4, an early blastocyst with poor inner cell mass definition is apparent; on day 5, the conceptus has developed into a good late blastocyst with a cohesive and multicellular trophectoderm, a slightly small inner cell mass, and possesses an extremely thin zona pellucida. This blastocyst was replaced along with one other that was less well developed (grade 2BB) and a pregnancy that started out with two gestational sacs was established; an ongoing singleton pregnancy with one fetal heart is now beyond 20 weeks; patient aged 40 years; (c) this conceptus, photographed on days 3, 4, and 5, possesses an abnormal zona pellucida. On day 3, a healthy appearing 12-cell preembryo was observed; on day 4, it had developed into a healthy appearing cavitating morula; by day 5, a blastocyst of mediocre quality has formed despite the persisting zona defect. This blastocyst was replaced, but pregnancy was not established. The patient shown here has undergone nine separate transfers between the ages of 24 and 31 years of age, twice with blastocysts, only achieving pregnancy one time with day-3 preembryos

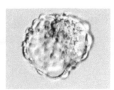

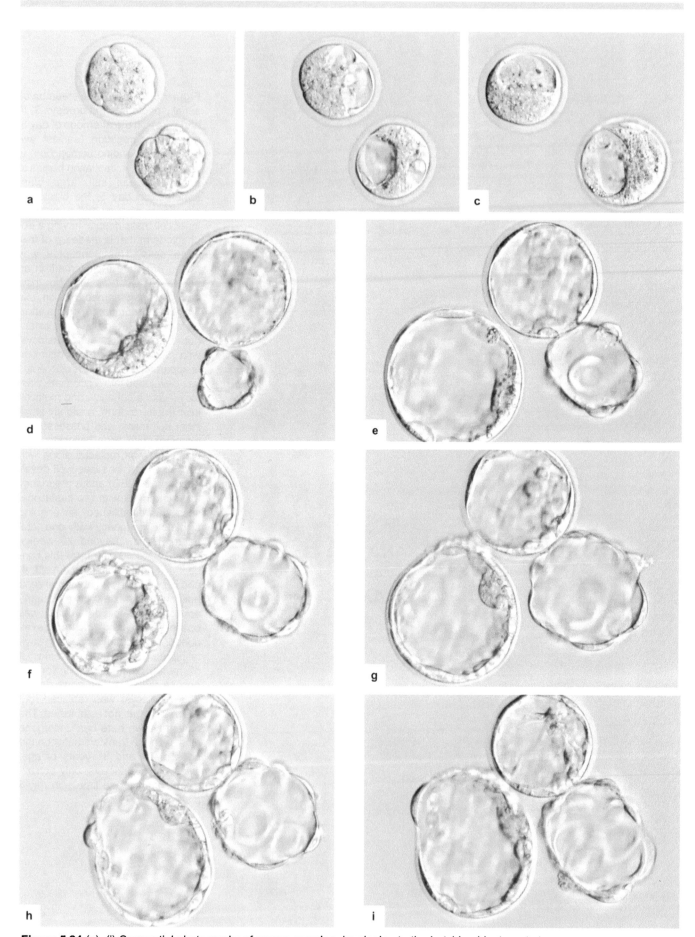

Figure 5.24 (a)–(i) Sequential photographs of mouse morulae developing to the hatching blastocyst stage

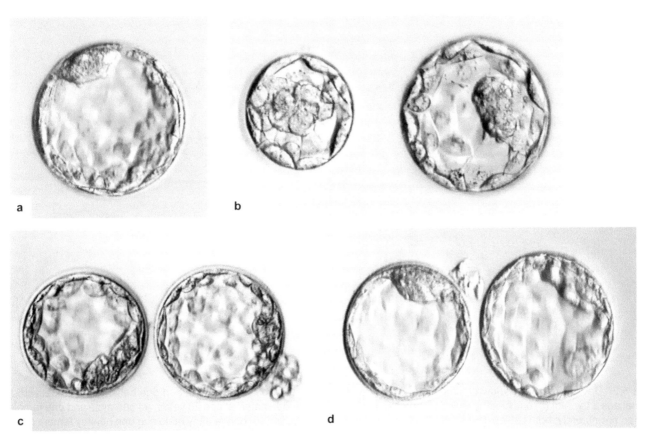

a   b

c   d

Figure 5.25 Day-5 blastocysts known to implant after their replacement. (a) One healthy female child delivered; maternal age 31 years; (b) two healthy female children delivered; maternal age 35 years; (c) two healthy male children delivered; maternal age 30 years; (d) two healthy female children delivered; maternal age 35 years

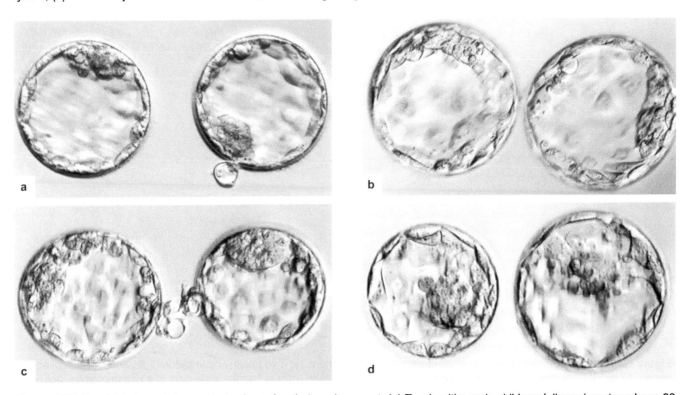

a   b

c   d

Figure 5.26 Day-5 blastocysts known to implant after their replacement. (a) Two healthy male children delivered; maternal age 28 years; (b) two healthy male children delivered; maternal age 38 years; (c) two healthy male children delivered; maternal age 33 years; (d) two healthy male children delivered; maternal age 30 years

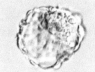

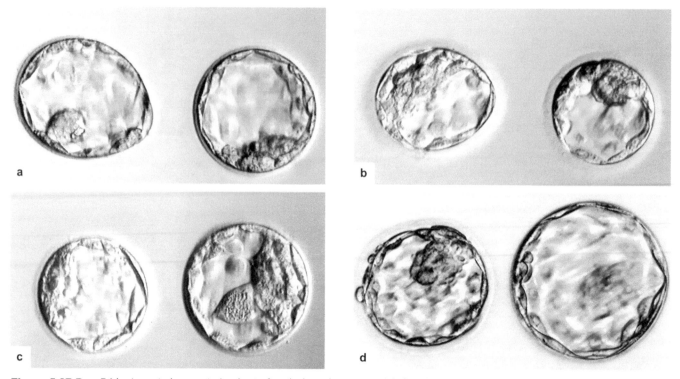

Figure 5.27 Day-5 blastocysts known to implant after their replacement. (a) One healthy male and one healthy female delivered; maternal age 31 years; (b) one healthy male and one healthy female delivered; maternal age 28 years; (c) one male and one female delivered prematurely; both babies died soon after birth; maternal age 32 years; (d) one healthy male and one healthy female delivered; maternal age 35 years

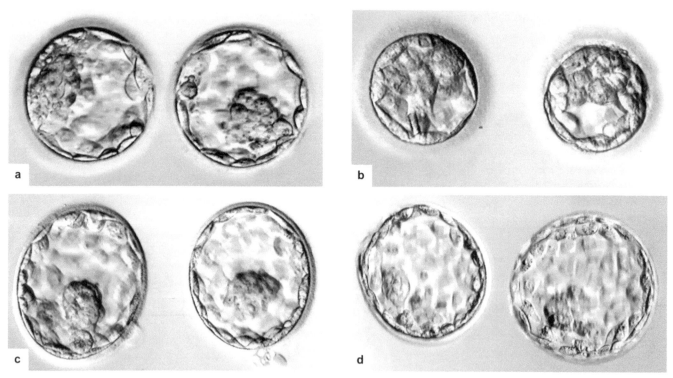

Figure 5.28 Day-5 blastocysts known to implant after their replacement. (a) Two healthy male children delivered; maternal age 30 years; (b) two healthy male children delivered; maternal age 35 years; (c) one healthy male and one healthy female delivered; maternal age 31 years; (d) two healthy male children delivered; maternal age 34 years

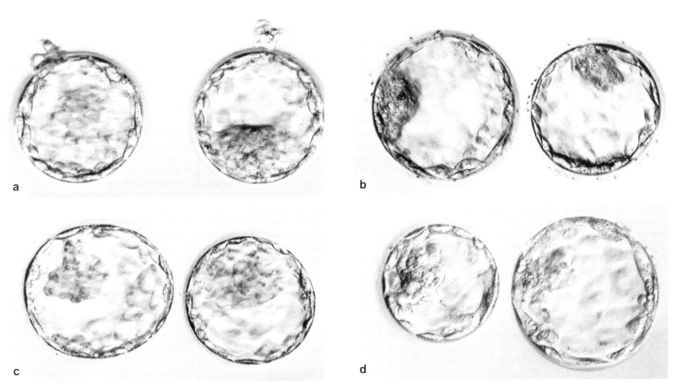

Figure 5.29 Day-5 blastocysts known to implant after their replacement. (a) Two healthy male children delivered; maternal age 38 years; (b) one healthy male and one healthy female delivered; maternal age 30 years; (c) two healthy female children delivered; maternal age 34 years; (d) two healthy female children delivered; maternal age 35 years

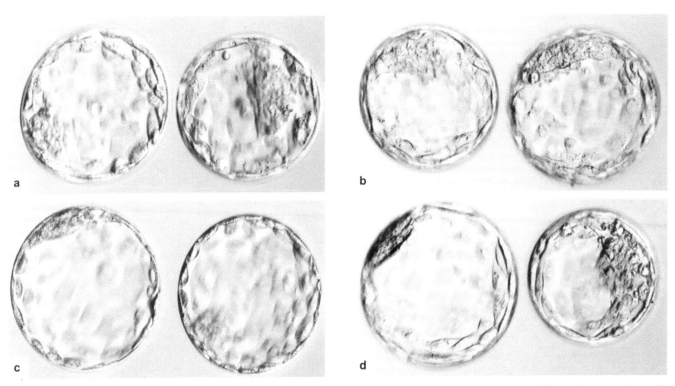

Figure 5.30 Day-5 blastocysts known to implant after their replacement. (a) Two healthy male children delivered; maternal age 30 years; (b) two healthy male children delivered; maternal age 31 years; (c) two healthy male children delivered; maternal age 32 years; (d) two healthy male children delivered; maternal age 38 years

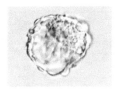

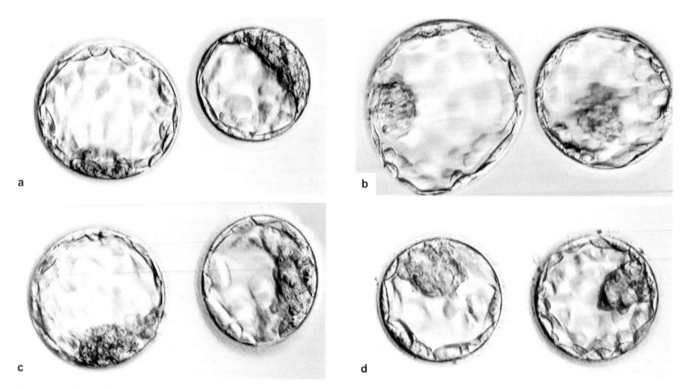

Figure 5.31 Day-5 blastocysts known to implant after their replacement. (a) One healthy male and one healthy female delivered; maternal age 32 years; (b) one healthy male and one healthy female delivered; maternal age 33 years; (c) two healthy males delivered; maternal age 35 years; (d) one healthy male and one healthy female delivered; maternal age 35 years

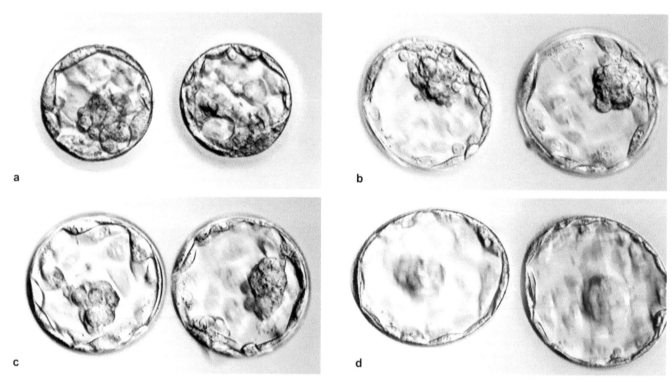

Figure 5.32 Day-5 blastocysts known to implant after their replacement. (a) One healthy male and one healthy female delivered; maternal age 29 years; (b) two fetal heart pregnancy; one healthy male ultimately delivered; maternal age 25 years; (c) two healthy females delivered; maternal age 42 years (oocyte donation); (d) two healthy females delivered; maternal age 45 years (oocyte donation)

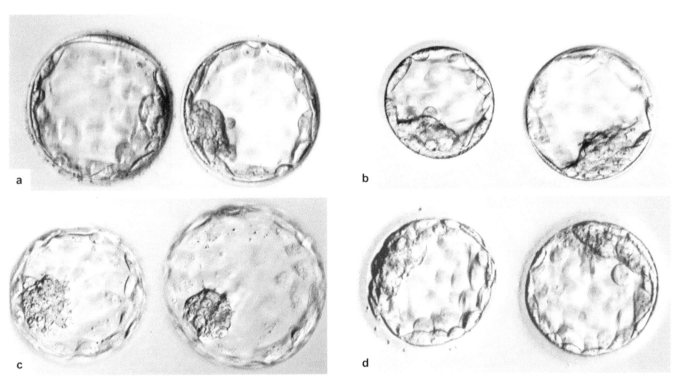

Figure 5.33 Day-5 blastocysts known to implant after their replacement. (a) Two healthy males delivered; maternal age 38 years; (b) two healthy females delivered; maternal age 29 years; (c) two fetal heart pregnancy ongoing greater than 30 weeks; maternal age 53 years (oocyte donation); (d) two fetal heart pregnancy ongoing greater than 30 weeks; maternal age 32 years (oocyte donation)

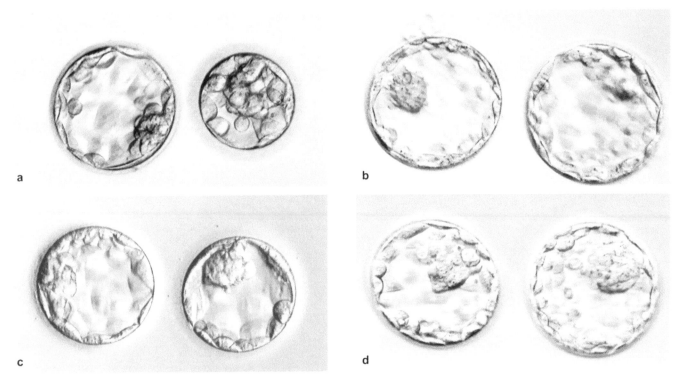

Figure 5.34 Day-5 blastocysts known to implant after their replacement. (a) Two fetal heart pregnancy ongoing greater than 20 weeks; maternal age 29 years; (b) two fetal heart pregnancy ongoing greater than 20 weeks; maternal age 33 years; (c) two fetal heart pregnancy ongoing greater than 20 weeks; maternal age 31 years; (d) two fetal heart pregnancy ongoing greater than 12 weeks; maternal age 31 years

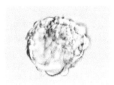

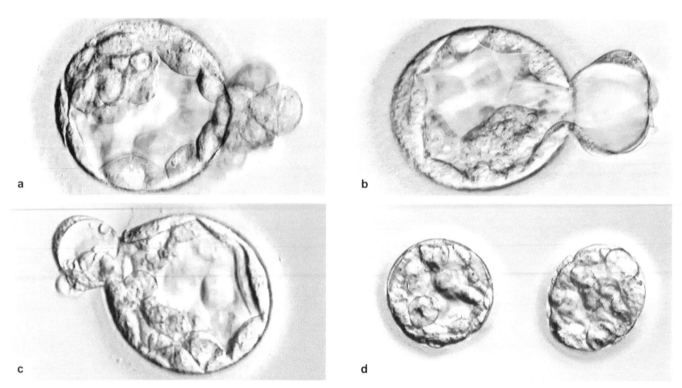

Figure 5.35 Day-5 blastocysts known to implant after PGD. (a) Ongoing singleton pregnancy greater than 20 weeks; maternal age 38 years; (b) ongoing singleton pregnancy greater than 12 weeks; maternal age 33 years; (c) ongoing singleton pregnancy greater than 12 weeks; maternal age 41 years; (d) ongoing twin pregnancy greater than 12 weeks; maternal age 38 years

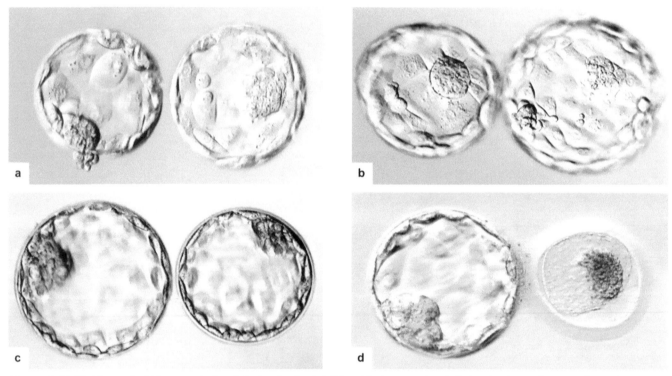

Figure 5.36 Highly graded blastocysts that failed to implant. (a)Two blastocysts that failed to implant after transfer to the uterine cavity; patient age 33 years; (b) two blastocysts that failed to implant after transfer to the uterine cavity; patient age 36 years; (c) two blastocysts that failed to implant after transfer to the uterine cavity; patient age 29 years; (d) blastocyst exhibiting a zona pellucida that is conjoined to the zona of a degenerative oocyte. After separation of the two, the healthy appearing blastocyst was transferred but failed to implant; patient age 36 years

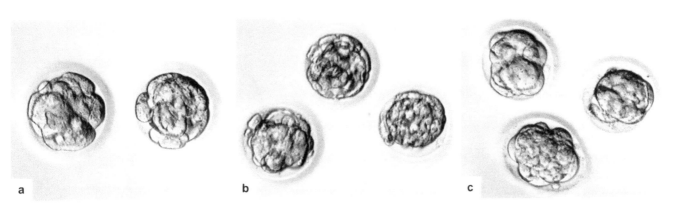

Figure 5.37 Poorly graded day-5 conceptuses that led to ongoing pregnancy. (a) These compacting morulae were transferred on day 5 to a 33-year-old woman; one implanted and a healthy male child was subsequently delivered; (b) three cavitating morulae on day 5 which were replaced in a 42-year-old woman and led to the birth of a healthy female child; (c) three morulae that were transferred on day 5 to a 47-year-old oocyte donation recipient and gave rise to two gestational sacs by ultrasound; ultimately, one healthy female child was delivered

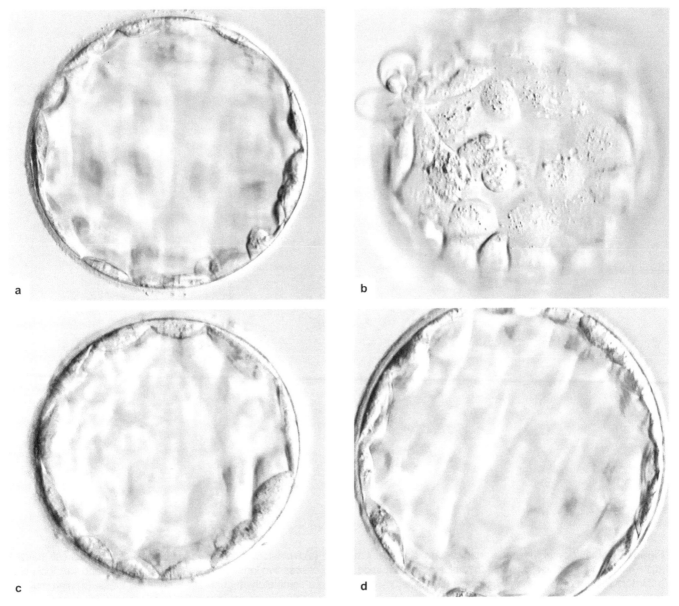

Figure 5.38 (a)–(d) Blastocysts without visible inner cell masses

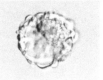

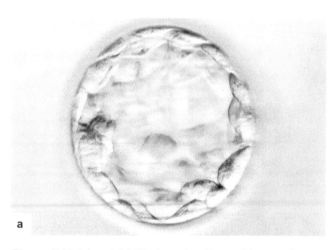
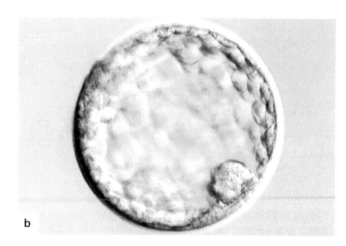

Figure 5.39 (a) and (b) Blastocysts with small inner cell masses

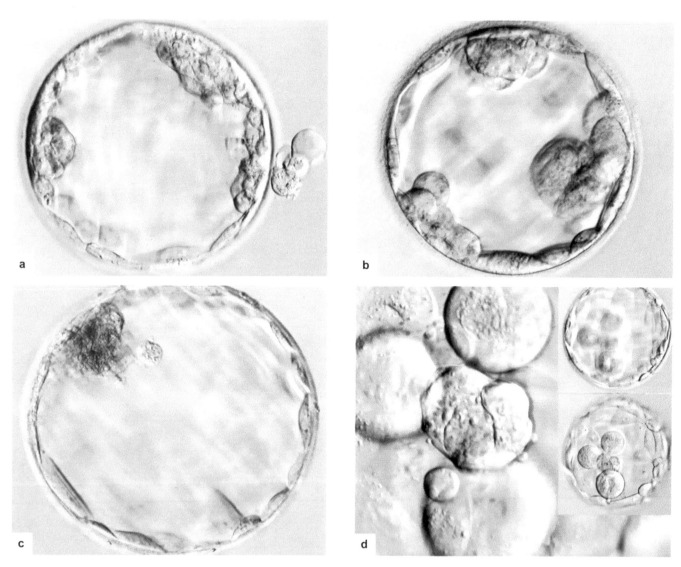

Figure 5.40 Blastocysts with apparently abnormal inner cell masses. (a) A blastocyst that appears to possess two inner cell masses at 1 o'clock and 9 o'clock positions; (b) a blastocyst that appears to possess two inner cell masses at 12 o'clock and 4 o'clock, plus a third thickening of TM cells at 7 o'clock; (c) a blastocyst exhibiting a completely degenerative inner cell mass; (d) high magnification of a blastocyst with three large cells surrounding a small, compacted inner cell mass; the two inserts to the right show the same blastocyst using different focal planes on lower magnification

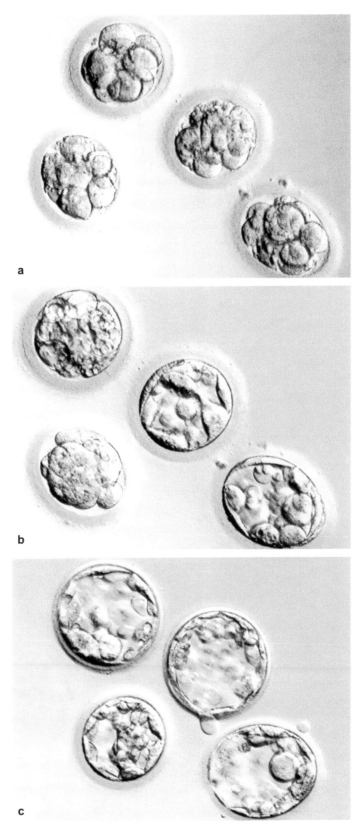

a

b

c

Figure 5.41 Sequential photographs of vacuolated conceptuses on days 3, 4, and 5 of development (preembryo/morula/blastocyst stages). (a)–(c) No vacuolization was noted in any of the three preembryos on day 3 of development. On day 4, the upper left morula exhibited extensive vacuolization. On day 5, the same conceptus (upper left) developed into a relatively healthy appearing expanded blastocyst; note small vacuoles in cells of the TM. The patient did not become pregnant after replacement of the upper-middle blastocyst. Same patient as in Figure 5.23(c) who failed to achieve pregnancy in eight of nine transfer attempts

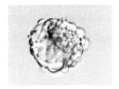

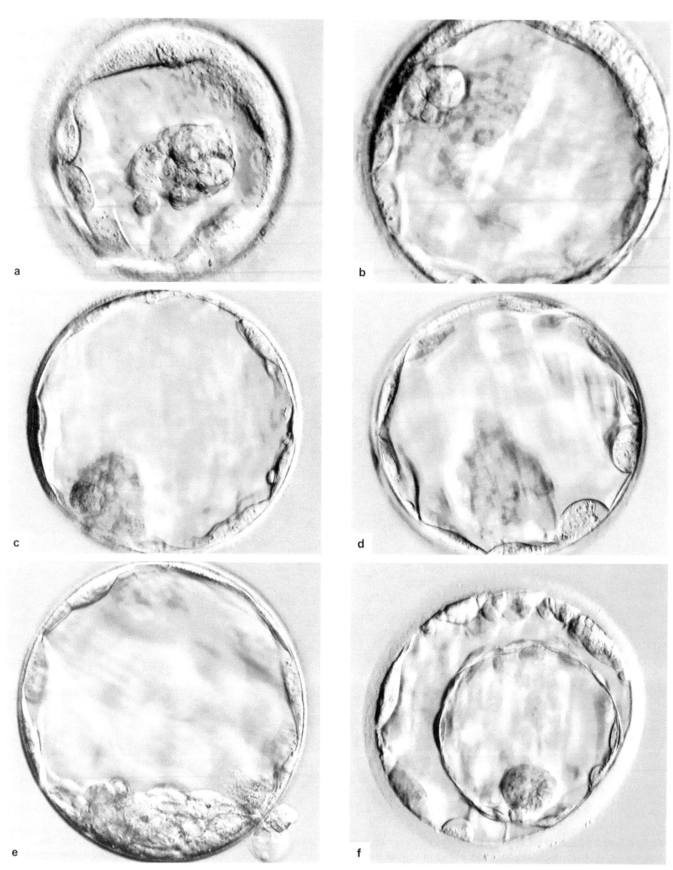

Figure 5.42 Abnormal trophectoderm. (a) Appears to have one large cell pushed to the upper and right sides; (b) single, unhealthy appearing cell pushed to the upper and right sides; (c) few cells make up this thin and unhealthy appearing trophectoderm; (d) while generally healthy in appearance, the trophectoderm is comprised of few cells; (e) despite a developing inner cell mass, the trophectoderm of this conceptus is made up of few cells; (f) this highly interesting blastocyst appears to have a second ring of TM cells within its blastocoele

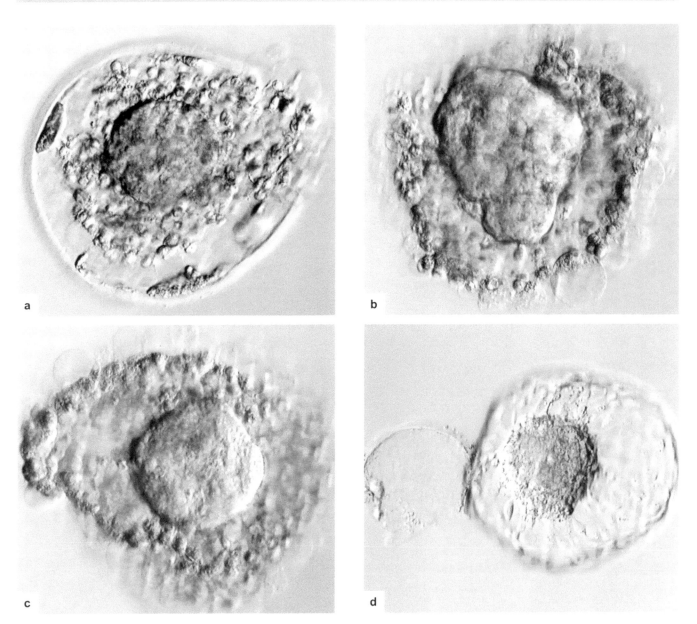

Figure 5.43 (a)–(d) Degenerating trophectoderm associated with inner cell mass proliferation and enlargement

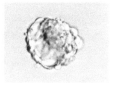

6 Preembryo selection and blastocyst quality: how to choose the optimal conceptus for transfer

Reducing the incidence of multiple pregnancy

Through the application of extended culture techniques, we have been given the opportunity to offer more responsible medical care to our patients by reducing the number of preembryos for transfer. Unfortunately, selective reduction of one or more fetuses is all too often necessary when higher-order gestations are established, and the procedure itself carries obvious medical and emotional risks[1-4]. Multifetal gestations are the largest single cause of poor obstetrical outcome and subsequent neonatal difficulties, these pregnancies being associated with increased incidences of pre-eclampsia, gestational diabetes, pregnancy-induced hypertension, preterm labor, low birth weight and extensive neonatal care (Figure 6.1)[5].

Patients and health-care professionals often present differing perspectives on the concept of establishing a multiple pregnancy[6]. When patients, embryologists and clinicians were given a questionnaire soliciting views on the potential risks and benefits of blastocyst culture and multiple pregnancy, it was discovered that patients were far more accepting of multiple pregnancy as a prospective outcome than those involved in their treatment, especially multiple pregnancy involving twins[7]. This greater acceptance was demonstrated despite an awareness of the concrete risks associated with multiple gestation. It is uncertain, however, how many patients would take the same view retrospective to actually experiencing a high-order gestation. It must be assumed that few would embrace the potential ordeal without reservation.

History of day-3 and day-5 transfer

Until the late 1990s, preembryos were routinely cultured until only day 2 or 3 before being transferred to the uterus. The primary impedance to culturing for longer periods involved the lack of an appropriate culture medium to sustain the viability of compaction and blastocyst development. In an effort to optimize clinical pregnancy rates under those conditions, clinics felt compelled to replace up to four day-3 preembryos, or even more, in women over the age of 35 or 40 years. The downside to this replacement strategy was that too many women were placed at risk of having triplet or quadruplet gestations (Figure 6.2).

Researchers then found that better than acceptable clinical pregnancy rates could be achieved with extended culture using specialized media and replacement of only two conceptuses that had grown to the blastocyst stage (Figure 6.3). The identification of key regulators and recognition of changing physiological requirements over the course of 5 days of preembryo growth led these researchers to refine the basic culture media used during critical days, and to develop what are now commonly referred to as 'sequential' media[8,9]. Because extended culture selects for preembryos with high implantation potential, clinical pregnancy and implantation rates after the replacement of only one or two day-5 conceptuses has been demonstrated to be quite high in selected patient populations, without the associated risk of high-order multiple births.

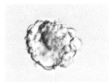

Advantages of day-5 transfer

Additional days of culture clearly single out preembryos with high implantation potential; those likely to result in viable offspring continue developing until day 5 of culture, forming healthy-appearing blastocysts with compacted inner cell masses and proliferating trophectoderm, highly suitable for replacement (Figure 6.4). Conversely, those arresting in culture may be selectively excluded from replacement.

In the Cornell program, 328 day-5 transfers carried out on selected *in vitro* fertilization (IVF) patients (age range 24–44 years) from late 1999 to mid-2002 yielded the following results: clinical pregnancy 71%, implantation 55%. The average number of day-5 preembryos replaced was 2.09. Recipients of donor oocytes fared even better (average age 42 years): 82% clinical pregnancy and 66% rate of implantation. Although most patients described here were selected for blastocyst transfer based on number and quality of their conceptuses on days 1–3, some were included because of the medical necessity to transfer only a single preembryo or because transfer had to be delayed, and others because they fervently desired extended culture. Those patients who selected themselves for day-5 transfer despite the laboratory's recommendations were often those who failed in the effort.

Unfortunately, the transfer of two blastocysts in our program resulted in a twinning rate per pregnancy of 52%. This means that over one-half of the women undergoing day-5 transfer in an effort to reduce their chances for multiple pregnancy actually ended up with precisely what they wished to avoid. The finding of excessive rates of twinning despite a conservative approach to the number of blastocysts being transferred has been demonstrated by other investigators outside of the Cornell program[10].

Very similar to our results, David Gardner and colleagues described a prospective randomized trial of selected patients (good responders to ovarian stimulation) in which day-5 transfers achieved 71% pregnancy and 51% implantation with an average of 2.2 blastocysts replaced[11]. While the pregnancy rate for matched day-3 transfers was not significantly different (66%), the implantation rate was lower (30%), despite a higher number of preembryos being replaced per transfer (3.7).

Schoolcraft and co-workers, in a multicenter trial, reported a 66% ongoing pregnancy rate and 48% implantation rate in 174 selected women undergoing day-5 transfer[12]. An average of 2.2 blastocysts was replaced per transfer. In a separate publication, Schoolcraft and Gardner described 229 oocyte recipients who established an 88% clinical pregnancy and a 66% implantation rate with 2.1 blastocysts replaced per transfer[13]. Oocyte recipients have been noted by other investigators to be particularly good candidates for extended culture, their rates of pregnancy and implantation exceeding those of non-donor day-5 transfers, even after controlling for donor age[14].

In 2000, Milki and associates reported a 68% pregnancy rate and 47% implantation rate (average number transferred 2.4), which surpassed the 46% pregnancy and 20% implantation observed in a similar patient population with transfer on day 3 (average number transferred 4.6)[15]. In this study, all patients were under the age of 40 and possessed at least three 8-cell preembryos on day 3.

For those IVF programs attempting blastocyst transfer in every patient walking through the door, there may be evidence of clinical advantage as well. An increase was reported by Marek and colleagues in ongoing pregnancy from 36% for day-3 transfer (in about 1997) to 44% for day-5 transfer (in about 1998) in non-selected women[16]. Not surprisingly, implantation rates were also significantly higher for day-5 transfers (23% vs. 34%) as a result of fewer conceptuses being transferred (3.0, day 3 and 2.5, day 5). Although this retrospective analysis of clinical data involved distinctly separate time periods and the use of different culture media between groups, it clearly demonstrates no detrimental effect after applying day-5 protocols for all patients. Similarly, Wilson and associates reported an increase in clinical and ongoing pregnancy rates in unselected patients with blastocyst transfer, particularly those under the age of 35 years, but also for their program as a whole[17].

Unfortunately, the management of an extended culture program is not as simple as purchasing new media and delaying transfer for 2 days. Minute deficiencies in gas regulation, temperature control or other environmental conditions affecting pH or resulting in premature amino acid degradation, barely recognizable with short-term culture, may be exacerbated by prolonged culture. In addition, variability in lots of some purchased media has been shown to contribute to mutable outcomes. As a result, many programs have experienced difficulty in maintaining high pregnancy rates with blastocyst transfer, and have ultimately dropped the procedure altogether. Their frustrations are often expressed on internet mail forums and during scientific exchange at meetings.

Comparisons of day-3 and day-5 transfer

Prospective and retrospective comparisons of day-3 versus day-5 results are rife with potential grouping mismatches. All too often, patients opt for one procedure or the other based upon what they have read, their previous experiences, what has happened to their friends or their desire for singleton births. As well, embryologists often convert a potential blastocyst transfer to day 3 because of concern over preembryo quality or quantity. A more appropriate means of comparing results would involve prospective application of blastocyst transfer to all even-numbered cycles and day-3 transfer to all odd-numbered cycles, and not to sway from this position until a very large number of patients had been treated without bias (same time period, same media, same incubators and environment, same embryologists). Regrettably, neither our internal review boards nor our well-educated patients would accept this sort of mandate, and we are therefore forced to draw conclusions from non-randomized populations. Comparing smaller, but similar, groups does not always take into account the differences in changing laboratory technique and personnel, preembryo fragmentation, zona pellucida characteristics, number of previous attempts or impact of gynecological history, uterine anomalies, transfer difficulties or other important clinical features that ultimately affect outcomes.

When one seeks to review the scientific literature on the issue of day-3 versus day-5 transfer, reports are varied. Some investigators have found no differences in either clinical pregnancy or implantation rate after day-5 replacement[18-24], some have noted a better implantation rate only[11,25-29] and yet others have experienced a general overall improvement in implantation and pregnancy rates in patients who have had blastocyst transfer[13-17,30,31]. In some programs, it has been suggested that blastocyst transfer may be detrimental for women demonstrating poor preembryo quality on day 3, or at least detrimental in unselected patient populations[27]. Another publication suggests that pregnancy and implantation rates decline dramatically in repeated cycles of blastocyst transfer

following one or more unsuccessful blastocyst attempts[32]. One report describes the experience of extended culture resulting in an almost 50% decrease in implantation and pregnancy rates[33].

At Cornell, we elected to pursue blastocyst transfer because of the disturbingly high triplet rate in good-responding patients with at least one morphologically optimal preembryo (grade 1 or 1.5) on day 3. Examination of our data identified 139 women, aged [24-39], with three preembryos replaced on day 3 who would have been automatic candidates for day-5 transfer if the technology had been available. In these cycles, the clinical pregnancy rate was 88.5%, the implantation rate was 61% and the multiple rate was 62.6%, 19% of which were triplets. Undoubtedly, transferring only two preembryos in these cycles would have proved reasonable, probably producing similar clinical pregnancy results without triplets. Now, after more than 2 years of working with blastocysts, we are seeing pregnancy and implantation rates not significantly different after day-5 transfer in the same type of patient (71% and 55%, respectively), with only two blastocysts transferred in most cases.

With the confidence of these results, we instigated a protocol to transfer electively only two preembryos on day 3 for consenting patients who met criteria for blastocyst transfer. Again, this study was not completely randomized since it required patient consent rather than assignment. Nonetheless, results of elective transfer of two preembryos on day 3 looked extremely similar to two blastocysts on day 5 when patient populations were closely matched. In our first investigation, 24 patients elected to accept two, rather than three, preembryos; 17/24 established clinical pregnancy (71%), and a 56% implantation rate was realized. It is rather surprising how close these numbers are to our current day-5 transfer results. Moreover, doing a simple computer search of all patients treated during the past year under the age of 40 who elected to have two preembryos replaced on day 3, despite the fact that they had more than two available, yielded similar results. Fifty-nine patients achieved a 68% clinical pregnancy rate and a 49% implantation rate. In an effort to elucidate further the differences between day-3 and day-5 transfers in selected patient populations, we will continue to accumulate numbers for this investigation.

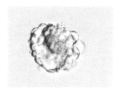

Experience of the United Kingdom

Other programs have published large studies finding no difference in clinical pregnancy rates when two, rather than three, preembryos were transferred[34–41]. In a massive analysis of outcome data from the United Kingdom, elective transfer of two preembryos was demonstrated to maintain that country's current standards in pregnancy rates, compared favorably to having three replaced and served to reduce the multiple pregnancy rate[42]. The group studied risk factors in 44 236 transfer cycles involving 25 240 women. They examined age, cause and duration of infertility, number of previous attempts, number of previous live births, number of oocytes fertilized and number of preembryos replaced. It was determined that only previous live birth could be shown to be correlated with a significantly higher birth rate after IVF. Conversely, older age, tubal infertility, longer duration of infertility and a greater number of previous attempts was associated with significantly lower birth and multiple birth rates. Interestingly, it was shown that when more than four oocytes were fertilized, there was no difference at all in the birth rate whether two or three preembryos were replaced. However, there was a considerable increase in the multiple birth rate with three (Figure 6.5).

Developments in selection criteria for day-3 transfer

The quest to look for markers of preembryo viability at early stages of development continues. If such markers can be easily identified without invasion or trauma to the conceptus, we will not need to depend on growth characteristics alone to select the lowest number of conceptuses for transfer.

Pronuclear distribution and alignment

Despite the fact that human preembryos are usually selected for transfer using morphology criteria on days 2 and 3, earlier morphological indicators may assist in predicting implantation and pregnancy potential. One group has examined the relationship between pronuclear morphology and subsequent blastocyst development[43]. In this study, prezygotes were scored according to distribution and size of nucleoli within each pronucleus (Figure 6.6). Those displaying equalities between the nuclei demonstrated 49.5% blastocyst formation, while those with unequal sizes, numbers or

distribution of nucleoli formed blastocysts only 28% of the time[44]. Cleaving preembryos that were selected initially by zygote morphology and secondarily by morphology on day 3 demonstrated increased pregnancy and implantation (31% and 57%, respectively), compared with those selected by morphology alone (19% and 33%, respectively; $p < 0.01$). Furthermore, the authors demonstrated that there was a significant difference between prezygote-scored and non-scored cycles on day 3 (pregnancy, 57% vs. 33%; implantation, 31% vs. 19%) and on day 5 (pregnancy, 73% vs. 58%; implantation, 52% vs. 39%). Other investigators have reported similar improvements in pregnancy after incorporating pronuclear assessment into their selection criteria[45–51].

In contrast, the Cornell program was unable to demonstrate the value of assessing either nucleolar distribution or alignment after extensive data were collected from more than 2000 fertilized oocytes[52]. We sought to determine whether the morphology of pronuclear-stage oocytes could be used to assess subsequent development. A retrospective evaluation of 2187 prezygotes from 258 patients was performed. Prezygotes were graded according to their pattern of nucleolar distribution: PZ1 (nucleoli in both pronuclei were aligned at pronuclear junctions); PZ2 (one pronucleus had aligned nucleoli but the second pronucleus exhibited scattered nucleoli); PZ3 (both pronuclei possessed scattered nucleoli); or PZ4 (one or both pronuclei had only 1–2 nuclei) (Figure 6.7). In addition, each prezygote was graded according to the orientation of pronuclei relative to the polar bodies: PB+ pronuclei were perpendicular to polar bodies and PB- pronuclei were parallel to polar bodies (Figure 6.8). Prezygotes were later assessed for cleavage at 24 h, day-3 preembryo quality (cell number and fragmentation) and day-5 development to the blastocyst stage. Of the 2187 conceptuses assessed after fertilization, 20% were classified as PZ1, 34% PZ2, 38% PZ3 and 8% PZ4. In addition, 70% were categorized as PB+ and 30% were PB-. Few differences were observed in any subgroup according to their cleavage status at 24 h (either still pronuclear, in syngamy or at the 2-cell stage). A slightly higher proportion of PZ3 zygotes cleaved by 24 h ($p < 0.03$), while differences were not found among other subgroups. In addition, the proportion of prezygotes developing into good-quality preembryos on day 3 (8-cell stage, < 20% fragmentation) was slightly higher ($p = 0.047$) in the PZ1 subgroup as compared to the other subgroups, although the clinical relevance of this statistical difference was questionable

(24% PZ1; 20% PZ2; 17% PZ3; 20% PZ4; 20% PB+; 20% PB-). Nor were any significant differences found in the capability of the various prezygote subgroups to develop to the blastocyst stage by day 5 of culture (PZ1 30%; PZ2 26%; PZ3 30%; PZ4 30%; PB+ 31%; PB- 25%). From these data, we concluded that no clinically relevant differences between any of these prezygote subgroups could be deemed beneficial for prediction of subsequent preembryo or blastocyst quality.

Timeliness of first cleavage and subsequent cleavage rate

Another indicator of preembryo viability involves the assessment of sperm-penetrated oocytes at 24 h after intracytoplasmic sperm injection (ICSI), or 26 h after insemination. Break-points of 24 and 26 h were chosen based on studies demonstrating that oocytes fertilized through ICSI procedures tended to undergo the first cleavage 2–3 h earlier than those produced through insemination[53].

It has been observed by us and others that oocytes undergoing a timely first cleavage (by 24–26 h) often produce more 8-cell conceptuses on day 3 and healthier-appearing blastocysts on day 5[54-56]. In one study from Cornell, it was demonstrated that a higher proportion of blastocysts on day 5 originated from 2-cell preembryos at 24/26 h when compared to those that were in syngamy or pronuclear stages (Figure 6.9), and the stage at 24/26 h in combination with the cleavage stage on the morning of day 3 proved extremely useful in predicting blastocyst development on day 5[55]. It was notable that the predictive value of day 3 morphology was dependent on evaluating preembryos by about 66 h after insemination or ICSI (mornings). Delaying day-3 evaluations until 72 h (afternoons) diluted the predictive correlation of the assessment. Furthermore, fewer than eight, or more than eight, blastomeres on the morning of day 3 had a significantly negative association with normal blastocyst development, a finding closely confirmed by other investigators (Figure 6.10)[57]. While it was not surprising to note that low blastomere numbers on day 3 were suboptimal, it was extremely interesting to verify the growing suspicion that preembryos with 12 or 14 blastomeres were not particularly better because of their advanced growth. It has become apparent that preembryos continuing to cleave beyond the 8-cell stage without undergoing compaction are less likely to develop normally to the blastocyst stage. Failure to undergo the compaction process at the appropriate stage

indicates that the internal 'clock' regulating sequential developmental events is faulty.

In the course of these investigations, it was also observed that an occasional oocyte began fragmenting even before the first cleavage (Figure 6.11). When fragmentation occurred so early, severely impaired development followed. In contrast, compromised development was not noted when minor or moderate fragmentation (< 20%) first occurred during or after the first cleavage.

Based on the results described above, we can now predict that a fertilized oocyte exhibiting two cells at 24 h with less than 20% fragmentation, followed by eight cells on the morning of day 3, will have a very high chance (>50%) of forming a viable blastocyst by day 5. We routinely look at conceptuses at 24/26 h to assist in identifying potential elective transfers of two conceptuses on day 3, as well as identifying potential extended culture candidates. Criteria used in our program to aid in selecting patients for blastocyst transfer include at least four syngamous or cleaved preembryos at the 24/26-h investigation, at least three 8-cell or six 7–9-cell preembryos on the morning of day 3 and fragmentation levels less than 20% in all preembryos meeting these conditions. We have proposed a model, suitable for our program, that describes a time line for optimal development to the blastocyst stage (see Table 5.3 and Figure 5.18).

Several other programs use slightly different criteria for selecting patients for blastocyst transfer. In the early work of Gardner and colleagues, normal basal follicle stimulating hormone (FSH) levels and ten follicles > 12 mm on the day of human chorionic gonadotropin (hCG) administration were required for inclusion in day-5 protocols[11]. The group of Milki and Behr required at least three 8-cell preembryos on day 3 to go forward with extended culture[15]. Similarly, Racowsky and co-workers used eight or more fertilized prezygotes to select patients for blastocyst transfer, and concluded that a minimum of three 8-cell preembryos on day 3 was necessary in order to realize improved outcomes with blastocyst protocols[27].

Cytoplasmic fragmentation and multinucleation

In addition to cleavage rates, Alikani and colleagues examined the degree of fragmentation on day 3, specific fragmentation pattern and blastomere multinucleation in relation to the success of blastocyst formation[57]. They discovered that more than 15% fragmentation on day 3

(Figure 6.12a) resulted in lower blastocyst formation on day 5 (16.5% vs. 33.3% with 1–15% fragmentation). Furthermore, type IV fragmentation (large, randomly distributed fragments, often necrotic and associated with uneven blastomeres; Figure 6.12b) led to a significant reduction in the percentage of blastocysts formed (14.7%) as compared to type I, II or III patterns (small and associated with a single blastomere, localized to the perivitelline space, or small and scattered: 38.6%, 32.9% and 32.4% respectively). The presence of multinucleated blastomeres (Figure 6.13) also had a negative impact on further development, only 15.9% of preembryos displaying multinucleation in one or more cells giving rise to a healthy blastocyst (versus 31.9% without multinucleation). Collectively, these data suggest that early cleavage anomalies significantly reduce the ability of preembryos to proceed with normal development to days 5 and 6.

Value of day-3 morphology as a single assessment

Several investigators have reported a very inexact correlation between a day-3 evaluation alone and subsequent normal blastocyst development[58,59] (Figures 6.14 and 6.15. A recent publication describes a study wherein the best two preembryos chosen on day 3 were cultured separately from the others for an additional 2 days[60]. These were preembryos that would have been transferred had replacement been carried out on day 3. On day 5, the two most advanced blastocysts were chosen for transfer. Examining associations between the choices on day 3 and the blastocysts chosen for transfer on day 5 revealed that both choices from day 3 were transferred only 23% of the time. At least one of those chosen on day 3 was transferred 38% of the time and 39% of the cycles had neither choice transferred. However, after extending culture to day 6, it was noted that 68% of the 'picks' on day 3 ended up being either transferred on day 5 or of a quality sufficient to be frozen on day 5 or 6.

Blastocyst development and chromosomal abnormalities

Human preembryos cultured in vitro present high rates of chromosomal anomalies. These anomalies may be numerical (e.g. trisomies or aneuploidy) or structural (e.g. translocations). The incidence of chromosomal abnormalities in cleaved preembryos after fluorescence in situ hybridization (FISH) analysis ranges between 15

and 85%, depending on the number and specificity of probes used. A high percentage of aberrant preembryos exhibit mosaic or chaotic abnormalities[61]. Chromosomal anomalies are even higher in arrested preembryos, suggesting that preembryo selection may exclude some abnormalities before implantation. For this reason it has been proposed that culturing preembryos to blastocyst stages will select chromosomally normal conceptuses. Another possibility represents selective allocation of aneuploid cells to the trophectoderm. This hypothesis was questioned recently after mosaicism was demonstrated in the inner cell mass of the human blastocyst[62]. The overall frequency of mosaicism has been shown to increase from 15% at the 2–4-cell stage to 49% at the 5–8-cell, 58% at the morula and up to 90% at the blastocyst stage[39]. On the other hand, certain forms of mosaicism, e.g. chaotic mosaicism and diploid–aneuploid mosaicism, were reduced at the blastocyst stage. The highest rates of mosaicism seen in blastocysts have been reported to be 2n-polyploid mosaicism, usually diploid/tetraploid[63,64]. It has also been shown that aneuploid cell lines from cleavage stages may persist to the blastocyst stage, but their incidence is very low[65]. Most polyploid cells in the blastocyst are thought to arise during blastocyst formation and are probably precursors of trophoblast differentiation[66].

Sandalinas and colleagues sought to correlate which chromosomal abnormalities were compatible with prolonged development in vitro[67]. This group took preembryos assessed as abnormal following preimplantation genetic diagnosis (PGD) analysis, allowed them to grow in culture until day 5 or 6 and correlated which abnormalities were associated with subsequent blastocyst formation. They found that extensive mosaicism could be detected in some blastocysts developing in vitro and that 37% of trisomic preembryos reached the blastocyst stage of development. They further reported that only monosomies X and 21, monosomies compatible with development into the first trimester, were actually found in conceptuses reaching the blastocyst stage. The authors concluded that, although there was a strong selection bias against chromosomally abnormal preembryos with extended culture, the selective potential was limited in its ability to exclude many clinically relevant aberrations, especially the trisomies.

Magli and associates reported similar findings[65]. Fifty-nine per cent of day-3 aneuploid preembryos did not reach the morula or blastocyst stages of development *in vitro*. Nonetheless, 40% of blastocysts studied by FISH techniques were shown to possess aneuploid cells, and a significant number of preembryos diagnosed as aneuploid on day 3 produced blastocysts with inner cell mass mosaicism. These data suggest that euploid cells are not necessarily preferentially allocated to inner cell masses, and that aneuploid cells are not necessarily preferentially allocated to the trophectoderm of affected blastocysts. A high concordance between day-3 aneuploidy diagnosis and inner cell mass lineage was observed with trisomies (97%), while a reduced concordance was found with monosomies (65%) and haploidies (18%). Further studies will be needed to correlate the chromosomal status of the blastocyst cultured in vitro with blastocyst morphology and implantation potential.

Blastocysts have been noted to form after a single pronculeus was observed at 18 h post-insemination, suggesting that this feature alone does not indicate developmental incompetence[68]. The Cornell group has similarly observed this type of outcome after documentation of a monopronuclear status (Figure 6.16). It has been suggested that all inseminated oocytes displaying a single pronucleus should be rechecked within 2–6 h to confirm pronuclear number. One report where investigators did this revealed that 25% of repeat observations led to the visualization of two pronuclei rather than one[69]. Such a finding suggests that developmental asynchrony between male and female pronuclei may not be a rare event.

A single pronucleus can form and persist after *in vitro* insemination or sperm injection, resulting in a gynogenic or rare androgenic haploid prezygote. Human oocytes displaying a single pronucleus have been observed to continue growth to blastocyst stages, and some of these have been shown actually to be diploid. One such study describes removing the pronucleus from single-pronucleate oocytes after conventional insemination. Of 16 pronuclei examined, six were diploid, four of which contained XY chromosomes[70]. This suggests that sperm and oocyte nuclei can associate to form a single diploid pronucleus, as opposed to simply being asynchronous in development. It has further been shown that preembryos developing from monopronucleate oocytes after IVF insemination are most often fertilized and diploid, while those forming from activated ICSI oocytes are almost always haploid parthenotes[69,71,72]. For this reason, preembryos developing from inseminated oocytes displaying one pronucleus may be replaced, although not preferentially; those developing after ICSI should not be transferred. Since it has been described that diploid pronuclei are often larger than usual owing to their double amount of DNA[73], this characteristic may be favorable in monopronculeate oocytes after *in vitro* insemination.

When should we transfer only a single conceptus?

Research from our program suggests that when a fertilized oocyte displays two cells at the 24/26-h observation, grows to an 8-cell stage by the morning of day 3 and possesses less than 20% fragmentation, it has a very high implantation potential. Add the situation where it develops into a high-grade blastocyst, and it has a greater than 70% chance of implanting in the uterine cavity (Figure 6.17). These conceptuses should probably be replaced alone, as the twinning rate is unacceptably high with two. Additionally, it has been proposed by other groups that elective transfer of a single blastocyst would benefit patients with poor obstetrical outcomes after previous high-order gestations[74].

Should we be transferring blastocysts for all patients?

We must first acknowledge that extended culture will not turn a poor-quality day-3 preembryo into a healthy blastocyst. The value of this technology is to provide better selection criteria when educated choices must be made. Neither will extended culture confer any special advantage to a woman with only one or two oocytes at harvest, at least not at this time.

Our data show that with good-responding patients, transferring two preembryos on day 3 serves the same purpose as using blastocysts in terms of clinical pregnancy and reduction of high-order gestation. The efforts described here with our own day-3 and day-5 trials, and those reported by most others, are primarily dealing with this type of patient.

For programs unable to carry out blastocyst transfer, unhappy with the variability in media or results, or unwilling to extend culture to day 5, options are available for the selection of appropriate preembryos on day 3. Such programs should consider examining fertilized oocytes at 24/26 h to assess for timely cleavage, and then evaluate preembryos on the morning of day 3,

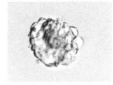

keeping in mind that the predictive value for blastocyst development may be lost if one waits until the afternoon. If the first cleavage has occurred by 24 h and at least two 8-cell day-3 preembryos of good quality (< 20% fragmentation) are available, one should consider replacing only two conceptuses in women under the age of 40 years.

Keep in mind that, whichever stage is chosen for carrying out transfer, a clinic's ultimate goal should be to help produce a single, healthy baby. Transfer of one conceptus alone will effectively eliminate all possibilities for multiple gestation, excluding identical twins. As responsible investigators and care-givers, our quest for the future must follow this direction.

References

1. Melgar CA, Rosenfeld DL, Rawlinson K, Greenberg M. Perinatal outcome after multifetal reduction to twins compared with nonreduced multiple gestations. *Obstet Gynecol* 1991;78:763–7

2. Groutz A, Yovel I, Amit A, Yaron Y, Azem F, Lessing JB. Pregnancy outcome after multifetal pregnancy reduction to twins compared with spontaneously conceived twins. *Hum Reprod* 1996;11:1334–6

3. Garel M, Salobir C, Blondel B. Psychological consequences of having triplets: a 4-year follow-up study. *Fertil Steril* 1997;67:1162–5

4. Elster N. Less is more: the risks of multiple births. The Institute for Science, Law, and Technology Working Group on Reproductive Technology. *Fertil Steril* 2000;74:617–23

5. Skupski DW, Nelson S, Kowalik A, et al. Multiple gestations from in vitro fertilization: successful implantation alone is not associated with subsequent pre-eclampsia. *Am J Obstet Gynecol* 1996;175:1029–32

6. Gleicher N, Campbell DP, Chan CL, et al. The desire for multiple births in couples with infertility problems contradicts present practice patterns. *Hum Reprod* 1995;10:1079–84

7. Hartshorne GM, Lilford RJ. Different perspectives of patients and health care professionals on the potential benefits and risks of blastocyst culture and multiple embryo transfer. *Hum Reprod* 2002;17:1023–30

8. Gardner DK, Lane M. Culture of viable human blastocysts in defined sequential serum-free media. *Hum Reprod* 1998;13(Suppl 3):148–59; discussion 160

9. Behr B, Pool TB, Milki AA, Moore D, Gebhardt J, Dasig D. Preliminary clinical experience with human blastocyst development *in vitro* without co-culture. *Hum Reprod* 1999;14:454–7

10. Gorrill MJ, Sadler-Fredd K, Patton PE, Burry KA. Multiple gestations in assisted reproductive technology: can they be avoided with blastocyst transfers? *Am J Obstet Gynecol* 2001;184:1471–5; discussion 1475–7

11. Gardner DK, Schoolcraft WB, Wagley L, Schlenker T, Stevens J, Hesla J. A prospective randomized trial of blastocyst culture and transfer in *in-vitro* fertilization. *Hum Reprod* 1998;13:3434–40

12. Schoolcraft WB, Gardner DK, Lane M, Schlenker T, Hamilton F, Meldrum DR. Blastocyst culture and transfer: analysis of results and parameters affecting outcome in two *in vitro* fertilization programs. *Fertil Steril* 1999;72:604–9

13. Schoolcraft WB, Gardner DK. Blastocyst culture and transfer increases the efficiency of oocyte donation. *Fertil Steril* 2000;74:482–6

14. Shapiro BS, Richter KS, Harris DC, Daneshmand ST. Implantation and pregnancy rates are higher for oocyte donor cycles after blastocyst-stage embryo transfer. *Fertil Steril* 2002;77:1296–7

15. Milki AA, Hinckley MD, Fisch JD, Dasig D, Behr B. Comparison of blastocyst transfer with day 3 embryo transfer in similar patient populations. *Fertil Steril* 2000;73:126–9

16. Marek D, Langley M, Gardner DK, Confer N, Doody KM, Doody KJ. Introduction of blastocyst culture and transfer

for all patients in an in vitro fertilization program. *Fertil Steril* 1999;72:1035–40

17. Wilson M, Hartke K, Kiehl M, Rodgers J, Brabec C, Lyles R. Integration of blastocyst transfer for all patients. *Fertil Steril* 2002;77:693–6

18. Coskun S, Hollanders J, Al-Hassan S, Al-Sufyan H, Al-Mayman H, Jaroudi K. Day 5 versus day 3 embryo transfer: a controlled randomized trial. *Hum Reprod* 2000;15:1947–52

19. Huisman GJ, Fauser BC, Eijkemans MJ, Pieters MH. Implantation rates after in vitro fertilization and transfer of a maximum of two embryos that have undergone three to five days of culture. *Fertil Steril* 2000;73:117–22

20. Toledo AA, Wright G, Jones AE, *et al*. Blastocyst transfer: a useful tool for reduction of high-order multiple gestations in a human assisted reproduction program. *Am J Obstet Gynecol* 2000;183:377–9; discussion 380–2

21. Lin G, Gong F, Lu C. [Preliminary study on application of blastocyst culture and day 5 transfer in patients with low oocyte number.] *Zhonghua Fu Chan Ke Za Zhi* 2001;36:536–8

22. Blake D, Proctor M, Johnson N, Olive D. Cleavage stage versus blastocyst stage embryo transfer in assisted conception (Cochrane Review). *Cochrane Database Syst Rev* 2002:CD002118

23. Kovacic B, Vlaisavljevic V, Reljic M, Gavric Lovrec V. Clinical outcome of day 2 versus day 5 transfer in cycles with one or two developed embryos. *Fertil Steril* 2002;77:529–36

24. Lundqvist M, Rova K, Simberg N, Lundkvist O. Embryo transfer after 2 or 5 days of IVF culture: a retrospective comparison. *Acta Obstet Gynecol Scand* 2002;81:126–32

25. Hsieh YY, Tsai HD, Chang FC. Routine blastocyst culture and transfer: 201 patients' experience. *J Assist Reprod Genet* 2000;17:405–8

26. Plachot M, Belaisch-Allart J, Mayenga JM, Chouraqui A, Serkine AM, Tesquier L. Blastocyst stage transfer: the real benefits compared with early embryo transfer. *Hum Reprod* 2000;15(Suppl 6):24–30

27. Racowsky C, Jackson KV, Cekleniak NA, Fox JH, Hornstein MD, Ginsburg ES. The number of eight-cell embryos is a key determinant for selecting day 3 or day 5 transfer. *Fertil Steril* 2000;73:558–64

28. Vidaeff AC, Racowsky C, Rayburn WF. Blastocyst transfer in human in vitro fertilization. A solution to the multiple pregnancy epidemic. *J Reprod Med* 2000;45:529–39, discussion 539–40

29. Karaki RZ, Samarraie SS, Younis NA, Lahloub TM, Ibrahim MH. Blastocyst culture and transfer: a step toward improved in vitro fertilization outcome. *Fertil Steril* 2002;77:114–18

30. Cruz JR, Dubey AK, Patel J, Peak D, Hartog B, Gindoff PR. Is blastocyst transfer useful as an alternative treatment for patients with multiple in vitro fertilization failures? *Fertil Steril* 1999;72:218–20

31. Van Der Auwera I, Debrock S, Spiessens C, *et al*. A prospective randomized study: day 2 versus day 5 embryo transfer. *Hum Reprod* 2002;17:1507–12

32. Shapiro BS, Richter KS, Harris DC, Daneshmand ST. Dramatic declines in implantation and pregnancy rates in patients who undergo repeated cycles of in vitro fertilization with blastocyst transfer after one or more failed attempts. *Fertil Steril* 2001;76:538–42

33. Levron J, Shulman A, Bider D, Seidman D, Levin T, Dor J. A prospective randomized study comparing day 3 with blastocyst-stage embryo transfer. *Fertil Steril* 2002;77:1300–1

34. Fujii S, Fukui A, Yamaguchi E, Sakamoto T, Sato S, Saito Y. Reducing multiple pregnancies by restricting the number of embryos transferred to two at the first embryo transfer attempt. *Hum Reprod* 1998;13:3550–4

35. Devreker F, Emiliani S, Revelard P, Van den Bergh M, Govaerts I, Englert Y. Comparison of two elective transfer policies of two embryos to reduce multiple pregnancies without impairing pregnancy rates. *Hum Reprod* 1999;14:83–9

36. Devreker F, Emiliani S, Revelard P, Govaerts I, Vannin AS, Englert Y. [Diminishing the risk of multiple pregnancies in in vitro fertilization: from selective transfer of two embryos to that of one blastocyst?] *Rev Med Brux* 1999;20:A463–7

37. Matson PL, Browne J, Deakin R, Bellinge B. The transfer of two embryos instead of three to reduce the risk of multiple pregnancy: a retrospective analysis. *J Assist Reprod Genet* 1999;16:1–5

38. Dean NL, Phillips SJ, Buckett WM, Biljan MM, Tan SL. Impact of reducing the number of embryos transferred from three to two in women under the age of 35 who produced three or more high-quality embryos. *Fertil Steril* 2000;74:820–3

39. Ludwig M, Schopper B, Katalinic A, Sturm R, Al-Hasani S, Diedrich K. Experience with the elective transfer of two embryos under the conditions of the German embryo protection law: results of a retrospective data analysis of 2573 transfer cycles. *Hum Reprod* 2000;15:319–24

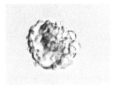

40. Licciardi F, Berkeley AS, Krey L, Grifo J, Noyes N. A two-versus three-embryo transfer: the oocyte donation model. *Fertil Steril* 2001;75:510–13

41. Ng EH, Lau EY, Yeung WS, Ho PC. Transfer of two embryos instead of three will not compromise pregnancy rate but will reduce multiple pregnancy rate in an assisted reproduction unit. *J Obstet Gynaecol Res* 2001;27:329–35

42. Templeton A, Morris JK. Reducing the risk of multiple births by transfer of two embryos after *in vitro* fertilization. *N Engl J Med* 1998;339:573–7

43. Scott LA, Smith S. The successful use of pronuclear embryo transfers the day following oocyte retrieval. *Hum Reprod* 1998;13:1003–13

44. Scott L, Alvero R, Leondires M, Miller B. The morphology of human pronuclear embryos is positively related to blastocyst development and implantation. *Hum Reprod* 2000;15:2394–403

45. Tesarik J, Greco E. The probability of abnormal preimplantation development can be predicted by a single static observation on pronuclear stage morphology. *Hum Reprod* 1999;14:1318–23

46. Tesarik J, Junca AM, Hazout A, et al. Embryos with high implantation potential after intracytoplasmic sperm injection can be recognized by a simple, non-invasive examination of pronuclear morphology. *Hum Reprod* 2000;15:1396–9

47. Balaban B, Urman B, Isiklar A, Alatas C, Aksoy S, Mercan R, et al. The effect of pronuclear morphology on embryo quality parameters and blastocyst transfer outcome. *Hum Reprod* 2001;16:2357–61

48. Fisch JD, Rodriguez H, Ross R, Overby G, Sher G. The Graduated Embryo Score (GES) predicts blastocyst formation and pregnancy rate from cleavage-stage embryos. *Hum Reprod* 2001;16:1970–5

49. Montag M, van der Ven H. Evaluation of pronuclear morphology as the only selection criterion for further embryo culture and transfer: results of a prospective multicentre study. *Hum Reprod* 2001;16:2384–9

50. Rienzi L, Ubaldi F, Iacobelli M, et al. Day 3 embryo transfer with combined evaluation at the pronuclear and cleavage stages compares favourably with day 5 blastocyst transfer. *Hum Reprod* 2002;17:1852–5

51. Zollner U, Zollner KP, Hartl G, Dietl J, Steck T. The use of a detailed zygote score after IVF/ICSI to obtain good quality blastocysts: the German experience. *Hum Reprod* 2002;17:1327–33

52. Clarke RN, Zaninovic N, Berrios R, Veeck LL. The relationship between human prezygote morphology and subsequent preembryo (PE) development in culture. Presented at the *57th Annual Meeting of the American Society for Reproductive Medicine*, Orlando, FL, October 2001

53. Nagy ZP, Janssenswillen C, Janssens R, et al. Timing of oocyte activation, pronucleus formation and cleavage in humans after intracytoplasmic sperm injection (ICSI) with testicular spermatozoa and after ICSI or *in-vitro* fertilization on sibling oocytes with ejaculated spermatozoa. *Hum Reprod* 1998;13:1606–12

54. Sakkas D, Shoukir Y, Chardonnens D, Bianchi PG, Campana A. Early cleavage of human embryos to the two-cell stage after intracytoplasmic sperm injection as an indicator of embryo viability. *Hum Reprod* 1998;13:182–7

55. Zaninovic N, Veeck LL, Clarke RN, Rosenwaks Z. Early assessment of human preembryos as in indicator for potential blastocyst development. Presented at the *56th Annual Meeting of the American Society for Reproductive Medicine*, San Diego, CA, 2000

56. Fenwick J, Platteau P, Murdoch AP, Herbert M. Time from insemination to first cleavage predicts developmental competence of human preimplantation embryos *in vitro*. *Hum Reprod* 2002;17:407–12

57. Alikani M, Calderon G, Tomkin G, Garrisi J, Kokot M, Cohen J. Cleavage anomalies in early human embryos and survival after prolonged culture *in-vitro*. *Hum Reprod* 2000;15:2634–43

58. Rijnders PM, Jansen CA. The predictive value of day 3 embryo morphology regarding blastocyst formation, pregnancy and implantation rate after day 5 transfer following *in-vitro* fertilization or intracytoplasmic sperm injection. *Hum Reprod* 1998;13:2869–73

59. Graham J, Han T, Porter R, Levy M, Stillman R, Tucker MJ. Day 3 morphology is a poor predictor of blastocyst quality in extended culture. *Fertil Steril* 2000;74:495–7

60. Milki AA, Hinckley MD, Gebhardt J, Dasig D, Westphal LM, Behr B. Accuracy of day 3 criteria for selecting the best embryos. *Fertil Steril* 2002;77:1191–5

61. Munne S, Cohen J. Chromosome abnormalities in human embryos. *Hum Reprod Update* 1998;4:842–55

62. Evsikov S, Verlinsky Y. Mosaicism in the inner cell mass of human blastocysts. *Hum Reprod* 1998;13:3151–5

63. Bielanska M, Tan SL, Ao A. Chromosomal mosaicism throughout human preimplantation development *in vitro*: incidence, type, and relevance to embryo outcome. *Hum Reprod* 2002;17:413–19

64. Ruangvutilert P, Delhanty JD, Serhal P, Simopoulou M, Rodeck CH, Harper JC. FISH analysis on day 5 post-insemination of human arrested and blastocyst stage embryos. *Prenat Diagn* 2000;20:552–60

65. Magli MC, Jones GM, Gras L, Gianaroli L, Korman I, Trounson AO. Chromosome mosaicism in day 3 aneuploid embryos that develop to morphologically normal blastocysts *in vitro. Hum Reprod* 2000;15:1781–6

66. Benkhalifa M, Janny L, Vye P, Malet P, Boucher D, Menezo Y. Assessment of polyploidy in human morulae and blastocysts using co-culture and fluorescent *in-situ* hybridization. *Hum Reprod* 1993;8:895–902

67. Sandalinas M, Sadowy S, Alikani M, Calderon G, Cohen J, Munne S. Developmental ability of chromosomally abnormal human embryos to develop to the blastocyst stage. *Hum Reprod* 2001;16:1954–8

68. Gras L, Trounson AO. Pregnancy and birth resulting from transfer of a blastocyst observed to have one pronucleus at the time of examination for fertilization. *Hum Reprod* 1999;14:1869–71

69. Staessen C, Janssenswillen C, Devroey P, Van Steirteghem AC. Cytogenetic and morphological observations of single pronucleated human oocytes after *in-vitro* fertilization. *Hum Reprod* 1993;8:221–3

70. Levron J, Munne S, Willadsen S, Rosenwaks Z, Cohen J. Male and female genomes associated in a single pronucleus in human zygotes. *Biol Reprod* 1995;52:653–7

71. Palermo GD, Munne S, Colombero LT, Cohen J, Rosenwaks Z. Genetics of abnormal human fertilization. *Hum Reprod* 1995;10(Suppl 1):120–7

72. Sultan KM, Munne S, Palermo GD, Alikani M, Cohen J. Chromosomal status of uni-pronuclear human zygotes following *in-vitro* fertilization and intracytoplasmic sperm injection. *Hum Reprod* 1995;10:132–6

73. Austin CR. *The Mammalian Egg.* Oxford: Blackwell Scientific Publications, 1961

74. Damario MA, Phy JL, Tummon IS. Successful elective single blastocyst transfer in a patient with prior repetitive high-order multiple gestations. *J Assist Reprod Genet* 2002;19:205–8

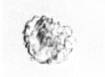

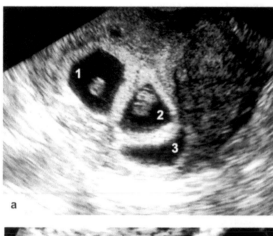

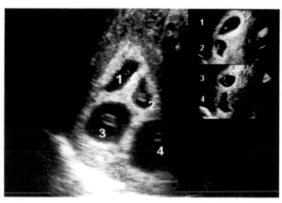

Figure 6.2 Ultrasound image of a quadruplet pregnancy. Inserts show individual embryos. Photograph courtesy of Isaac Kligman, Weill Medical College of Cornell University

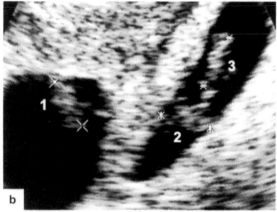

Figure 6.1 Ultrasound images of triplet pregnancies. Photographs courtesy of Steven Spandorfer, Weill Medical College of Cornell University. (a) Three individual sacs; (b) two sacs, three embryos (monozygotic twins)

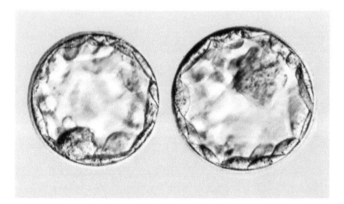

Figure 6.3 Human blastocysts replaced on day 5. High-graded blastocysts, each with a prominent ICM and cohesive TM

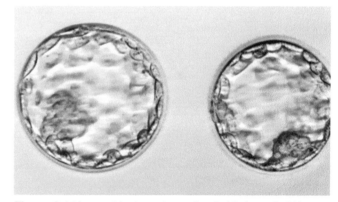

Figure 6.4 Human blastocysts on day 5. High-graded blastocysts suitable for replacement. In these cases only one blastocyst should be replaced as the implantation rate is quite high

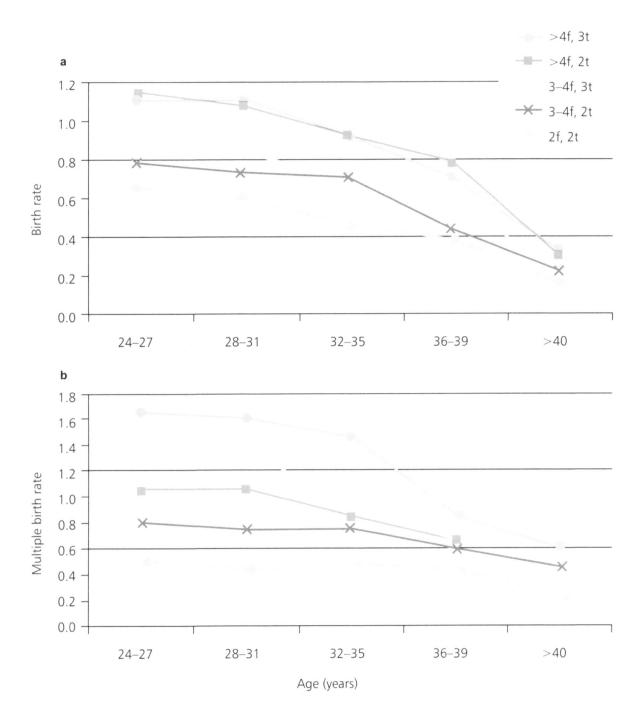

Legend:
- >4f, 3t
- >4f, 2t
- 3–4f, 3t
- 3–4f, 2t
- 2f, 2t

Figure 6.5 Odds of birth and multiple birth related to age, number of oocytes fertilized, and number of preembryos replaced (Templeton A, Morris JK. *N Engl J Med* 1998;339:573). The authors studied birth and multiple birth risk factors in 44 236 cycles (25 240 women) by examining age, cause and duration of infertility, number of previous attempts, number of previous live births, number of oocytes fertilized, and number of preembryos transferred. They found that older age, tubal infertility, longer duration of infertility, and greater number of previous attempts correlated with significantly lower birth and multiple birth rates while previous live birth correlated with significantly higher birth rate (but not multiple birth rate). (a) When more than four oocytes were fertilized, there was no difference in the birth rate whether two or three preembryos were replaced. The odds of a birth were calculated as compared with those of a 30-year-old woman with more than four oocytes fertilized and two preembryos replaced (odds for such a woman, 1.0); (b) there was, however, a considerable increase in the multiple birth rate when three were replaced. The odds of a multiple birth were calculated as compared with those of a 30-year-old woman with more than four oocytes fertilized and two preembryos replaced (odds for such a woman, 1.0)

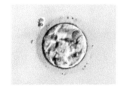

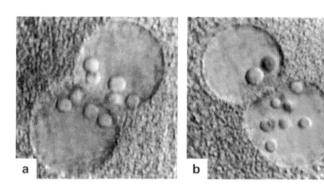

Figure 6.6 Nucleolar distribution in human male and female pronuclei approximately 18 hours post-insemination. (a) Nucleoli are nearly equal in number and size and are closely aligned at pronuclear junctions, an example of a good pronuclear score; (b) unequal number and size of nucleoli with scattered distribution; a poor pronuclear score

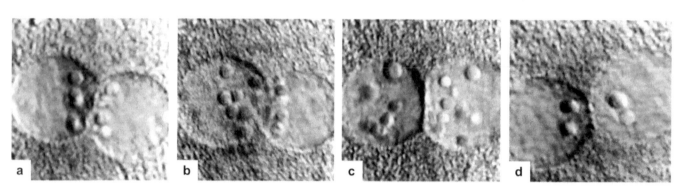

Figure 6.7 Pronuclear grading system according to pattern of nucleolar distribution. (a) PZ1: both pronuclei have aligned nucleoli; (b) PZ2: one pronucleus with aligned nucleoli, the other exhibiting scattered nucleoli; (c) PZ3: both pronuclei possess scattered nucleoli; (d) PZ4: few nucleoli in one or both pronuclei (in this instance, both)

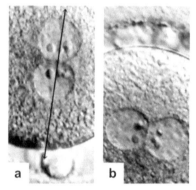

Figure 6.8 Orientation of pronuclei in relation to polar body (PB) position. (a) PB+: pronuclei are perpendicular to PB, in correct position for syngamy and the first cleavage. (b) PB-: pronuclei are parallel to PB, necessitating rotation before syngamy

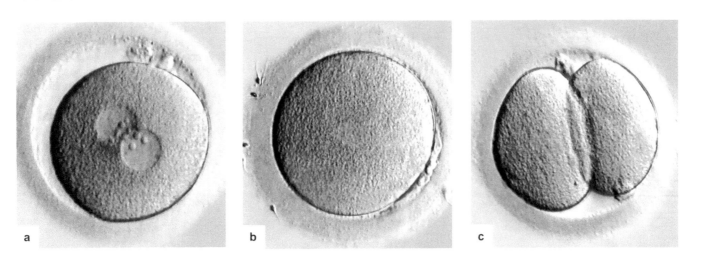

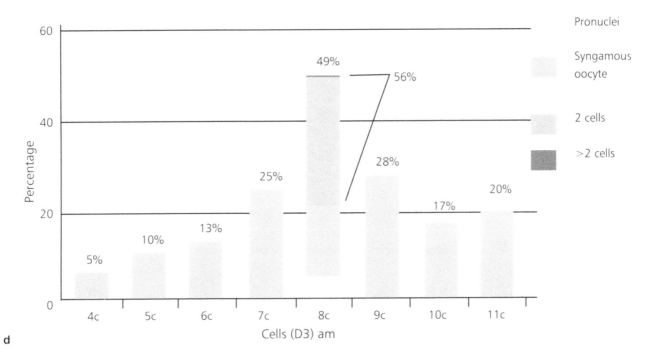

Figure 6.9 Assessment of preembryo development at 24/26 hours post-ICSI/insemination. (a) At 24 hours post-injection, this prezygote possesses two pronuclei (2PN); (b) at 26 hours post-insemination, no PN are seen in this syngamous oocyte; (c) 2-cell conceptus at 24 hours after ICSI; (d) graph depicting how blastocyst development on day 5 correlates to the number of blastomeres observed on the morning (am) of day 3. The 8-cell stage, on the morning of day 3, is optimal for blastocyst development on day 5. The majority of 8-cell preembryos that develop into blastocysts on day 5 arise from those that possessed two cells at 24/26 hours (approximately 56%). It is interesting to note that preembryos with more than eight cells on the morning of day 3 form blastocysts at lower rates than those with exactly eight cells

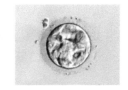

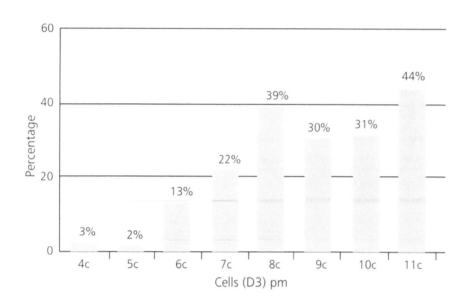

Figure 6.10 Predictive criteria for day-5 blastocyst development were lost if pre-embryos were not evaluated until the afternoon of day 3. Some conceptuses with fewer than eight cells in the morning developed to eight cells by the afternoon (pm), yet their ability to form blastocysts was impaired

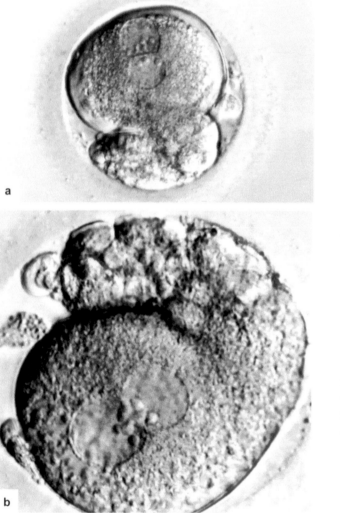

Figure 6.11 Fragmentation before the first cleavage. (a) and (b) Pronuclear oocytes with excessive fragmentation 24 hours after injection. Such fragments are not reincorporated into the zygote and developmental arrest generally follows

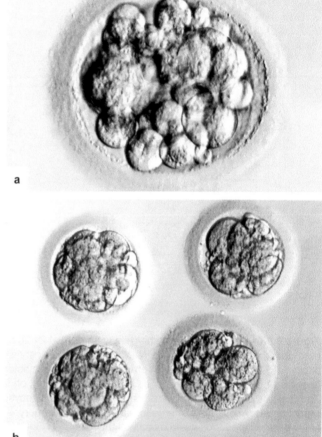

Figure 6.12 (a) Day-3 preembryo exhibiting two to three blastomeres surrounded by multiple cytoplasmic fragments. Due to the reduction of available cytoplasm for cleavage, these are usually unable to develop further; (b) type IV fragmentation (per Alikani et al.[58]), with large, randomly distributed fragments and associated with unevenly sized and shaped blastomeres; these are associated with a significant decrease in subsequent blastocyst formation

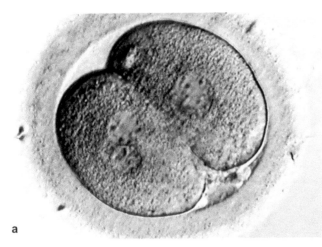
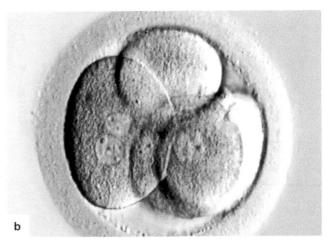

a   b

Figure 6.13 Multinucleation. (a) Multinucleated blastomere in a day-2 2-cell preembryo. The blastomere to the left possesses three nuclei; there are two nuclei in the blastomere to the right (overlapping from this angle). Multinucleation of all blastomeres in a 2-cell conceptus is associated with impaired blastocyst development; (b) multinucleated blastomere in a day-2 4-cell preembryo. The blastomere to the left presents with at least two nuclei. There is less negative impact on subsequent development when multinucleation first occurs in a single blastomere in preembryos possessing four or more cells

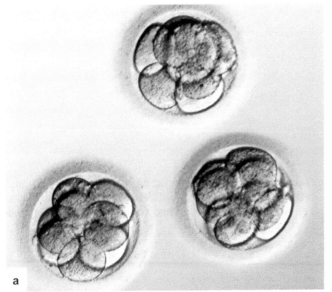
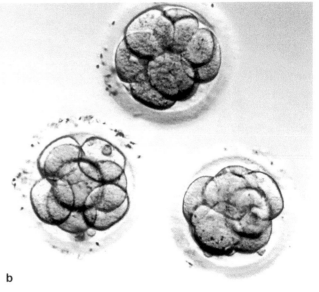

a   b

Figure 6.14 (a) and (b) Preembryos with good morphology on day 3 that subsequently failed to form viable blastocysts

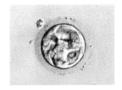

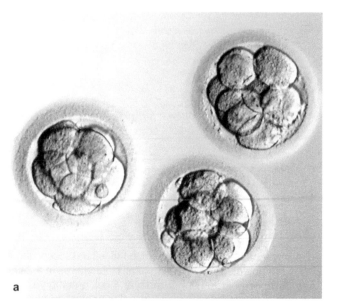
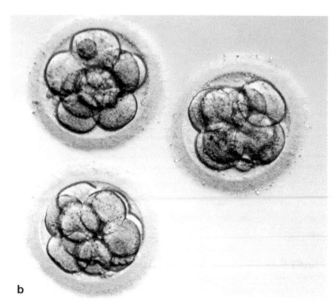

a   b

Figure 6.15 (a) and (b) Day-3 preembryos exhibiting good morphology, but which failed to reach the blastocyst stage of development after continued culture. Each possesses 8–10 blastomeres and none are associated with more than very minor cytoplasmic fragmentation. Unfortunately, correlation between day-3 morphology and subsequent blastocyst development is not precise

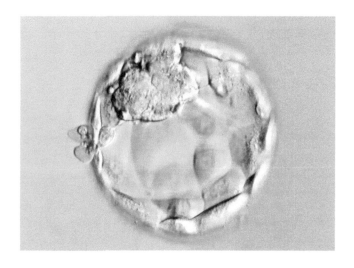

Figure 6.16 Human blastocyst on day 5, developed from a prezygote displaying one pronucleus (1PN) after insemination. The ICM is well-developed and compacting; the TM is made up of large, but healthy, cells

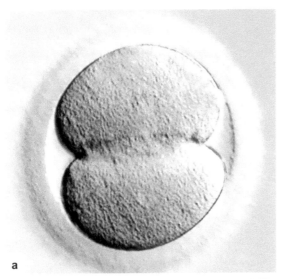

a

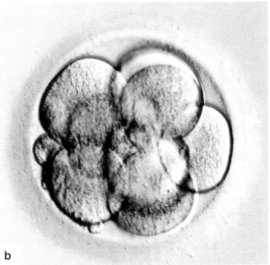

b

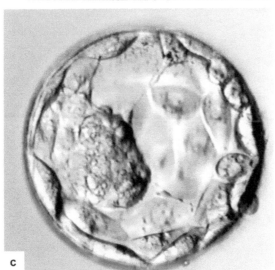

c

Figure 6.17 A 2-cell conceptus at 24/26 hours that grows to eight cells by the morning of day 3 and then subsequently develops into a healthy appearing blastocyst, which possesses an extremely high implantation potential, exceeding 70%. Single blastocyst replacement is recommended under these growth and development conditions. (a) Two-cell stage at 24 hours after ICSI; (b) eight blastomeres on the morning of day 3; (c) high-graded blastocyst on day 5

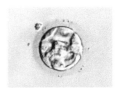

7   Blastocyst hatching

The zona pellucida is a glycoprotein layer that surrounds oocytes and preembryos during the preimplantation period. A number of authors have demonstrated that the human zona is composed of three acidic glycoproteins called ZP1, ZP2 and ZP3[1-3]. The zona has various possible roles in preimplantation development: prevention of polyspermy, protecting the preembryo from physical or immunological damage and preserving its integrity during cleavage. Although the zona is sometimes described as having roles in sperm binding, in induction of the acrosome reaction and as a matrix for sperm penetration, these last phenomena may be the simple consequence of its presence around the oocyte (personal communication, Michael Bedford). After compaction and formation of cell junctions, this protective coat is no longer necessary for the developing human preembryo, at least under *in vitro* culture conditions. *Hatching* is a process that involves blastocyst escape through the zona pellucida, a prerequisite for normal implantation. In the human, implantation is initiated by trophoblastic invasion of the uterine endometrium.

As the blastocyst expands, there is a gradual accumulation of fluid in the blastocoel, resulting in increased pressure on both trophectoderm and the zona pellucida. At the same time, cells of the trophectoderm proliferate rapidly to form a cohesive monolayer[4]. It is not entirely clear whether the concomitant thinning of the zona pellucida results from physical pressures exerted by blastocyst expansion and trophectoderm proliferation, or whether thinning is primarily the effect of lytic enzymes produced by the developing preembryo, or both[5]. There is some evidence to support the involvement of enzymes, since viable preembryos demonstrate very gradual thinning of the zona pellucida, or at least show variations in zona thickness, even before blastocyst expansion[6]. In contrast, arrested preembryos do not[7]. Because the overall size of the preembryo does not increase until cavitation, it can be deduced that at least some aspects of zona pellucida thinning are related to enzymes released from the preembryo.

While the process of hatching is well characterized in the mouse, it is less well understood in the human. It is possible that some or all of the mechanisms involved are similar. In the mouse, the *in vitro* hatching mechanism involves, at the least, a trypsin-like proteinase, called strypsin[8]. Before hatching, strypsin is found in mural trophectoderm cells, presumably at the site where hatching will occur. After hatching, strypsin is again identified around the opening from which the blastocyst emerges. But proof of trypsin-like protease involvement in mouse hatching comes from studies of inhibitors. Yamazaki and colleagues showed that hatching was suppressed in 83% of murine embryos by a synthetic trypsin inhibitor with no adverse effect on subsequent blastocyst development[9]. A potential substrate for the trypsin-like protease action may be ZP3[10]. Experiments utilizing an antihatching mouse model support the theory of embryo-produced enzyme involvement[11]. Furthermore, *in vivo* hatching studies also reveal zona lysis activity during the peri-implantation period. It is possible that non-embryonic uterine enzymes are at least partly responsible for the complete shedding of the zona pellucida *in vivo*[12].

At the onset of hatching, the mouse blastocyst generates greater than ten times the amount of superoxide anion radicals than in the pre- and post-hatching stages. In fact,

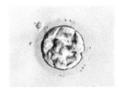

adding superoxides to cultured zonae induces thinning and hatching within a matter of seconds, the result of superoxides disrupting the glycosilic bonds of zona glycoproteins[13]. Interestingly, hatching can occur in the absence of an inner cell mass, supporting the primary importance of the trophectoderm for this process[11,14,15].

In the mouse, hatching occurs in areas adjacent to mural trophectoderm opposite to the inner cell mass[16]. Although more variable in the human, the hatching site usually develops relatively close to the inner cell mass in proximity to the polar trophectoderm (Figures 7.1–7.4). In human blastocysts cultured *in vitro*, small membrane blebs or vesicles frequently protrude through the zona pellucida before hatching occurs (Figures 7.5 and 7.6). Contrary to popular belief, they do not always indicate the precise location of subsequent hatching. After the zona pellucida has begun to rupture (Figure 7.7), the ultimate size of the opening created is roughly between one-quarter and one-third of the circumference of the zona pellucida, permitting easy and rapid blastocyst escape (Figures.7.8 and 7.9).

Once an opening is created, the blastocyst begins to protrude through the zona. After this, several mechanisms may be involved in the completion of hatching. If lytic enzymes and blastocoelic tension are primarily responsible for zona pellucida rupture, then another mechanism must be responsible for complete extrusion and escape of the blastocyst. It has been suggested that actin polymerization plays a role in this regard, since actin filaments are heavily concentrated on trophectoderm cells, especially so at the site of hatching. The initial protrusion is probably mediated through continuous actin polymerization of trophectoderm cell microfilaments. When cytochalasin-B, an inhibitor of actin polymerization, is added to mouse blastocyst culture medium, hatching will not occur even when the zona pellucida is open. This inhibition is reversible once blastocysts are transferred to cytochalasin-B-free medium, indicating the importance of actin filament activity during the protrusion/extrusion processes[17].

As blastocysts hatch *in vitro*, small *trophectoderm projections* can be observed outside the zona pellucida. These projections exhibit ameboid movement before and after hatching is completed (Figure 7.10). Such projections have been observed in several species including mouse, human and bovine, but only at the late blastocyst stage of development[16,18]. Trophectoderm projections are not simple artifacts of *in vitro* culture; they have been noted in mouse blastocysts that have developed and hatched *in vivo*[12,19]. The length of these projections in the human averages 27 μm, and they have been suggested to serve as a first contact between blastocyst and uterus since they are localized to the precise region of the blastocyst that will ultimately attach to uterine epithelium.

Blastocysts studied *in vitro* typically undergo repeated expansion and collapse before hatching is accomplished[20,21] (Figures 7.11 and 7.12). Collapse is rapid, occurring in less than 5 min, whereas complete re-expansion requires several hours. It has been observed in our laboratory that human blastocyst collapse often occurs just before complete and final extrusion through an already ruptured zona pellucida (Figure 7.13). However, collapse of the blastocyst can be induced by mechanical, chemical, osmotic or temperature-related stress, suggesting that it is particularly susceptible to environmental conditions and requires careful handling. It is not known whether *in vivo*-produced human blastocysts collapse and re-expand in the same manner *in utero*.

In vitro, hatching of healthy human blastocysts is typically observed on day 6 or 7 of culture, or by day 5 if the zona has been manipulated. Left in culture, blastocysts delayed in their growth may hatch as late as day 9. Because intrauterine transfer is almost always carried out by day 6 in clinical settings, it is unclear whether these are capable of implantation and subsequent normal development.

In some hybrid strains of the mouse, the rate of blastocyst development rate *in vitro* approaches 100% and hatching rates exceed 90%, percentages far higher than the human rates of approximately 50% and 25%, respectively. Whether such differences reflect dissimilar effects of culture or different mechanisms of growth and hatching is not clear. Culture media for human *in vitro* fertilization almost always include protein supplements, e.g. whole serum, purified albumin or another substance which ultimately provides protein macromolecules. While considered undefined and therefore potentially toxic by some investigators, these substances have been used successfully over the years, and are held to contribute to softening and/or pliability of the zona. Conversely, culturing human preembryos in totally protein-free media has not led to widespread success, and in a number of species, including the human, adding growth factors to *serum-free* culture media increases blastocyst developmental and hatching rates[22-24]. Heparin-binding epidermal growth factor (HB-EGF) has been demonstrated to promote human blastocyst development significantly *in vitro*, in that blastocyst hatching rates double (45–80%), possibly through enhanced blastocyst expansion and/or by simulating preembryonic enzymes[25]. While human blastocysts do not express HB-EGF, it is expressed in the uterine endometrium and so may contribute to *in vivo* hatching success[26]. One must be prudent about adding these growth factors to culture media in clinical settings, however, as their effects may be harmful[27]. Interestingly, human blastocysts do not demonstrate remarkably higher rates of hatching when cocultured on endometrial cells, their rate of implantation after intrauterine transfer being higher than their rate of hatching *in vitro*[28].

After sperm entry into the oocyte, the zona pellucida hardens. This natural hardening helps to prevent polyspermy and serves to protect the developing preembryo. It has been speculated that the zona pellucida hardens spontaneously during *in vitro* culture, leading to impairment of blastocyst hatching[29]. To overcome this problem, various assisted hatching techniques have been developed (for review, see reference 30). Creating a slit in the zona pellucida of unfertilized oocytes by means of mechanical tearing was initially used to enhance fertilization for couples experiencing male factor infertility. However, after the creation of such a small and narrow opening, blastocysts were often observed to become trapped during subsequent hatching, leaving part inside and part outside[31]. This trapping phenomenon may be implicated as an occasional consequence of intracytoplasmic sperm injection (ICSI) as well (Figure 7.14). It is generally held that such an abnormal hatching process can split the inner cell mass and result in monozygotic twinning[32]. Therefore, acidic Tyrode's (AT) solution has been used for assisted hatching procedures in order to create a larger opening in the zonae of day-3 preembryos. The 15–20 μm opening this creates allows the blastocyst to hatch more freely (Figure 7.15). The consequences of AT treatment and a larger hole include: no thinning of the zona pellucida as the blastocoel enlarges, no blastocyst expansion and hatching occurring 1 day earlier than in controls. In addition, there is some evidence that these conceptuses implant slightly earlier than zona-intact ones[33]. Thus, the size of the opening and the method used to create it (mechanical vs. chemical) determine whether or not the zona pellucida thins during *in vitro* development and whether or not the resulting blastocyst expands (Figure 7.16). It has been

our experience that preembryos undergoing assisted hatching or biopsy on day 3 demonstrate premature hatching through a thick zona on day 5 (Figure 7.17). Blastocysts whose zonae have been manipulated in these ways demonstrate extrusion wherever an artificial hole has been made, taking a path of least resistance (Figure 7.18).

Initial reports of assisted hatching on day 3 followed by blastocyst transfer on day 5 demonstrate higher pregnancy and implantation rates compared to day 5 transfers with zona-intact blastocysts[34]. Patients with zona abnormalities, advanced maternal age, excessive cytoplasmic fragmentation or multiple previous failures have been suggested as candidates for this treatment combination[35]. However, these techniques often result in a smaller zona opening than after natural hatching, and therefore may result in abnormal hatching (Figure 7.19).

Blastocysts cultured *in vitro* can demonstrate a variety of problems including the inability to hatch and excessive expansion without hatching (Figure 7.20), resulting ultimately in their collapse and degeneration (Figure 7.21). One also sees variants of partial hatching wherein blastocysts fail to complete the process and subsequently arrest and die (Figure 7.22). Occasionally, hatching occurs at more than one site, probably associated with zona damage or multiple cracks brought on by freezing and thawing procedures (Figure 7.23). To eliminate hatching problems altogether, complete removal of the zona pellucida has been attempted at various stages[21]. This can be accomplished through global exposure to weak AT solution or by using pronase. The AT method is rarely used because of its potential toxicity. On the other hand, pronase is widely used, the length of exposure to it depending on zona pellucida thickness. At Cornell, expanded blastocysts are exposed to 10 IU/ml of pronase (Sigma, St. Louis, MO, USA) for no more than 1 min and then washed extensively (Figure 7.24). While treatment in this manner does not appear to interfere with subsequent development or implantation, longer exposure to pronase is extremely detrimental, bringing about trophectoderm blebbing, blastocyst collapse and extensive vacuolization after 5 min[36].

In summary, the human hatching process *in vitro* involves thinning and rupture of the zona pellucida, possibly mediated by preembryonic enzymes and certainly by blastocyst expansion, followed by complete zona shedding. *In vivo*, uterine enzymes probably play a complementary role.

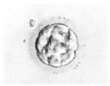

References

1. Moos J, Faundes D, Kopf GS, Schultz RM. Composition of the human zona pellucida and modifications following fertilization. *Hum Reprod* 1995;10:2467–71

2. Sacco AG, Yurewicz EC, Subraminian MG, DeMayo FJ. Zona pellucida composition: species cross reactivity and contraceptive potential of antiserum to a purified pig zona antigen (PPZA). *Biol Reprod* 1981;25:997–1008

3. Shabanowitz RB, O'Rand MG. Characterization of the human zona pellucida from fertilized and unfertilized eggs. *J Reprod Fertil* 1988;82:151–61

4. Hardy K, Handyside AH, Winston RM. The human blasto cyst: cell number, death and allocation during late preimplantation development *in vitro*. *Development* 1989;107:597–604

5. Schiewe MC, Araujo E Jr, Asch RH, Balmaceda JP. Enzymatic characterization of zona pellucida hardening in human eggs and embryos. *J Assist Reprod Genet* 1995;12:2–7

6. Wright G, Wiker S, Elsner C, *et al.* Observations on the morphology of pronuclei and nucleoli in human zygotes and implications for cryopreservation. *Hum Reprod* 1990;5:109–15

7. Chan PJ. Developmental potential of human oocytes according to zona pellucida thickness. *J In Vitro Fertil Embryo Transf* 1987;4:237–41

8. Perona RM, Wassarman PM. Mouse blastocysts hatch *in vitro* by using a trypsin-like proteinase associated with cells of mural trophectoderm. *Dev Biol* 1986;114:42–52

9. Yamazaki K, Suzuki R, Hojo E, *et al.* Trypsin-like hatching enzyme of the mouse blastocyst: evidence for its participation in the hatching process before zona shedding of embryos. *Dev Growth Differ* 1994;36:149–54

10. Wassarman PM. Profile of a mammalian sperm receptor. *Development* 1990;108:1–17

11. Schiewe MC, Hazeleger NL, Sclimenti C, Balmaceda JP. Physiological characterization of blastocyst hatching mechanisms by use of a mouse antihatching model. *Fertil Steril* 1995;63:288-94

12. Lin SP, Lee RK, Tsai YJ. *In vivo* hatching phenomenon of mouse blastocysts during implantation. *J Assist Reprod Genet* 2001;18:341–5

13. Thomas M, Jain S, Kumar GP, Laloraya M. A programmed oxyradical burst causes hatching of mouse blastocysts. *J Cell Sci* 1997;110:1597–602

14. Ansell JD, Snow MH. The development of trophoblast *in vitro* from blastocysts containing varying amounts of inner cell mass. *J Embryol Exp Morphol* 1975;33:117–85

15. Spindle AI, Pedersen RA. Hatching, attachment, and out growth of mouse blastocysts *in vitro*: fixed nitrogen requirements. *J Exp Zool* 1973;186:305–18

16. Gonzales DS, Jones JM, Pinyopummintr T, *et al.* Trophectoderm projections: a potential means for locomotion, attachment and implantation of bovine, equine and human blastocysts. *Hum Reprod* 1996;11:2739–45

17. Cheon YP, Gye MC, Kim CH, *et al.* Role of actin filaments in the hatching process of mouse blastocyst. *Zygote* 1999;7:123–9

18. Gonzales DS, Boatman DE, Bavister BD. Kinematics of trophectoderm projections and locomotion in the peri-implantation hamster blastocyst. *Dev Dyn* 1996;205:435–44

19. McRae AC, Church RB. Cytoplasmic projections of trophectoderm distinguish implanting from preimplanting and implantation-delayed mouse blastocytes. *J Reprod Fertil* 1990;88:31–40

20. Gonzales DS, Jones JM, Bavister BD, Shapiro SS. Human embryo development *in vitro*. *Hum Reprod Update* 1995;1(item 5: video)

21. Fong CY, Bongso A, Ng SC, Kumar J, Trounson A, Ratnam S. Blastocyst transfer after enzymatic treatment of the zona pellucida: improving *in-vitro* fertilization and understanding implantation. *Hum Reprod* 1998;13:2926–32

22. Dunglison GF, Barlow DH, Sargent IL. Leukaemia inhibitory factor significantly enhances the blastocyst formation rates of human embryos cultured in serum-free medium. *Hum Reprod* 1996;11:191–6

23. Harvey MB, Kaye PL. Insulin-like growth factor-1 stimulates growth of mouse preimplantation embryos *in vitro*. *Mol Reprod Dev* 1992;31:195–9

24. Sargent IL, Martin KL, Barlow DH. The use of recombinant growth factors to promote human embryo development in serum-free medium. *Hum Reprod* 1998;13 (Suppl 4):239–48

25. Martin KL, Barlow DH, Sargent IL. Heparin-binding epidermal growth factor significantly improves human blastocyst development and hatching in serum-free medium. *Hum Reprod* 1998;13:1645–52

26. Yoo HJ, Barlow DH, Mardon HJ. Temporal and spatial regulation of expression of heparin-binding epidermal

growth factor-like growth factor in the human endometrium: a possible role in blastocyst implantation. *Dev Genet* 1997;21:102–8

27. Hardy K, Spanos S. Growth factor expression and function in the human and mouse preimplantation embryo. *J Endocrinol* 2002;172:221–36

28. Mercader A, Simon C, Galan A, *et al*. An analysis of spontaneous hatching in a human endometrial epithelial coculture system: is assisted hatching justified? *J Assist Reprod Genet* 2001;18:315–19

29. De Vos A, Van Steirteghem A. Zona hardening, zona drilling and assisted hatching: new achievements in assisted reproduction. *Cells Tissues Organs* 2000;166:220–7

30. Zaninovic N. Assisted hatching and fragment removal. In Veeck LL, ed. *An Atlas of Human Gametes and Conceptuses: an Illustrated Reference for Assisted Reproductive Technology*. Carnforth, UK: Parthenon Publishing, 1999:86–96

31. Cohen J, Elsner C, Kort H, *et al*. Impairment of the hatching process following IVF in the human and improvement of implantation by assisting hatching using micromanipulation. *Hum Reprod* 1990;5:7–13

32. Van Langendonckt A, Wyns C, Godin PA, Toussaint-Demylle D, Donnez J. Atypical hatching of a human blastocyst leading to monozygotic twinning: a case report. *Fertil Steril* 2000;74:1047–50

33. Liu HC, Cohen J, Alikani M, Noyes N, Rosenwaks Z. Assisted hatching facilitates earlier implantation. *Fertil Steril* 1993;60:871–5

34. Graham MC, Hoeger KM, Phipps WR. Initial IVF–ET experience with assisted hatching performed 3 days after retrieval followed by day 5 embryo transfer. *Fertil Steril* 2000;74:668–71

35. Sagoskin AW, Han T, Graham JR, Levy MJ, Stillman RJ, Tucker MJ. Healthy twin delivery after day 7 blastocyst transfer coupled with assisted hatching. *Fertil Steril* 2002;77:615–17

36. Fong CY, Bongso A, Sathananthan H, Ho J, Ng SC. Ultrastructural observations of enzymatically treated human blastocysts: zona-free blastocyst transfer and rescue of blastocysts with hatching difficulties. *Hum Reprod* 2001;16:540–6

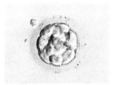

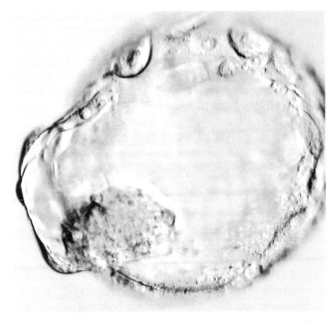

Figure 7.1 Initiation of hatching in a human blastocyst on day 6. The hatching site is very near the ICM; the TM is of poor quality (low cell number)

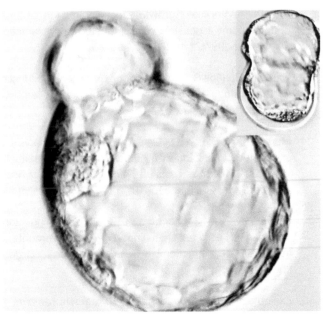

Figure 7.2 Initiation of hatching in a human blastocyst on day 6. In the human, the hatching site develops in close proximity to the ICM, while in the mouse hatching occurs in an area of the mural trophectoderm, opposite to the ICM (insert)

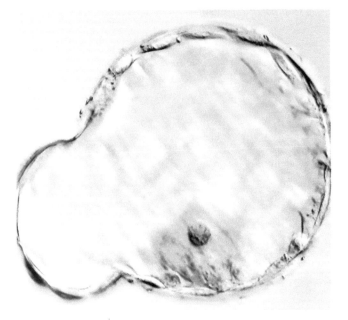

Figure 7.3 Hatching on day 7. The ICM is adjacent to the hatching site (ICM out of focus)

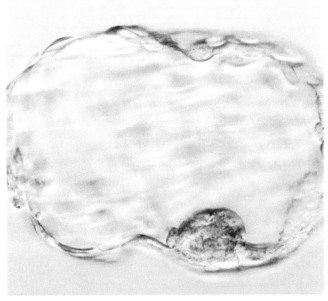

Figure 7.4 Hatching of the human blastocyst on day 6. The ICM is clearly visible at six o'clock, in close proximity to the hatching site. One-third to one-half of the thin zona pellucida (ZP) is opened during the hatching process

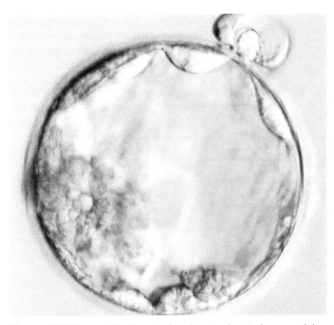

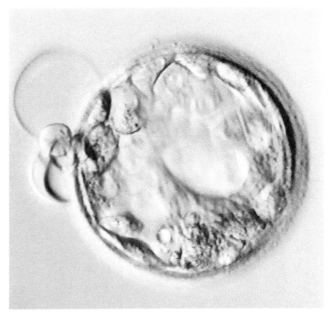

Figure 7.5 Human blastocyst showing trophectoderm vesicles (blebs) at a 1 o'clock position. These vesicles do not necessarily indicate the future hatching site and are frequently observed in ICSI-derived blastocysts (possible location of needle penetration for ICSI)

Figure 7.6 Trophectoderm vesicles in morphologically poor human blastocyst. An undeveloped ICM and TM can be seen. This blastocyst still possesses a somewhat thickened zona pellucida and is not yet ready to hatch. Such membrane protrusions do not indicate the onset of hatching

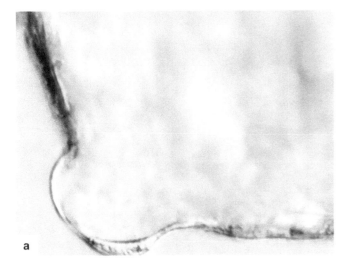

a

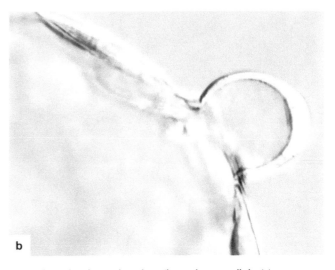

b

Figure 7.7 (a) and (b) Beginnings of the hatching process. The trophectoderm begins to herniate through a small, but true, opening (not a simple crack or vesicle breach). These blastocysts are fully expanded as indicated by their thin zona pellucidae

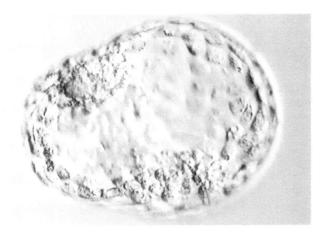

Figure 7.8 Human blastocyst in the process of hatching. The size of the opening is between one-third to one-quarter of the circumference of the zona pellucida. The ICM is closely associated with the hatching site

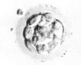

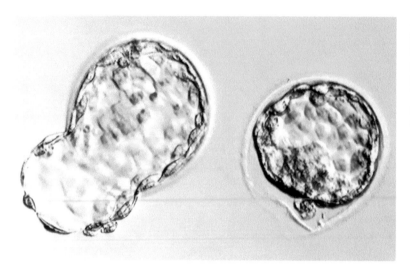

Figure 7.9 Two sibling human blastocysts in the process of hatching. The left blastocyst exhibits a large opening in the zona pellucida and subsequently escaped easily. The one to the right possesses an already ruptured zona pellucida at a 7 o'clock position; the blastocyst itself is in a slightly contracted state just before final expansion and escape

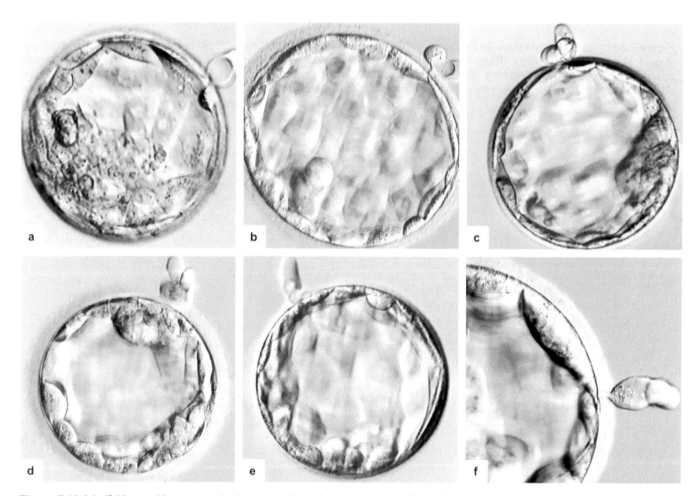

Figure 7.10 (a)–(f) Human blastocysts displaying small trophectoderm projections. These projections display amoeboid-like movement, suggesting they seek an implantation site. Their presence before hatching may represent the first contact between blastocyst and uterine lining. Trophectoderm projections are morphologically different to the vesicles and blebs seen in Figures 7.5 and 7.6

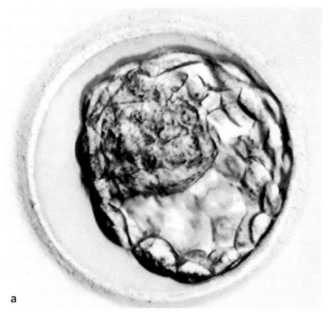
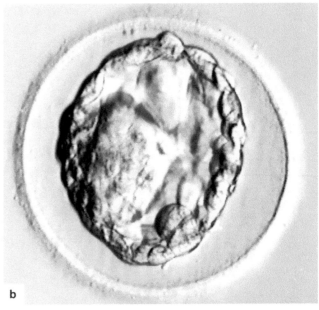

a b

Figure 7.11 (a) and (b) Human blastocysts showing partial collapse of the blastocoele. During collapse, the morphology of the ICM and TM remains unchanged. Collapse occurs frequently in *in vitro* cultured blastocysts, a process alternatively termed 'blastocyst breathing'

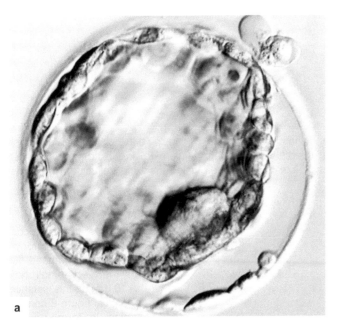
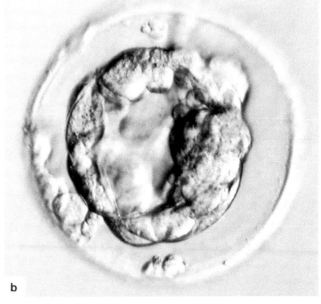

a b

Figure 7.12 (a) and (b) Partial collapse of the human blastocyst. The blastocyst is susceptible to environmental conditions (physical, chemical, temperature-related, or osmotic) and requires careful handling. Fragments inside the zona pellucida do not participate in blastocyst development

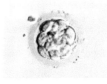

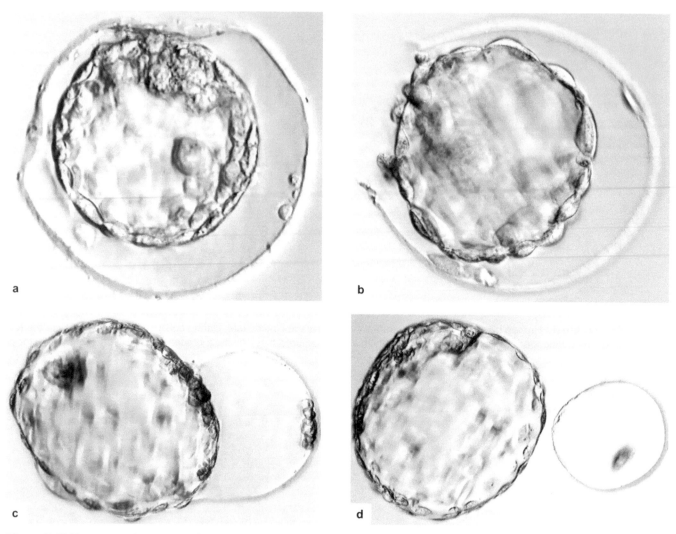

Figure 7.13 Blastocysts that collapsed, re-expanded, and subsequently hatched *in vitro*. (a) Collapsing blastocyst just before hatching; the zona pellucida is irregular at the hatching site (9 o'clock); (b) partial collapse before final extrusion. Note the large hatching opening; (c) blastocyst in the last stage of the hatching process. Note fragments left inside the zona pellucida; (d) hatched blastocyst. Note the increase in blastocyst size once free

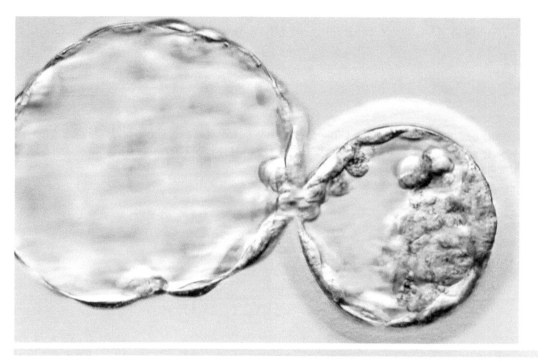

Figure 7.14 ICSI-derived blastocyst in the process of hatching. Blastocyst can become trapped due to the very small hole (<10 μm). In this instance, a typical figure-8 configuration is formed which may lead to trapping or hatching delay

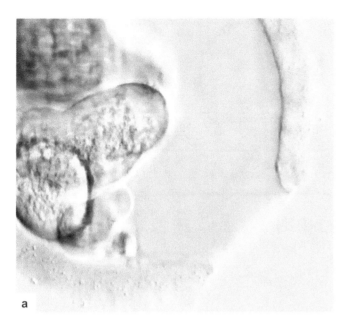
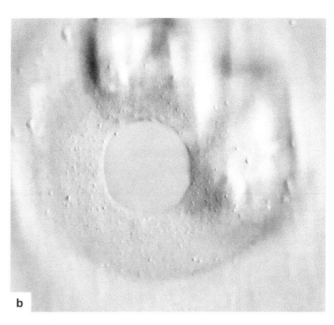

Figure 7.15 High-power magnification of a hole made through an assisted hatching (AHA) procedure. (a) Side view of the opening made with acidic Tyrode's solution; the round and very smooth hole was noted after blastocyst hatching. Note the large fragments remaining inside the zona pellucida; (b) frontal view of the opening. The size of the opening is between 15 and 20 µm

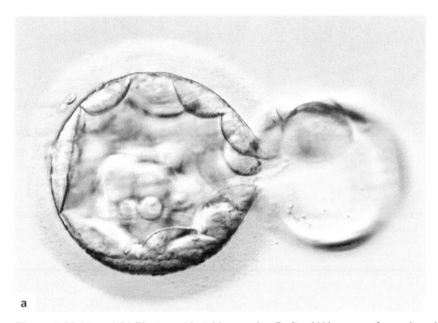
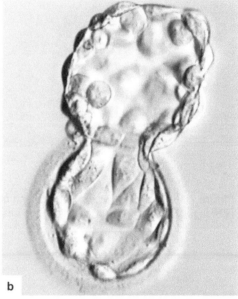

Figure 7.16 (a) and (b) Blastocyst hatching on day 5 after AHA was performed on day 3. No thinning of the zona pellucida occurred and blastocysts hatched earlier than usual

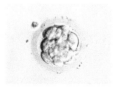

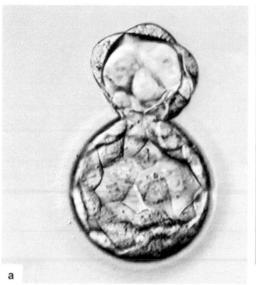
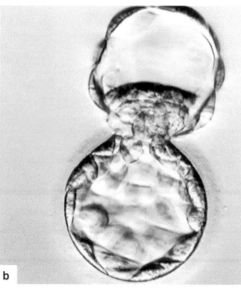

Figure 7.17 Blastocyst hatching on day 5 after blastomere biopsy for preimplantation genetic diagnosis on day 3. (a) Because an artificial hole was made, very little or no thinning of the zona pellucida occurred, resulting in the hatching of a non-expanded blastocyst; (b) in this case, the ICM was in the first section of the blastocyst to extrude through the biopsy hole

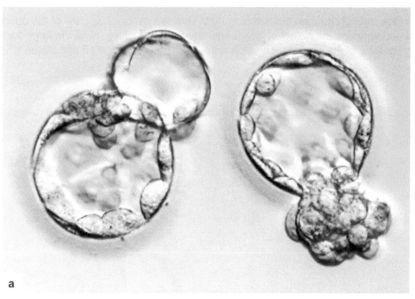
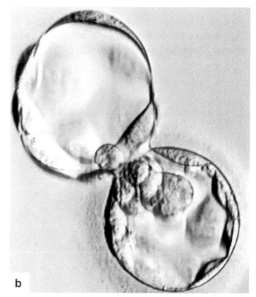

Figure 7.18 (a) and (b) Blastocyst hatching of zonae-manipulated preembryos. The blastocyst will hatch through artificially made openings in the zona pellucida, taking a course of least resistance. Zonae remain thick

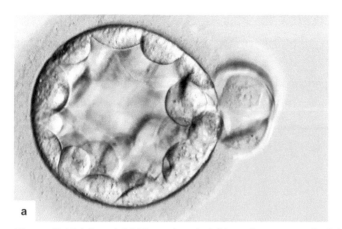
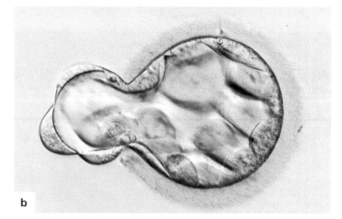

Figure 7.19 (a) and (b) Premature hatching of zonae-manipulated preembryos. Due to artificial openings in the zonae, undeveloped blastocysts will hatch passively as early as late on day 4. Cell numbers in the TM are low and ICM formations are unclear. These undeveloped blastocysts will be exposed prematurely to the uterine environment

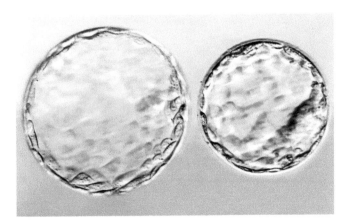

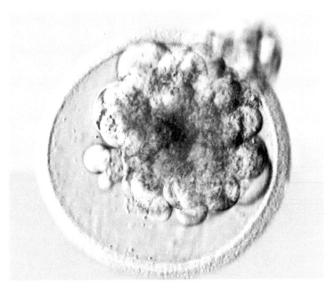

Figure 7.20 To the left, a very expanded human blastocyst on day 6 compared to a normally sized blastocyst to the right. The blastocyst to the left possesses an extremely thin zona pellucida without displaying any evidence of impending hatching (no rupture sites, no trophectoderm projections, not even trophectoderm vesicles). Unfortunately, these types of blastocysts often collapse and perish within their zonae, an indication for proactive zona pellucida removal

Figure 7.21 Collapsed human blastocyst on day 7 showing degenerative changes in morphology. Inability to hatch completely resulted in blastocyst death

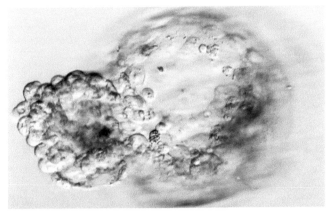

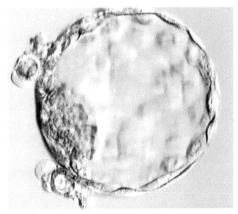

Figure 7.22 Human blastocyst that failed to complete hatching. Cells both outside and inside the zona pellucida show signs of impending degeneration

Figure 7.23 Human blastocyst showing multiple blebbing sites due to cracks in the zona pellucida. This can occur after freezing and thawing procedures

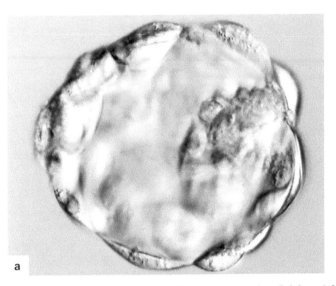

a

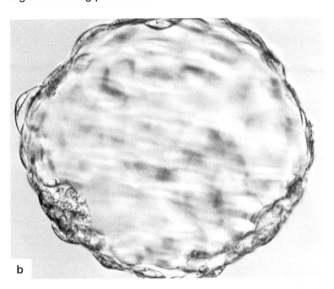

b

Figure 7.24 (a) and (b) Human blastocysts on day 5 (a) and 6 (b) after enzymatic zona pellucida removal using pronase for 1 minute. These blastocysts are suitable for either replacement or freezing and often result in live births

8 Blastocyst cryopreservation and thawing

Blastocysts have the advantage of possessing many cells. The loss of a few during freezing and thawing procedures will not compromise the integrity of the entire specimen. This may be one reason why blastocysts have been frozen and thawed so successfully over the years in domestic animals for both research and commercial purposes. Blastocyst cryopreservation in the human was first reported by Cohen and colleagues in 1985 using glycerol in a series of ten increasing concentrations[1]. Following that initial report, blastocyst freezing was only occasionally incorporated into clinical protocols because of the difficulties involved with maintaining high rates of blastocyst development *in vitro*.

Eighteen years have passed since that first thawed human blastocyst led to the birth of a child, and it is 20 years since the very first pregnancy from a thawed human preembryo was reported in the world[2]. During this time, most IVF programs have embraced cryobiology in order to augment clinical pregnancy from a single ovarian stimulation attempt. As ovulation-induction protocols have improved, allowing the recruitment of multiple healthy oocytes, so the need has grown to manage their numbers responsibly. It is usual today to harvest in excess of ten, or sometimes even 20, mature oocytes from a woman. Before freezing techniques were routinely used in the laboratory, a woman producing so many gametes would be forced either to limit the number inseminated or to risk having to discard healthy preembryos, since only three or four could be transferred safely to the uterus after fertilization. Neither was an attractive option. It is now apparent that pregnancy after thawing is nearly equal to the transfer of fresh preembryos, at least in some programs. When the cumulative effect of adding thawed pregnancies (only from cycles failing to become pregnant following fresh transfer) to fresh pregnancies is examined, delivery outcomes are significantly enhanced[3]. Additionally, patients at risk of ovarian hyperstimulation syndrome (OHSS) may be managed effectively by freezing all conceptuses up front, thereby reducing, although not eliminating, the likelihood of adverse clinical symptoms if a pregnancy is established[4].

The availability of sequential media has led to an increase in the practice of blastocyst freezing. Several groups have reported freezing blastocysts quite successfully, some of the earliest investigations using coculture systems to support preembryo growth[1,5,7]. Until the mid-1990s, most reports of clinical pregnancy after thawing fell in the range of 10–20% per transfer[8], results that were not significantly better as compared to thawing earlier stages. This situation has changed dramatically, and now pregnancy rates in the range of 40–60% are common for thawed blastocysts.

Cryobiology and the blastocyst

The primary goal in establishing an appropriate freezing protocol is to do as little damage as possible while exposing blastocysts to non-physiological ultralow temperatures. Popular protocols essentially *freeze-dry* or dehydrate blastocysts to prevent intracellular ice from forming.

The formation of intracellular ice crystals can mechanically damage specimens by disrupting and displacing organelles, or slicing through membranes. This is why freezing techniques use cryoprotective agents and

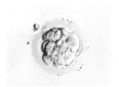

control ice formation at critical temperatures. It has been shown that when human cells are placed into a medium that contains an intracellular cryoprotective agent, intracellular water readily exits the cell as a result of the higher extracellular concentration of cryoprotectant. This causes some cell shrinkage until osmotic equilibrium is reached by the slower diffusion of the cryoprotectant into the cell[9]. Once equilibrium is reached, the cell resumes a normal appearance. The rate of permeation of cryoprotectant and water is dependent on temperature; equilibrium is achieved faster at higher temperatures. For this reason, we have chosen to add blastocysts to cryoprotective media containing glycerol and sucrose at room temperature. However, some cryoprotectants like dimethylsulfoxide (DMSO) are toxic at elevated concentrations, and must be used at lower temperatures to reduce adverse effects.

Cryoprotectants are also beneficial in their ability to lower the freezing point of a solution. Solutions may remain unfrozen at -5°C to -15°C because of *supercooling* (cooling to well below the freezing point without extracellular ice formation). When solutions supercool, cells do not dehydrate appropriately since there is no increase in osmotic pressure from the formation of extracellular ice crystals. To prevent supercooling, an ice crystal is introduced in a controlled fashion in a process call *seeding*. This contributes to intracellular dehydration as water leaves the cell to achieve equilibrium with the extracellular environment[9,10]. If the rate of cooling is too rapid, water cannot pass quickly enough from the cell, and as the temperature continues to drop, it reaches a point when the intracellular solute concentration is not high enough to prevent the formation of ice crystals. Blastocysts, which hold substantial intracellular water, are usually cooled at slow rates below the seeding temperature (0.3°C/min) to permit adequate dehydration.

Membrane permeability by cryoprotectants varies between developmental stages. As such, it has been found that some cryoprotective agents are more suitable for blastocyst freezing than others. While DMSO and 1,2 propanediol (PROH) are frequently used for freezing early cleavage stage preembryos, propylene glycol (glycerol) is commonly used for blastocysts. All three intracellular agents have fairly small molecules that permeate cell membranes easily. In addition to these, there are several extracellular substances that help dehydrate and protect cells. The most frequently used is sucrose, which possesses large, non-permeating molecules and exerts an osmotic effect to aid in accelerated cell dehydration. Sucrose cannot be used alone but is often used in conjunction with standard permeating, intracellular cryoprotectants.

During the freezing procedure, all chemical reactions within cells should be suspended. Under extremely cold liquid nitrogen storage conditions (-196°C), it is estimated that it would take hundreds of years before background ionizing radiation could cause significant damage to stored cells.

If cooling is terminated at relatively high temperatures (> -35°C), cells carry more intracellular ice than if cooled longer to lower temperatures (≤ -80°C). In order to protect cells, thawing must be carried out rapidly to induce rapid ice dispersal. Conversely, samples cooled to ≤ -80°C should be thawed more slowly to allow for gradual rehydration[11]. If water re-enters cells too rapidly, they may swell or burst. It is common to expose frozen specimens to progressively lower dilutions of cryoprotectant to ensure that it is slowly and gently removed.

Vitrification

The idea behind vitrification is to protect cells by completely avoiding all ice crystal formation. To accomplish this, cryoprotective solutes must be increased to 40% (wt/vol) or higher. DMSO is frequently used, but PROH, propylene glycol, ethylene glycol and other agents have been tested. Because high concentrations of these cryoprotectants are toxic at room temperature, blastocysts are generally exposed to them at 0°C. Samples may be plunged directly into liquid nitrogen without needing to introduce a seed; the viscosity is so great that solutions solidify into glasslike states. Vitrified specimens must be thawed in ice water, which is fairly inconvenient[12-14]. Although the procedure has been slow to gain acceptance for routine human blastocyst cryopreservation, several live births have recently been reported[15-19]. One novel modification to standard vitrification techniques has been to reduce the fluid content within the blastocoel before freezing[19]. Because the authors noted that the efficiency of their standard technique was negatively correlated to the expansion of the blastocoel, they postulated that ice crystal formation was damaging blastocysts during the cooling process. They then artificially reduced the blastocoelic volume before freezing by inserting a needle into the cavity until contraction occurred. Using this method, survival rates were much improved over those of controls, pregnancy rates showed a positive trend and implantation rates were significantly higher.

Slow freezing and thawing techniques

Most blastocyst freezing protocols employed today are based on the original work of Yves Menezo and co-workers, and use glycerol and sucrose as cryoprotectants[20,21]. The basic protocols for blastocyst freezing and thawing used by the Cornell program are illustrated in Figures 8.1 and 8.2. These are modifications of the original Menezo two-step protocols, amended in several ways to fit our current needs. Modifications include:

(1) Substitution of the same base medium as is used in our phase I sequential formulation, except that it is HEPES buffered;

(2) Addition of extra macromolecules (protein) in the form of 0.5 g/l human serum albumin (5% HSA solution) and 15% Plasmanate® (human plasma protein);

(3) Elevation of the freezing cryoprotectant concentration to 10%;

(4) Inclusion of several additional dilutions during the thawing process.

Frozen–thawed blastocysts are replaced in either natural or programmed cycles. Replacement regimes are detailed in Figures 8.3–8.6. Natural cycles are not supplemented with progesterone unless there is an overwhelming reason to do so, and all women are treated in a prophylactic manner for 4 days with antibiotics and corticosteroids.

Blastocyst expansion and contraction

Blastocysts with a high probability of survival after thaw act as perfect osmometers, shrinking, re-expanding and swelling in accordance with their osmotic environment[22]. One uneasy task immediately after thawing is to determine that a blastocyst has indeed survived, since it presents a contracted state for up to several hours after reincubation in standard culture medium (Figure 8.7). It has been our experience that blastocysts that shrink appropriately in response to cryoprotective agents and exhibit contracted, healthy-appearing cells after thaw do quite well in their ability to survive the rigors of freezing and thawing.

Zona-free blastocysts survive freezing and thawing without difficulty, indicating that the zona coat is not necessary for protective purposes during these procedures.

Pregnancy rates after blastocyst freezing and thawing

Of the many tribulations associated with running a cryopreservation program, one of the most frustrating is that embryologists cannot reap the fruits of their labor (pregnancy after thawing) until months or years have passed. It is common for patients to wait for some time before returning for a thawing attempt after a negative fresh cycle, or to delay 2 or more years after the birth of a child. This situation gives rise to special problems in tracking results during a given freezing period, and makes it difficult to identify the efficiency of a new protocol. Few reports have been published to date detailing the efficiency of blastocyst freezing after culture in sequential media. Langley and colleagues describe a comparison of day-3 versus blastocyst thawed transfer during a 30-month period[23]. In this study involving 72 thawed blastocyst cycles, the survival rate was higher for blastocysts as compared to preembryos and the implantation rate for blastocysts was doubled (21.9% vs. 10.1%). In 2002, Behr and associates reported a 36% clinical pregnancy rate and 16% implantation rate for thawed blastocysts from 64 cycles[24]. Given these few peer-reviewed reports, there may not be adequate evidence to support the concept that the blastocyst stage is optimal for freezing.

Nonetheless, the Cornell program has benefited greatly from the adoption of blastocyst freezing protocols. While acceptable clinical pregnancy rates in the range of 42% were realized after freezing and thawing cleavage stage preembryos in more than 800 cycles, much higher rates have been established using blastocysts (64%) without any concomitant drop in the number or proportion of patients having conceptuses frozen. Nearly one in four women under age 40 have had blastocysts frozen after undergoing day 3 transfers, and 60% of women undergoing day-5 transfers have had at least one blastocyst cryopreserved on day 5 or day 6. To date, 2000 blastocysts have been frozen. Less than one-fifth have been thawed, since so many of these patients became pregnant in their fresh cycles and have not yet returned to try for a second child.

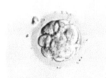

Most of the blastocysts frozen in the Cornell program are generated following the transfer of day-3 or day-5 conceptuses. After intrauterine transfer, remaining viable preembryos are examined each day for 1–3 additional days to evaluate their suitability for freezing. We have termed this the *post-transfer observation* period. Blastocysts forming on either day 5 (at least one grade 1BB) or day 6 (at least one grade 2BB) are cryopreserved for future use. Only rarely and under special circumstances have day-7 conceptuses been frozen.

The survival rate for thawed blastocysts in our program is very stable at 77%. Clinical pregnancy per cycle with blastocysts thawed and replaced is 64%; the ongoing or delivered rate is 54% and the implantation rate is 39%. Pregnancy rates are not different whether blastocysts are replaced in either natural or programmed cycles. Furthermore, pregnancy rates with blastocysts are stable across all maternal ages: 14/21 women (67%) over the age of 40 have established clinical pregnancies, although their miscarriage rate is more than double that observed for younger women (24% miscarriage, 43% ongoing).

Are there differences in the reproductive potentials of blastocysts frozen on day 5 and day 6?

It is generally assumed that blastocysts that develop in a timely manner *in vitro* are of better quality than those that develop more slowly. However, a retrospective review of blastocyst thaw outcomes from Cornell demonstrates otherwise. In our program, blastocysts have been frozen on either day 5 or day 6 depending on their speed of growth *in vitro*. Day-5 frozen blastocysts are thawed the day before transfer, while day-6 blastocysts are thawed in the morning when transfer is carried out.

We analyzed pregnancy outcomes in 84 patients returning for thawed blastocysts over a 2-year period. Thirty-nine patients received a transfer from day-5 frozen–thawed blastocysts and 45 patients underwent transfer with day-6 blastocysts. There were no significant group differences in patient age (34.0 vs. 34.8 years, respectively), average number of blastocysts transferred (2.3 vs. 2.0) or morphology of the blastocysts after thawing. No significant differences were found in the post-thaw survival rates (73.4% vs. 80.5%), clinical pregnancy rates (63.2% vs. 63.4%) or ongoing pregnancy rates (55.3% vs. 53.7%). Nor were differences observed in implantation rates (39.8% vs. 39.5%).

While it is more logical to assume that preembryos reaching the blastocyst stage faster (day 5) will be 'healthier' than their day-6 counterparts, these data and the data of others suggest that rate of development may not be crucial to subsequent post-thaw success[24]. Surprisingly, this is in direct conflict to reports of fresh transfer using day-5 and day-6 blastocysts, where pregnancy rate is observed to be significantly higher with faster-growing conceptuses[25]. Also, in contrast to our work, Marek and colleagues carried out a similar study, comparing outcomes from 127 thawed blastocyst cycles where blastocysts were frozen on day 5 or day 6[26]. Survival rates post-thawing were good for both groups, but the clinical pregnancy rate per thaw (50% vs. 29%, respectively), ongoing pregnancy rate per thaw (43% vs. 23%) and implantation rate (34% vs. 15%) were all significantly lower for day-6 blastocysts, a result quite different from what we describe.

Children born following cryopreservation and thawing

Cryopreservation has no apparent negative impact on perinatal outcome and does not appear to affect adversely the growth or health of children during infancy and early childhood[27]. The available data indicate that there is no elevation in the congenital malformation rate for children born after freeze–thaw procedures[28–30]. While it remains unclear whether freezing poses long-term risks to children so conceived or whether the freezing of blastocysts poses any additional risks over earlier stages, there is no direct evidence to raise concern.

Freezing the isolated inner cell mass

It is entirely possible to isolate and freeze selectively the inner cell mass of the mouse blastocyst, a procedure that has been carried out successfully at Cornell for mouse stem cell research. In the human, an occasional blastocyst presents a healthy-appearing inner cell mass but an abnormal or degenerative trophectoderm that is clearly incapable of further development and therefore possesses no implantation potential (Figure 8.8). Whether or not the cells from these specimens are truly normal would require culture and analysis by a panel of metabolic and genetic testing procedures. Similar to this situation, an occasional thawed blastocyst will exhibit a completely degenerated trophectoderm while possessing a surviving inner cell mass (Figure 8.9). As there is no implantation potential for such blastocysts, should they not be made available for approved study? It is surely not more appropriate to discard these precious pluripotent cells rather than to grow them for potential therapeutic use.

Blastocysts before freezing and after thawing

Figure 8.10 shows blastocysts with degenerative features after thaw. Figures 8.11–8.14 depict blastocysts as they appeared before freezing and again after thawing. Subsequent pregnancy outcomes are detailed.

Thawed blastocysts known to implant

Figures 8.15–8.22 show thawed blastocysts that are associated with implantation success. Pregnancy outcomes are detailed.

References

1. Cohen J, Simons RF, Edwards RG, Fehilly CB, Fishel SB. Pregnancies following the frozen storage of expanding human blastocysts. *J In Vitro Fertil Embryo Transf* 1985;2:59–64

2. Trounson A, Mohr L. Human pregnancy following cryopreservation, thawing and transfer of an eight-cell embryo. *Nature (London)* 1983;305:707–9

3. Veeck LL, Amundson CH, Brothman LJ, *et al*. Significantly enhanced pregnancy rates per cycle through cryopreservation and thaw of pronuclear stage oocytes. *Fertil Steril* 1993;59:1202–7

4. Queenan JT Jr, Veeck LL, Toner JP, Oehninger S, Muasher SJ. Cryopreservation of all prezygotes in patients at risk of severe hyperstimulation does not eliminate the syndrome, but the chances of pregnancy are excellent with subsequent frozen–thaw transfers. *Hum Reprod* 1997;12:1573–6

5. Hartshorne GM, Elder K, Crow J, Dyson H, Edwards RG. The influence of *in-vitro* development upon post-thaw survival and implantation of cryopreserved human blastocysts. *Hum Reprod* 1991;6:136–41

6. Kaufman RA, Menezo Y, Hazout A, Nicollet B, DuMont M, Servy EJ. Cocultured blastocyst cryopreservation: experience of more than 500 transfer cycles. *Fertil Steril* 1995;64:1125–9

7. Menezo YJ, Ben Khalifa M. Cytogenetic and cryobiology of human cocultured embryos: a 3-year experience. *J Assist Reprod Genet* 1995;12:35–40

8. Freitas S, Le Gal F, Dzik A, *et al*. Value of cryopreservation of human embryos during the blastocyst stage. *Contracept Fertil Sex* 1994;22:396–401

9. Mazur P. Freezing of living cells: mechanisms and implications. *Am J Physiol* 1984;247:C125–42

10. Whittingham DG. Some factors affecting embryo storage in laboratory animals. *Ciba Found Symp* 1977;52:97–127

11. Schneider U. Cryobiological principles of embryo freezing. *J In Vitro Fertil Embryo Transf* 1986;3:3–9

12. Friedler S, Shen E, Lamb EJ. Cryopreservation of mouse 2-cell embryos and ova by vitrification: methodologic studies. *Fertil Steril* 1987;48:306–14

13. Friedler S, Giudice LC, Lamb EJ. Cryopreservation of embryos and ova. *Fertil Steril* 1988;49:743–64

14. Quinn P, Kerin JF. Experience with the cryopreservation of human embryos using the mouse as a model to establish successful techniques. *J In Vitro Fertil Embryo Transf* 1986;3:40–5

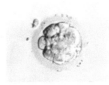

15. Choi DH, Chung HM, Lim JM, Ko JJ, Yoon TK, Cha KY. Pregnancy and delivery of healthy infants developed from vitrified blastocysts in an IVF–ET program. *Fertil Steril* 2000;74:838–9

16. Yokota Y, Sato S, Yokota M, *et al*. Successful pregnancy following blastocyst vitrification: case report. *Hum Reprod* 2000;15:1802–3

17. Yokota Y, Sato S, Yokota M, Yokota H, Araki Y. Birth of a healthy baby following vitrification of human blastocysts. *Fertil Steril* 2001;75:1027–9

18. Mukaida T, Nakamura S, Tomiyama T, Wada S, Kasai M, Takahashi K. Successful birth after transfer of vitrified human blastocysts with use of a cryoloop containerless technique. *Fertil Steril* 2001;76:618–20

19. Vanderzwalmen P, Bertin G, Debauche C, *et al*. Births after vitrification at morula and blastocyst stages: effect of artificial reduction of the blastocoelic cavity before vitrification. *Hum Reprod* 2002;17:744–51

20. Menezo Y, Nicollet B, Herbaut N, Andre D. Freezing cocultured human blastocysts. *Fertil Steril* 1992;58:977–80

21. Menezo YJ, Nicollet B, Dumont M, Hazout A, Janny L. Factors affecting human blastocyst formation *in vitro* and freezing at the blastocyst stage. *Acta Eur Fertil* 1993;24:207–13

22. Kaidi S, Donnay I, Lambert P, Dessy F, Massip A. Osmotic behavior of *in vitro* produced bovine blastocysts in cryoprotectant solutions as a potential predictive test of survival. *Cryobiology* 2000;41:106–15

23. Langley MT, Marek DM, Gardner DK, Doody KM, Doody KJ. Extended embryo culture in human assisted reproduction treatments. *Hum Reprod* 2001;16:902–8

24. Behr B, Gebhardt J, Lyon J, Milki AA. Factors relating to a successful cryopreserved blastocyst transfer program. *Fertil Steril* 2002;77:697–9

25. Shapiro BS, Richter KS, Harris DC, Daneshmand ST. A comparison of day 5 and day 6 blastocyst transfers. *Fertil Steril* 2001;75:1126–30

26. Marek DM, Langley MT, McKean C, Weiand L, Doody KM, Doody KJ. Frozen embryo transfer (FET) of day 5 blastocyst embryos compared to transfer of day 6 blastocyst embryos. *Fertil Steril* 2000;74 (Suppl 1):S52–3

27. Wennerholm UB, Albertsson-Wikland K, Bergh C, *et al*. Postnatal growth and health in children born after cryopreservation as embryos. *Lancet* 1998;351:1085–90

28. Wada I, Macnamee MC, Wick K, Bradfield JM, Brinsden PR. Birth characteristics and perinatal outcome of babies conceived from cryopreserved embryos. *Hum Reprod* 1994;9:543–6

29. Tarlatzis BC, Grimbizis G. Pregnancy and child outcome after assisted reproduction techniques. *Hum Reprod* 1999;14(Suppl 1):231–42

30. Wennerholm WB. Cryopreservation of embryos and oocytes: obstetric outcome and health in children. *Hum Reprod* 2000;15(Suppl 5):18–25

Blastocyst freezing

Planer biological freezer; freezing carried out in 10% glycerol/0.2 M sucrose in HEPES-based medium containing 0.5% HSA and 20% Plasmanate; use sterile 1.8 ml Nunc cryovials containing 0.3 ml freezing medium

- 5% glycerol solution for 10 min
- 10% glycerol/0.2 M sucrose solution for 10 min
- Load into cryovials
- Cool at rate of −2.0°C/min until −7.0°C
- Hold 5 min, manual seed, hold 10 min
- Continue cooling at −0.3°C/min until −38°C
- Plunge into liquid nitrogen

Figure 8.1 Blastocyst freezing protocol used in the Cornell program

Blastocyst thawing
30°C waterbath

- Thaw cryovial at room temperature for 60 s
- Warm cryovial in waterbath for 30–90 s (until all ice removed)
- 10% glycerol + 0.4 M sucrose for 30 s
- 5% glycerol + 0.4 M sucrose solution for 3 min
- 0.4 M sucrose solution for 3 min
- 0.2 M sucrose solution for 2 min
- 0.1 M sucrose solution for 1 min
- Wash well and incubate until transfer

Figure 8.2 Blastocyst thawing protocol used in the Cornell program

Natural cycle replacement

- Used for regular ovulatory cycles with normal luteal phase progesterone levels
- *Day 5 blastocysts:* Thaw 4 days after LH peak or 3 days after ovulation; transfer next day
- *Day 6 blastocysts:* Thaw 5 days after LH peak or 4 days after ovulation; transfer same day
- No supplemental progesterone unless indicated or after previous failure without supplementation
- Begin administering medrol and tetracycline on the day of the LH surge; continue for 4 days

Figure 8.3 Cornell replacement strategy for natural cycle thawed blastocyst transfer

Natural cycle replacement

Progesterone (if indicated):
200 mg micronized P4 vaginally b.i.d. or t.i.d.; continued until negative pregnancy test 14 days after replacement or through week 12 if pregnant (weaned down starting weeks 9–10)

Medrol:
16 mg/day for 4 days starting day of LH surge

Tetracycline:
250 mg q.i.d. for 4 days starting day of LH surge

Figure 8.4 Cornell replacement regimen for natural cycle thawed blastocyst transfer

Programmed replacement
(adequate suppression confirmed on day 2 of cycle)

- Luteal suppression with 0.2 mg GnRHa; drop to 0.1 mg starting on predetermined day 1 and maintain until day 15
- Transdermal estrogen patches:

Days 1–4   0.1 mg every other day

Days 5–8   0.2 mg every other day

Days 9–14   0.3–0.4 mg every other day (depending on E$_2$ levels)

Days 15+   0.2 mg (every other day until negative pregnancy test or for 7 weeks if pregnant)

- 50 mg P4 day 15 through 12 weeks gestation (weaned down starting week 9–10, depending on serum levels)
- Tetracycline + Medrol beginning day 15 for 4 days
Day 5 blastocysts: Thaw day 19, transfer next day
Day 6 blastocysts: Thaw day 20, transfer same day

Figure 8.5 Cornell replacement strategy for programmed cycle thawed blastocyst transfer

Programmed replacement

Estrogen patches:
Climara, 0.1 mg patch (every other day)

Progesterone:
50 mg/day i.m. beginning day 15; continued until negative pregnancy test or through week 12 if pregnant (weaned starting weeks 9–10)

Medrol:
16 mg/day for 4 days starting day 15

Tetracycline:
250 mg q.i.d. for 4 days starting day 15

Figure 8.6 Cornell replacement regime for programmed cycle thawed blastocyst transfer

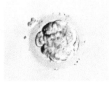

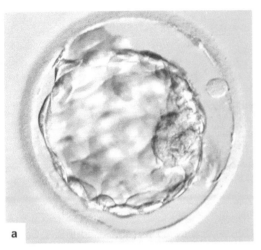
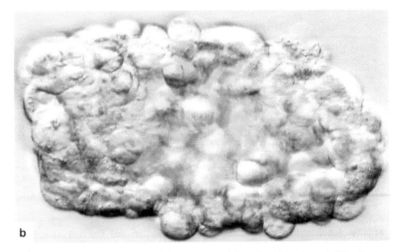

Figure 8.7 Thawed blastocysts. (a) Contracted blastocyst immediately after thawing; (b) contracted, hatched blastocyst 30 minutes after thawing

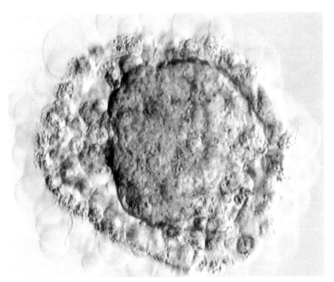

Figure 8.8 Non-surviving blastocyst exhibiting a degenerative trophectoderm immediately after thawing; inner cell mass appears viable

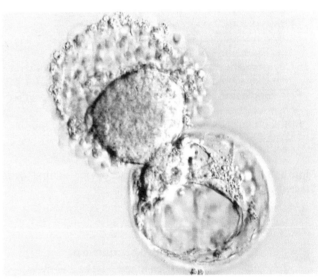

Figure 8.9 Viable and proliferating inner cell mass surrounded by a degenerating trophectoderm after thawing; the process of hatching is not completed and blastocyst appears trapped

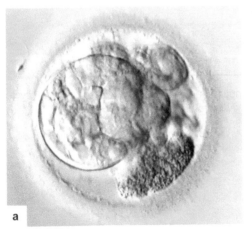
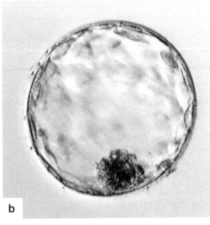

Figure 8.10 Degenerative features after thawing. (a) Contracted cavitating morula with degenerating fragments after thaw: (b) non-viable inner cell mass despite blastocoel re-expansion after thaw

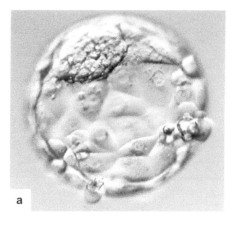
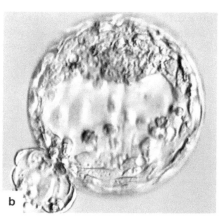

a

b

Figure 8.11 Before freezing and after thawing. Maternal age 39 years at time of freeze. (a) Expanded blastocyst immediately before freezing; (b) same blastocyst as in (a) after thawing 141 days later; membrane blebbing through the zona pellucida is seen, likely by virtue of subtle zona pellucida damage that occurred during thaw. This blastocyst was transferred, implanted, and a pregnancy with one fetal heart is on-going > 30 weeks

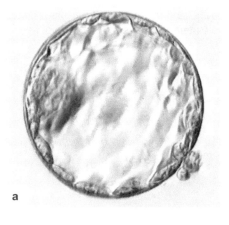
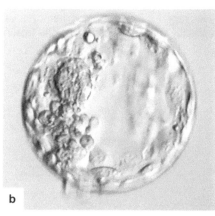

a

b

Figure 8.12 Before freezing and after thawing. Maternal age 31 years at time of freeze. (a) Expanded blastocyst immediately before freezing; (b) same blastocyst as in (a) after thawing 163 days later; inner cell mass appears intact but some cells of the trophecto-derm appear unhealthy. This blastocyst was transferred, implanted, but an early loss occurred after ultrasound evidence of one gestational sac

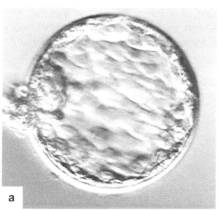
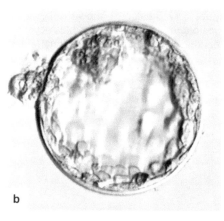

a

b

Figure 8.13 Before freezing and after thawing. Maternal age 22 years at time of freeze. (a) Expanded blastocyst immediately before freezing; prolifera-tive trophectoderm and smallish inner cell mass; (b) same blastocyst as in (a) after thawing 124 days later; most cells appear viable. This blastocyst was transferred, implanted, and a healthy male child was delivered at term

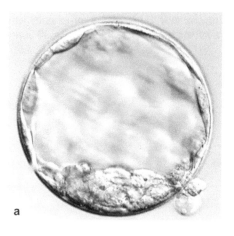
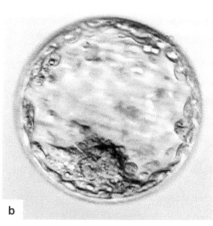

a

b

Figure 8.14 Before freezing and after thawing. Maternal age 37 years at time of freeze. (a) Expanded blastocyst immediately before freezing; inner cell mass is large and trophectoderm is sparse; (b) same blastocyst as in (a) after thawing 56 days later; most cells appear viable. This blastocyst was transferred, implanted, and a healthy female child was delivered. Note here that the blastocyst was thawed almost 1 full day before replacement and that the trophectoderm appears quite differ-ent after prolonged culture, being made up of many more cells

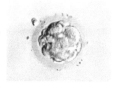

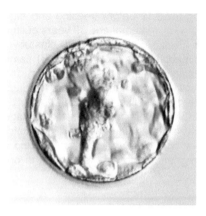

Figure 8.15 Blastocyst known to have implanted after freeze, thaw, and transfer. After cryostorage for 57 days, this blastocyst was thawed and led to the birth of a healthy female child. Maternal age 34 years at time of freeze

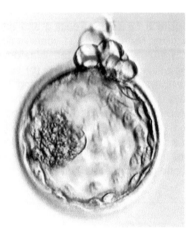

Figure 8.16 Blastocyst known to have implanted after freeze, thaw, and transfer. After cryostorage for 79 days, this blastocyst was thawed and transferred. A currently ongoing pregnancy was established with one fetal heart. Maternal age 26 years at time of freeze

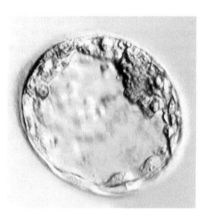

Figure 8.17 Blastocyst known to have implanted after freeze, thaw, and transfer. After cryostorage for 155 days, this blastocyst was thawed and transferred. A currently ongoing pregnancy was established with one fetal heart. Maternal age 41 years at time of freeze

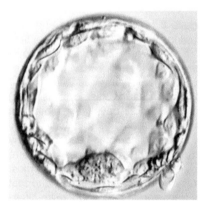

Figure 8.18 Blastocyst known to have implanted after freeze, thaw, and transfer. After cryostorage for 558 days, this blastocyst was thawed and transferred. A pregnancy was established with one fetal heart. One healthy male was delivered. Maternal age 30 years at time of freeze

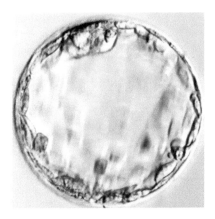

Figure 8.19 Blastocyst known to have implanted after freeze, thaw, and transfer. After cryostorage for 102 days, this blastocyst was thawed and transferred. A pregnancy was established with one fetal heart. One healthy female was delivered. Maternal age 34 years at time of freeze

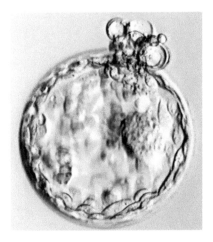

Figure 8.20 Blastocyst known to have implanted after freeze, thaw, and transfer. After cryostorage for 86 days, this blastocyst was thawed and transferred. A pregnancy was established with one fetal heart. One healthy male was delivered. Maternal age 39 years at time of freeze

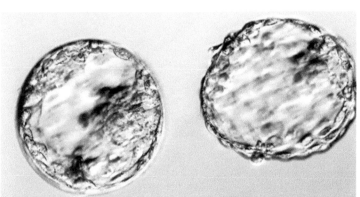

Figure 8.21 Two blastocysts known to have implanted after freeze, thaw, and transfer. After cryostorage for 84 days, these blastocysts were thawed and transferred. Two healthy male children were subsequently delivered. Maternal age 29 years at time of freeze

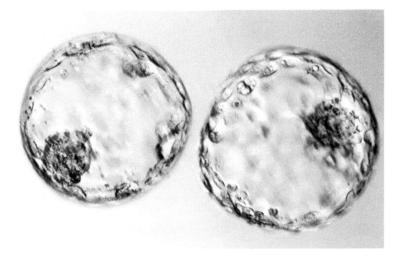

Figure 8.22 Two blastocysts known to have implanted after freeze, thaw, and transfer. After cryostorage for 68 days, these blastocysts were thawed and transferred. Two fetal hearts have been documented for this currently ongoing pregnancy. Maternal age 37 years at time of freeze

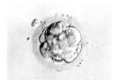

9 Cell death (apoptosis) in human blastocysts

Kate Hardy, Sophie Spanos and David L. Becker

INTRODUCTION

The orchestrated death of cells is fundamental for tissue and organ modelling during development[1-3]. Furthermore, the ability of cells to die without damaging adjacent cells is a vital component of the quality control and repair programs needed for maintaining healthy tissue. In this way, excess, damaged or unwanted cells can be safely and discreetly removed. These key concepts of developmental biology originated from a seminal article published in 1972 by Kerr and colleagues[4], who first observed and described the classic morphological features of this physiological mode of cell death, which they termed apoptosis.

Examples of developmental events that require extensive apoptosis include the sculpting of digits in the developing limb bud, and the removal of the Müllerian duct during development of the male[3]. During early rodent development, apoptosis plays a crucial role in amniotic cavity formation, soon after implantation[5]. Surprisingly, there is now increasing evidence that apoptosis occurs before implantation (for review, *see* reference 6).

Apoptotic nuclei have been seen in blastocysts from many mammalian species, including mouse[7-9], rat[10], cow[11-13], baboon[14], rhesus monkey[15-17] and human[11,18-22]. These dying cells are characterized by blebbing of the nuclear membrane, chromatin condensation, cytoplasmic vacuoles and the formation of both nuclear and cytoplasmic fragments.

APOPTOSIS

Morphological features of apoptosis

Cells can die either as a result of accidental injury or by design. Injury, such as physical trauma or ischemia, will result in the death of swathes of cells, which will undergo swelling and membrane rupture[2]. The cellular contents will spill into the extracellular spaces, invoking an inflammatory response in adjacent healthy tissue. This process is known as necrosis. However, cells also have mechanisms in place which allow them to control and contain their death, and to die without causing widespread chaos. Death by this mechanism is sufficiently neat and quick to be almost undetectable by classical histology, and it was only 30 years ago that the extent of this phenomenon, which came to be termed apoptosis, was recognized and described[4]. Apoptosis is the mechanism by which cells undergo a programmed and carefully orchestrated series of steps whereby the cellular contents are dismantled, packaged and disposed of, with no associated inflammation.

Apoptosis is characterized by a sequence of morphologically distinct phases, which distinguish it from necrosis (Figure 9.1). Apoptosis is heralded by cell rounding, indicating that changes in cell adhesion occur[2]. Initially, chromatin condenses into clumps on the inner nuclear membrane and the cytoplasm also condenses. The nuclear and cytoplasmic membranes become indented and the nucleus fragments. Finally, the whole cell blebs and fragments into membrane-bound apoptotic bodies, which may contain nuclear fragments. The production of membrane-bound apoptotic bodies prevents the release of intracellular contents from the

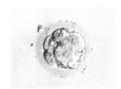

dying cell, which would result in damage to adjacent healthy cells and inflammation. These bodies are either dispersed in the intercellular tissue spaces and extruded from the tissue or phagocytosed by neighboring tissue cells. Apoptotic cells that are not phagocytosed, for example those shed from an epithelium into a duct lumen, undergo secondary necrosis. This classical sequence of events has been seen at the ultrastructural level in a wide variety of different cell types[2,23,24], and is under physiological control.

Regulation and execution of apoptosis

Apoptosis may result from activation of an endogenous developmental program, or be induced by a stimulus, such as DNA damage, cell surface ligand–receptor interactions, disruption of cell–cell or cell–matrix inter-actions, or growth factor deprivation. The signals that initiate apoptosis mediate their effects through distinct signal transduction pathways which trigger the apoptotic machinery via a variety of routes, but which all have the same end point: the death of the cell.

The co-ordinated dismantling of a cell by apoptosis involves a large family of death proteases known as the caspases. All caspase proteins exist normally in healthy cells as inactive proenzymes, which require proteolysis for enzymatic activation. Activation of these caspases results in the death of the cell. Caspases can be broadly subdivided into two groups: initiator caspases (caspase 8 and caspase 9), whose main function is to activate downstream caspases, and effector caspases (such as caspases 3, 6 and 7), which are responsible for dismantling cellular proteins critical for cell survival, including those involved in the cytoskeleton, DNA repair, nuclear envelope integrity and cell cycle control[23]. The activation of effector caspases results in the apoptotic morphology observed in cells, including the formation of fragmented nuclei and apoptotic bodies[25]. Effector caspases also activate endonucleases, resulting in the cleavage of DNA between nucleosomes into oligonucleosomal fragments[2,26,27].

The other major regulators of apoptosis are the bcl-2 family of mitochondrial proteins, various members of which promote (bad, bax, bak, bcl-x_s) and inhibit (bcl-2, bcl-w, bcl-x_L) apoptosis. It is thought that the ratio between pro- and antiapoptotic members determines whether the cell lives or dies[28]. The bcl-2 family is believed to regulate the release of proapoptotic factors

from mitochondria, which in turn leads to the activation of caspases[29].

Evidence for apoptosis in preimplantation embryos

The study of apoptosis in preimplantation human embryos is constrained by the limited number of embryos available for research, and in most studies the only embryos available are those which have arrested development or which are highly fragmented and unsuitable for cryopreservation. Furthermore, each embryo contains only between one and 100 or so cells. It is difficult to estimate the full extent of cell death in the mammalian embryo, as it is not known how long dead cells persist; therefore, current techniques provide only a 'snapshot' of the embryo at a specific time.

Historically, while it was evident from histological analysis that cell death was taking place in mammalian blastocysts, it was not clear whether the death was necrotic or apoptotic. As around 50% of human embryos fail to reach the blastocyst stage[22], and as the involvement of cell death in this developmental arrest is a possibility[30], the importance of understanding the causes and roles of these processes in the human embryo cannot be underestimated.

Membrane changes

Early apoptotic events involve changes in the cell membrane, which are controlled by initiator caspases. These include modifications of the plasma membrane itself, and alterations in the cytoskeleton leading to aberrant membrane behavior such as blebbing (reviewed in reference 31).

An early event of apoptosis is a redistribution of the phospholipid phosphatidylserine in the cell membrane. In healthy cells, phosphatidylserine is normally confined to the inner cytoplasmic leaflet of the membrane. In apoptotic cells this asymmetry is lost, with exposure of phosphatidylserine on the outer leaflet[32]. Annexin V (an anticoagulant protein) has a specific and high affinity for phosphatidylserine, and labelled annexin V is a classical marker for externalized phosphatidylserine, indicative of the early stages of apoptosis.

Annexin V labelling has been examined in early human embryos and oocytes[33–35], with conflicting results. Levy and colleagues[33] found extensive labelling in arrested and fragmented human embryos. However, the nuclei in these embryos also labelled with propidium iodide, indicating that the plasma membrane was permeable. Therefore, it was probable that these arrested embryos were undergoing secondary necrosis. In contrast, Antczak and Van Blerkom[35] found no annexin V or propidium iodide labelling in cleavage-stage human embryos with varying degrees of fragmentation, strongly suggesting that there is no correlation between fragmentation and apoptosis.

Video time-lapse cinematography is a useful tool for observing the kinetics of apoptosis. Using this technique, violent membrane blebbing in trophectoderm and inner cell mass cells over a time period of up to 1 h, followed by rupture of the cell and its contents into the blastocoel cavity, have been observed (Figure 9.2). Similar cytoplasmic blebbing has been seen in other cell types undergoing apoptosis using time-lapse cinematography[23,36]. In addition, small cytoplasmic blebs have been seen on the surface of the inner cell mass (e.g. Figure 9.3), which may either reflect these early membrane events, or be the final products of apoptosis in these cells.

Chromatin condensation

The earliest morphological change indicative of apoptosis, which in fact is a late event within the apoptosis cascade, is the condensation of chromatin on the inner nuclear membrane. Initially, this was detected by transmission electron microscopy in mouse embryos[7] and later in human embryos[20,37]. More recently, nuclei with clumped or condensed chromatin have been visualized in arrested cleavage stage embryos[33,38] and human blastocysts using propidium iodide or Hoescht staining and standard fluorescence microscopy[19] or laser scanning confocal microscopy[39] (Figures 9.4–9.8).

Condensed nuclei

With the same approach of labelling DNA, condensed and misshapen nuclei have been seen in fragmented arrested[20,33] and developing[21] human embryos. These may be precursors of fragmented nuclei (*see below*).

Nuclear fragmentation

Nuclear fragmentation, which is perhaps the most classical morphological feature of apoptosis, has been observed in human embryos using a variety of techniques. Fragmented nuclei have been described in paraffin-embedded sections of human embryos *in vivo*[40], providing unique evidence that apoptosis occurs *in vivo* during preimplantation human development. Fragmenting nuclei have also been visualized by fluorescence microscopy of blastocysts labelled with DNA-specific fluorochromes[19]. Apoptotic nuclei in both the trophectoderm and the inner cell mass can be identified as discrete clusters of fluorochrome-labelled nuclear fragments, which are smaller than intact healthy nuclei (Figures 9.7 and 9.8). More recently, confocal microscopy has allowed clear identification and quantification of fragmented nuclei at high resolution in human blastocysts[21,22] (Figures 9.9–9.11).

DNA fragmentation

Another classical feature of apoptosis is the degradation of DNA into oligonucleosomal fragments. The small numbers of cells in preimplantation embryos do not allow the use of electrophoretic techniques to look for DNA laddering typical of apoptotic nuclei. However, the development of terminal deoxynucleotidyl transferase-mediated dUTP nick-end labelling (TUNEL)[41] allows the assessment of nuclear DNA fragmentation *in situ*. This technique can be used on specimens with only a few cells, and is based on the fluorescent labelling of the 3' end of oligonucleosome fragments. This technique has the additional advantages of allowing both the localization and the quantification of the percentage of nuclei with DNA fragmentation[41].

The enzyme terminal deoxynucleotidyl transferase (TdT) binds to exposed 3'-OH ends of DNA single-strand breaks and catalyzes the addition of labelled deoxynucleotides that have been labelled with a marker such as fluorescein isothiocyanate (FITC), in which case TUNEL-positive nuclei will be clearly seen using fluorescent microscopy or laser scanning confocal microscopy (Figures 9.10–9.17).

Positive labelling of fragmented nuclei has been observed in arrested[20,33] and fragmented[42] cleavage-stage human embryos, and in human blastocysts[21,22], providing evidence that DNA is being degraded into oligonucleosomal fragments.

Where TUNEL labelling has been seen in arrested embryos, it is possible that DNA degradation is occurring in cells undergoing the early stages of secondary necrosis, rather than apoptosis.

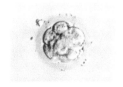

Certainly secondary necrotic changes with disrupted membranes and swollen organelles have been observed in cytoplasmic fragments[37]. During 'normal' development of non-arrested embryos *in vitro*, DNA fragmentation is only seen at the blastocyst stage in mice[43], after compaction in human embryos[22] and after the 8-cell stage in cow embryos[13].

Condensed cytoplasm

Condensed cytoplasm has been observed by transmission electron microscopy in arrested embryos[20,37,42].

Changes in expression of genes involved in regulation and execution of apoptosis

The classical morphological changes associated with apoptosis, including nuclear fragmentation, are a consequence of the action of active caspases, which in turn are regulated, at least in part, by the bcl-2 family of proteins.

Expression of mRNA and protein for members of the caspase and bcl-2 families of genes in preimplantation embryos have been studied using reverse transcriptase-polymerase chain reaction (RT-PCR) and immunohisto-chemistry, providing information about the timing of gene expression. Studies in mouse preimplantation embryos have shown that preimplantation oocytes and embryos of all stages express the relevant molecular machinery to undergo apoptosis[44,45]. In addition to members of the bcl-2 family, caspase expression has been detected in mouse embryos throughout preimplantation development[45]. Quantitative RT-PCR has been used to detect increased expression of bax mRNA in mouse embryos exposed to high glucose concentrations in the culture medium[46].

In human preimplantation embryos, mRNA for bax, bcl-2 and bad has also been detected by RT-PCR[47,48]. In addition, bax, bcl-2, bcl-x and bcl-w protein has been detected in human embryos using immunohisto-chemistry[35,39,48,49] (Figures 9.18 and 9.19).

The presence of active caspases within cells indicates that the execution phase of the apoptotic cascade is under way. Detection of active caspases currently involves the use of fluorescently tagged specific caspase inhibitors that bind only to active caspases. The cytoplasm of cells which contain active caspases, and are undergoing apoptosis, is fluorescently labelled. Healthy cells remain unlabelled. Using this approach, active caspases have not been detected in arrested or developing cleavage-stage human embryos, but have been seen in some (but not all) fragments[48,50]. However, following compaction, individual cells with cytoplasmic labelling for active caspases have been seen in morulae and blastocysts[48] (Figures 9.20 and 9.21). In particular, cells with fragmented nuclei are frequently positive for active caspases, suggesting that they play a role in the formation of the apoptotic morphology seen in human blastocysts.

Morphological changes

Excluded cells

The earliest events in apoptosis involve the cell membrane, with the apoptotic cell rounding up and separating from neighboring cells[23]. At the time of compaction and blastocyst formation, it is not uncommon to see excluded cells which lie between the developing embryo and the zona pellucida (Figures 9.22 and 9.23) or within the blastocoel cavity (Figure 9.24). Transmission electron microscopy and laser scanning confocal microscopy have often revealed extruded cells in the perivitelline space or blastocoel cavity[12,18].

Cytoplasmic fragmentation

Over 75% of human embryos generated following *in vitro* fertilization (IVF) have various degrees of cytoplasmic fragmentation (Figure 9.25). Fragmentation has also been seen in human embryos *in vivo*[40,51,52], indicating that fragmentation is not an *in vitro* artifact. Ultrastructural examination of fragmented embryos *in vitro* has shown that these membrane-bound fragments contain organelles and resemble apoptotic bodies[20,42]. The issue of whether cytoplasmic fragments are apoptotic bodies or not remains contentious, with no clear consensus. Some workers have shown that features of apoptosis are present in fragments; either fragmented DNA[20], active caspases[48,50] or ultrastructural features[20]. In contrast, others have failed to demonstrate either TUNEL labelling (indicating DNA fragmentation) or annexin V labelling (indicating phosphatidylserine redistribution in the plasma membrane)[35], leading these workers to postulate that fragmentation was not part of, or a consequence of, apoptosis.

It is not known how long fragments have been present, and whether they arose during the previous cleavage division or during earlier ones. If the fragments have persisted for some time it is possible that the DNA has fragmented during secondary necrosis. Furthermore, fragmentation is not inhibited by caspase inhibitors[53], providing further evidence that the mechanisms involved in fragment formation do not invariably involve apoptosis.

Cytoplasmic vacuoles

Translucent vacuoles are frequently associated with cytoplasmic condensation typical of cells undergoing apoptosis[2]. Vacuoles are a common feature of human preimplantation embryos and have been seen by light[38] (Figures 9.4 and 9.26), electron[7,54] and laser scanning confocal[38] microscopy.

Cell corpses

Cell corpses have been observed by transmission electron microscopy, lying between cells[11,37].

Phagocytosis

Further degeneration results in the formation of extracellular debris[2], with the presence of mitochondria and nuclear remnants confirming its cellular origin, for example, in arrested human embryos[20]. Confocal microscopy of human and cow blastocysts has shown cells being engulfed by neighboring cells[38,55] (Figure 9.27). Autophagic vacuoles have been seen at the ultrastructural level using transmission electron microscopy in human[11], cow[55], rhesus[16] and mouse blastocysts[7]. However, while it appears that many dead cells are cleared by phagocytosis within the blastocyst, other apparently arrested cells simply persist. In other cell types, apoptotic cells formed in single-layered epithelia may be extruded into lumina, and thus escape phagocytosis[2,24]. This process appears to occur in human blastocysts, with isolated cells being observed in the blastocoel cavity or between the trophectoderm and the zona pellucida[18,39] (Figures 9.22–9.24). These cells and fragments are excluded from normal development. These isolated cells in the blastocoel cavity have been shown to be TUNEL labelled[39], as have similar cells in mouse blastocysts[43]. In some cases, these cells are large, and this, coupled with the lack of intercellular junctions, poorly differentiated mitochondria and paucity of rough endoplasmic reticulum, suggests that these cells originated during early cleavage. It is possible that such cells lack cell surface markers which would promote their ingestion by neighboring cells, causing them to persist throughout preimplantation development.

Furthermore, cell corpses with condensed chromatin and cytoplasm were not phagocytosed[37].

Timing of apoptosis

In human embryos which are non-arrested and developing on schedule, apoptosis (as quantified by DNA and nuclear fragmentation) has not been seen in early cleavage stages[22,42]. Nuclear fragmentation was observed rarely before compaction and at increasing levels during blastocyst formation. TUNEL labelling was seen only after compaction, and the proportion of nuclei with DNA fragmentation increased during blastocyst formation to around 10%[22].

This is consistent with studies of rodent, bovine and porcine embryos, where apoptosis is not observed until the morula and blastocyst stages[9,10,12,43,56]. It has been proposed that upstream death inducers or downstream death effectors are either absent or suppressed during early cleavage stages[12]. As it has been shown that most components of the apoptotic machinery are present in mouse[44,45] and human[48] embryos throughout development, the most likely scenario is that apoptosis is suppressed during early cleavage stages.

Incidence of apoptosis

In the human blastocyst, cell death is present equally in the trophectoderm and the inner cell mass, with approximately 10% of nuclei in each lineage showing evidence of apoptosis. The incidence appears to be correlated with embryo quality, with embryos of poor morphology having higher levels of apoptosis[19].

Role of apoptosis

In addition to cell division and differentiation within the preimplantation embryo, it is now clear that cell death by apoptosis is common, even *in vivo*[9]. Within a blastocyst, the percentage of dying cells is sufficiently high (10–20%) to suggest that apoptosis is playing a developmental role, which has not yet been elucidated. It is possible that the higher levels of apoptosis seen in the inner cell mass of the mouse blastocyst are to remove cells that retain the potential to form trophectoderm[57], which could lead to ectopic expression of trophectoderm cells in the germ layers during later development. In addition, levels of apoptosis can be modulated by environmental factors. Apoptosis in preimplantation embryos is increased in suboptimal

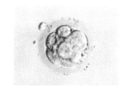

culture media[58], in the presence of high concentrations of glucose[46,59] and in the absence of specific growth factors[21,43,60,61]. Furthermore, apoptosis has been associated with increased levels of reactive oxygen species thought to result from high oxygen tension during culture[42], exposure to high concentrations of sperm during human IVF and increased maternal age[62]. Finally, nuclear[63] and chromosomal[64,65] abnormalities are common in human embryos, and it has been suggested

that one role of apoptosis may be to remove such defective cells[6].

In conclusion, apoptosis occurs in human embryos following compaction. The reasons for certain cells undergoing apoptosis are unclear, the role during preimplantation development remains unknown and the early signalling events that trigger apoptosis require elucidation.

References

1. Glücksmann A. Cell death in normal development. *Arch Biol* 1965;76:419–37

2. Wyllie AH, Kerr JF, Currie AR. Cell death: the significance of apoptosis. *Int Rev Cytol* 1980;68:251–306

3. Meier P, Finch A, Evan G. Apoptosis in development. *Nature (London)* 2000; 407:796-801

4. Kerr JF, Wyllie AH, Currie AR. Apoptosis: a basic biological phenomenon with wide-ranging implications in tissue kinetics. *Br J Cancer* 1972;26:239–57

5. Coucouvanis E, Martin GR. Signals for death and survival: a two-step mechanism for cavitation in the vertebrate embryo. *Cell* 1995;83:279–87

6. Hardy K. Cell death in the mammalian blastocyst. *Mol Hum Reprod* 1997;3:919–25

7. El-Shershaby AM, Hinchliffe JR. Cell redundancy in the zona-intact preimplantation mouse blastocyst: a light and electron microscope study of dead cells and their fate. *J Embryol Exp Morphol* 1974;31:643–54

8. Copp AJ. Interaction between inner cell mass and trophectoderm of the mouse blastocyst. I. A study of cellular proliferation. *J Embryol Exp Morphol* 1978;48:109–25

9. Handyside AH, Hunter S. Cell division and death in the mouse blastocyst before implantation. *Roux's Arch Dev Biol* 1986;195:519–26

10. Pampfer S, De Hertogh R, Vanderheyden I, Michiels B, Vercheval M. Cell allocation to the inner cell mass and the trophectoderm in rat embryos during *in vivo* preimplantation development. *Roux's Arch Dev Biol* 1990;198:257–63

11. Mohr LR, Trounson AO. Comparative ultrastructure of hatched human, mouse and bovine blastocysts. *J Reprod Fertil* 1982;66:499–504

12. Matwee C, Betts DH, King WA. Apoptosis in the early bovine embryo. *Zygote* 2000;8:57–68

13. Byrne AT, Southgate J, Brison DR, Leese HJ. Analysis of apoptosis in the preimplantation bovine embryo using TUNEL. *J Reprod Fertil* 1999;117:97–105

14. Enders AC, Lantz KC, Schlafke S. Differentiation of the inner cell mass of the baboon blastocyst. *Anat Rec* 1990;226:237–48

15. Hurst PR, Jefferies K, Eckstein P, Wheeler AG. An ultra structural study of preimplantation uterine embryos of the rhesus monkey. *J Anat* 1978;126:209–20

16. Enders AC, Schlafke S. Differentiation of the blastocyst of the rhesus monkey. *Am J Anat* 1981;162:1–21

17. Enders AC, Hendrickx AG, Binkerd PE. Abnormal development of blastocysts and blastomeres in the rhesus monkey. *Biol Reprod* 1982;26:353–66

18. Lopata A, Kohlman DJ, Kellow GN. The fine structure of human blastocysts developed in culture. In *Embryonic Development, Part B: Cellular Aspects*. New York: Alan R Liss, 1982:69–85

19. Hardy K, Handyside AH, Winston RM. The human blastocyst: cell number, death and allocation during late preimplantation development *in vitro*. *Development* 1989;107:597–604

20. Jurisicova A, Varmuza S, Casper RF. Programmed cell death and human embryo fragmentation. *Mol Hum Reprod* 1996;2:93–8

21. Spanos S, Becker DL, Winston RM, Hardy K. Anti-apoptotic action of insulin-like growth factor-I during human preimplantation embryo development. *Biol Reprod* 2000;63:1413–20

22. Hardy K, Spanos S, Becker D, Iannelli P, Winston RM, Stark J. From cell death to embryo arrest: mathematical models of human preimplantation embryo development. *Proc Natl Acad Sci USA* 2001;98:1655–60

23. Wyllie AH. Apoptosis: an overview. *Br Med Bull* 1997;53:451–65

24. Harmon BV, Winterford CM, O'Brien BA, Allan DJ. Morphological criteria for identifying apoptosis. In Celis JE, ed. *Cell Biology: A Laboratory Handbook*, 2nd edn. San Diego: Academic Press, 1998;1:327–40

25. Earnshaw WC, Martins LM, Kaufmann SH. Mammalian caspases: structure, activation, substrates, and functions during apoptosis. *Annu Rev Biochem* 1999;68:383–424

26. Nagata S. Apoptotic DNA fragmentation. *Exp Cell Res* 2000;256:12–18

27. Arends MJ, Wyllie AH. Apoptosis: mechanisms and roles in pathology. *Int Rev Exp Pathol* 1991;32:223–54

28. Oltvai ZN, Milliman CL, Korsmeyer SJ. Bcl-2 heterodimerizes *in vivo* with a conserved homolog, Bax, that accelerates programmed cell death. *Cell* 1993;74:609–19

29. Adams JM, Cory S. Life-or-death decisions by the Bcl-2 protein family. *Trends Biochem Sci* 2001;26:61–6

30. Jurisicova A, Varmuza S, Casper RF. Involvement of programmed cell death in preimplantation embryo demise. *Hum Reprod Update* 1995;1:558–66

31. Huppertz B, Frank HG, Kaufmann P. The apoptosis cascade – morphological and immunohistochemical methods for its visualization. *Anat Embryol (Berl)* 1999;200:1–18

32. Martin SJ, Reutelingsperger CP, McGahon AJ, *et al*. Early redistribution of plasma membrane phosphatidylserine is a general feature of apoptosis regardless of the initiating stimulus: inhibition by overexpression of Bcl-2 and Abl. *J Exp Med* 1995;182:1545–56

33. Levy R, Benchaib M, Cordonier H, Souchier C, Guerin JF. Annexin V labelling and terminal transferase-mediated DNA end labelling (TUNEL) assay in human arrested embryos. *Mol Hum Reprod* 1998;4:775–83

34. Van Blerkom J, Davis PW. DNA strand breaks and phosphatidylserine redistribution in newly ovulated and cultured mouse and human oocytes: occurrence and relationship to apoptosis. *Hum Reprod* 1998;13:1317–24

35. Antczak M, Van Blerkom J. Temporal and spatial aspects of fragmentation in early human embryos: possible effects on developmental competence and association with the differential elimination of regulatory proteins from polarized domains. *Hum Reprod* 1999;14:429–47

36. Collins JA, Schandi CA, Young KK, Vesely J, Willingham MC. Major DNA fragmentation is a late event in apoptosis. *J Histochem Cytochem* 1997;45:923–34

37. Jurisicova A, Varmuza SL, Casper RF. Developmental consequences of programmed cell death in human preimplantation embryos. In Tilly J, ed. *Cell Death in Reproductive Physiology*. New York: Springer Verlag, 1997:34–47

38. Hardy K, Warner A, Winston RM, Becker DL. Expression of intercellular junctions during preimplantation development of the human embryo. *Mol Hum Reprod* 1996;2:621–32

39. Hardy K. Apoptosis in the human embryo. *Rev Reprod* 1999; 4:125–34

40. Hertig AT, Rock J, Adams EC, Mulligan WJ. On the preimplantation stages of the human ovum: a description of four normal and four abnormal specimens ranging from the second to fifth day of development. *Contrib Embryol* 1954;35:199–220

41. Gavrieli Y, Sherman Y, Ben-Sasson SA. Identification of programmed cell death *in situ* via specific labeling of nuclear DNA fragmentation. *J Cell Biol* 1992;119:493–501

42. Yang HW, Hwang KJ, Kwon HC, Kim HS, Choi KW, Oh KS. Detection of reactive oxygen species (ROS) and apoptosis in human fragmented embryos. *Hum Reprod* 1998;13:998–1002

43. Brison DR, Schultz RM. Apoptosis during mouse blastocyst formation: evidence for a role for survival factors including transforming growth factor α. *Biol Reprod* 1997;56:1088–96

44. Jurisicova A, Latham KE, Casper RF, Casper RF, Varmuza SL. Expression and regulation of genes associated with cell death during murine preimplantation embryo development. *Mol Reprod Dev* 1998;51:243–53

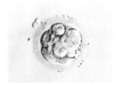

45. Exley GE, Tang C, McElhinny AS, Warner CM. Expression of caspase and BCL-2 apoptotic family members in mouse preimplantation embryos. *Biol Reprod* 1999;61:231–9

46. Moley KH, Chi MM, Knudson CM, Korsmeyer SJ, Mueckler MM. Hyperglycemia induces apoptosis in pre-implantation embryos through cell death effector pathways. *Nat Med* 1998;4:1421–4

47. Warner CM, Cao W, Exley GE, *et al.* Genetic regulation of egg and embryo survival. *Hum Reprod* 1998;13 (Suppl 3):178–90, discussion 191–6

48. Spanos S, Rice S, Karagiannis P, *et al.* Caspase activity and expression of cell death genes during development of human preimplantation embryos. *Reproduction* 2002;124:353–63

49. Brison DR. Apoptosis in mammalian preimplantation embryos: regulation by survival factors. *Hum Fertil* 2000;3:36–47

50. Martinez F, Rienzi L, Iacobelli M, *et al.* Caspase activity in preimplantation human embryos is not associated with apoptosis. *Hum Reprod* 2002;17:1584–90

51. Pereda J, Croxatto HB. Ultrastructure of a seven-cell human embryo. *Biol Reprod* 1978;18:481–9

52. Buster JE, Bustillo M, Rodi IA, *et al.* Biologic and morphologic development of donated human ova recovered by nonsurgical uterine lavage. *Am J Obstet Gynecol* 1985;153:211–17

53. Xu J, Cheung T, Chan ST, Ho P, Yeung WS. The incidence of cytoplasmic fragmentation in mouse embryos *in vitro* is not affected by inhibition of caspase activity. *Fertil Steril* 2001;75:986–91

54. Sathananthan AH, Wood C, Leeton JF. Ultrastructural evaluation of 8–16 cell human embryos cultured *in vitro*. *Micron* 1982;13:193–203

55. Plante L, King WA. Light and electron microscopic analysis of bovine embryos derived by *in vitro* and *in vivo* fertilization. *J Assist Reprod Genet* 1994;11:515–29

56. Long CR, Dobrinsky JR, Garrett WM, Johnson LA. Dual labeling of the cytoskeleton and DNA strand breaks in porcine embryos produced *in vivo* and *in vitro*. *Mol Reprod Dev* 1998;51:59–65

57. Pierce GB, Lewellyn AL, Parchment RE. Mechanism of programmed cell death in the blastocyst. *Proc Natl Acad Sci USA* 1989;86:3654–8

58. Devreker F, Hardy K. Effects of glutamine and taurine on preimplantation development and cleavage of mouse embryos *in vitro*. *Biol Reprod* 1997;57:921–8

59. Pampfer S, Vanderheyden I, McCracken JE, Vesela J, De Hertogh R. Increased cell death in rat blastocysts exposed to maternal diabetes in utero and to high glucose or tumor necrosis factor-α *in vitro*. *Development* 1997;124:4827–36

60. Herrler A, Krusche CA, Beier HM. Insulin and insulin-like growth factor-I promote rabbit blastocyst development and prevent apoptosis. *Biol Reprod* 1998;59:1302–10

61. O'Neill C. Autocrine mediators are required to act on the embryo by the 2-cell stage to promote normal development and survival of mouse preimplantation embryos *in vitro*. *Biol Reprod* 1998;58:1303–9

62. Jurisicova A, Rogers I, Fasciani A, Casper RF, Varmuza S. Effect of maternal age and conditions of fertilization on programmed cell death during murine preimplantation embryo development. *Mol Hum Reprod* 1998;4:139–45

63. Hardy K, Winston RM, Handyside AH. Binucleate blastomeres in preimplantation human embryos *in vitro*: failure of cytokinesis during early cleavage. *J Reprod Fertil* 1993;98:549–58

64. Jamieson ME, Coutts JR, Connor JM. The chromosome constitution of human preimplantation embryos fertilized *in vitro*. *Hum Reprod* 1994;9:709–15

65. Munné S, Alikani M, Tomkin G, Grifo J, Cohen J. Embryo morphology, developmental rates, and maternal age are correlated with chromosome abnormalities. *Fertil Steril* 1995;64:382–91

66. Hardy K, Spanos S. Growth factor expression and function in the human and mouse preimplantation embryo. *J Endocrinol* 2002;172:221–36

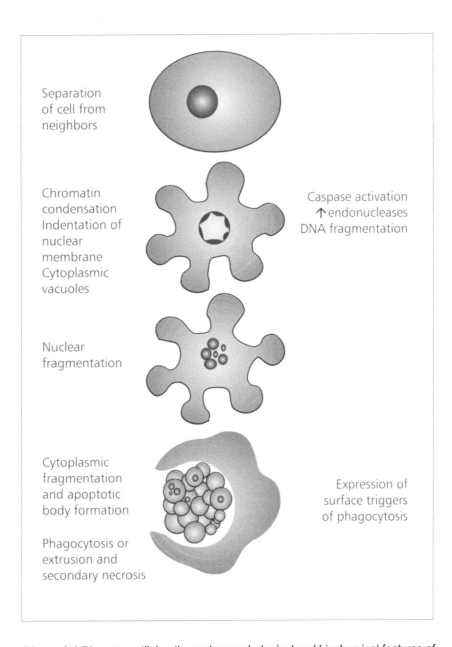

Separation of cell from neighbors

Chromatin condensation
Indentation of nuclear membrane
Cytoplasmic vacuoles

Caspase activation
↑ endonucleases
DNA fragmentation

Nuclear fragmentation

Cytoplasmic fragmentation and apoptotic body formation

Phagocytosis or extrusion and secondary necrosis

Expression of surface triggers of phagocytosis

Figure 9.1 Diagram outlining the main morphological and biochemical features of apoptosis. Reproduced with permission from Hardy K. Apoptosis in the human embryo. *Rev Reprod* 1999;4:125–34

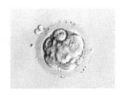

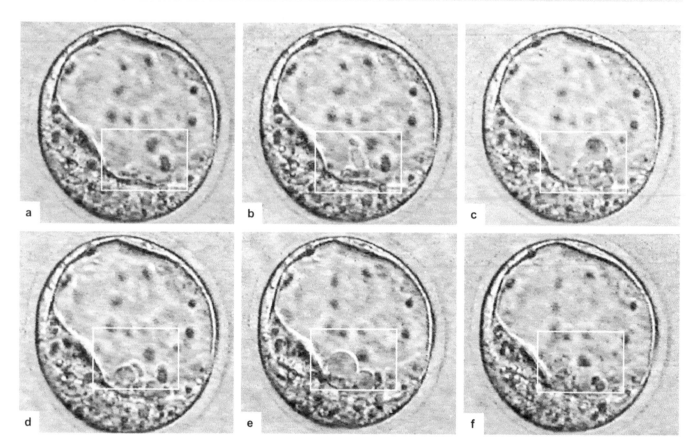

Figure 9.2 Frames from video time-lapse of cells blebbing and exploding on the surface of the inner cell mass of an expanded mouse blastocyst

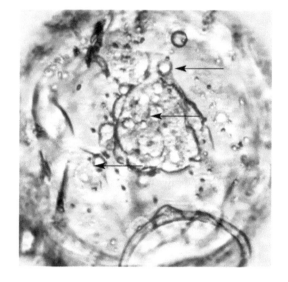

Figure 9.3 Small cytoplasmic blebs (arrowed) on the surface of the inner cell mass of a human blastocyst

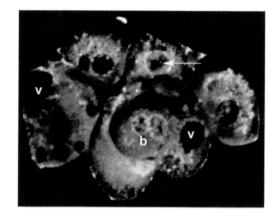

Figure 9.4 Confocal micrograph of a day-4 10-cell embryo with condensed chromatin (arrowed), vacuoles (v) and a binucleate cell (b). Nuclei are labeled with propidium iodide. Reproduced with permission from Hardy K. Apoptosis in the human embryo. *Rev Reprod* 1999;4:125–34

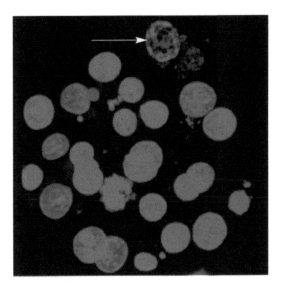

Figure 9.5 Confocal micrograph of a day-6 early human blastocyst with condensed chromatin (arrowed) and a metaphase. Nuclei are labeled with 4',6-diamidino-2-phenylindole (DAPI)

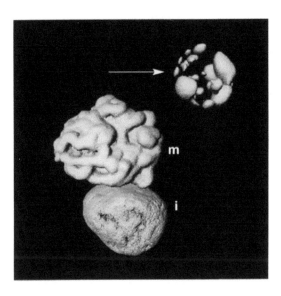

Figure 9.6 Three-dimensional confocal reconstruction of nuclei from a day-6 blastocyst showing nucleus with condensed chromatin (arrow), healthy interphase nucleus (i) and a nucleus in mitosis (m). Nuclei are labeled with DAPI. Reproduced with permission from Hardy K. Apoptosis in the human embryo. *Rev Reprod* 1999;4:125–34

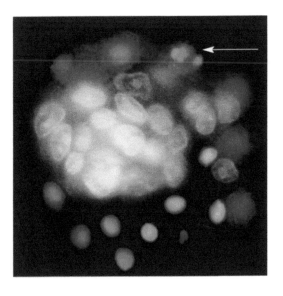

Figure 9.7 Whole mount of a differentially labeled human blastocyst (labeled as described in reference 19), with the trophectoderm nuclei in orange (labeled with propidium iodide and DAPI) and the inner cell mass nuclei in green (labeled with DAPI alone). Note the fragmenting trophectoderm nucleus (arrowed)

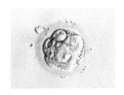

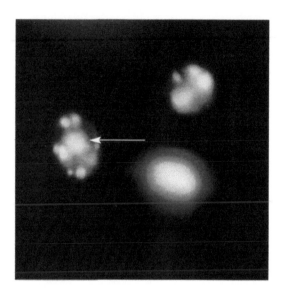

Figure 9.8 Two fragmented inner cell mass nuclei (arrowed) from a mouse blastocyst

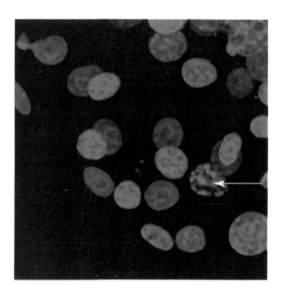

Figure 9.9 Confocal micrograph of a fragmented nucleus (arrowed) in a day-6 human blastocyst with 110 nuclei. Nuclei are labeled with DAPI (high-power view of Figure 9.15)

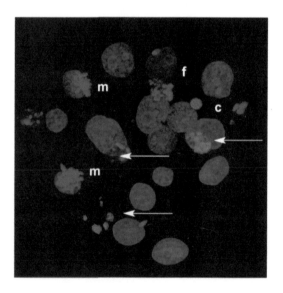

Figure 9.10 Confocal micrograph of a day-6 early human blastocyst with 26 nuclei, seven of which are showing clear morphological evidence of apoptosis. The DNA is fragmented in terminal deoxynucleotidyl transferase-mediated dUTP nick-end labeled (TUNEL) nuclei (pink) and intact in DAPI-labeled nuclei (blue). Fragmented nuclei with (arrowed) and without (f) TUNEL labeling are clearly shown, as is a condensed nucleus with TUNEL labeling (c), and two nuclei undergoing mitosis (m)

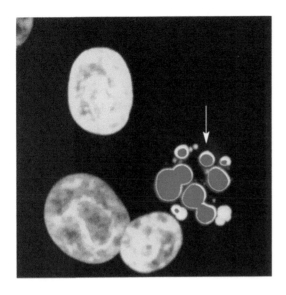

Figure 9.11 Confocal micrograph of a fragmented, TUNEL-labeled, nucleus (arrowed, pink) and healthy interphase nuclei (green). Reproduced with permission from Hardy K. Apoptosis in the human embryo. *Rev Reprod* 1999;4:125–34, and from Hardy K, *et al*. From cell death to embryo arrest: mathematical models of human preimplantation embryo development. *Proc Natl Acad Sci USA* 2001;98:1655–60
© 2001, National Academy of Sciences, USA

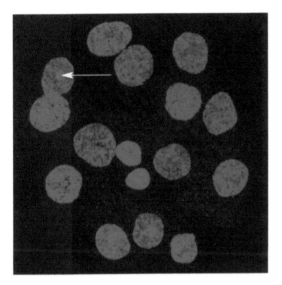

Figure 9.12 Confocal micrograph of a day-4 uncompacted human embryo with 14 cells (and 16 nuclei). Only the polar body is TUNEL-labeled (pink, arrowed), showing DNA fragmentation. Nuclei with intact DNA are labeled with DAPI (blue)

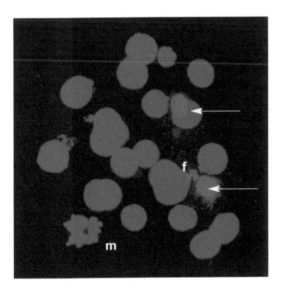

Figure 9.13 Confocal micrograph of a day-5 human morula with 29 nuclei. Two condensed nuclei are TUNEL-labeled (pink, arrowed), one fragmented nucleus is TUNEL-labeled (f) and one nucleus is in mitosis (m). Nuclei with intact DNA are labeled with DAPI (blue)

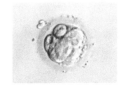

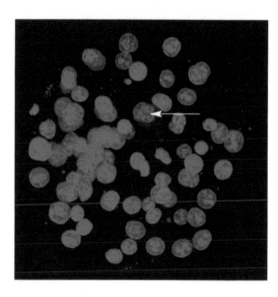

Figure 9.14 Confocal micrograph of a day-5 human blastocyst with 82 nuclei. Only one nucleus is TUNEL-labeled (pink, arrowed). Nuclei with intact DNA are labeled with DAPI (blue)

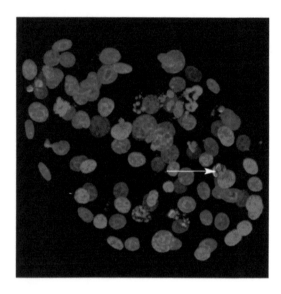

Figure 9.15 Confocal micrograph of a day-6 hatching human blastocyst with 95 nuclei, 11 of which are TUNEL-labeled (pink, arrowed). Nuclei with intact DNA are labeled with DAPI (blue)

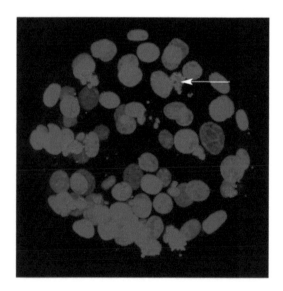

Figure 9.16 Confocal micrograph of a day-6 human blastocyst with 89 nuclei, 14 of which are TUNEL-labeled (pink, arrowed). Nuclei with intact DNA are labeled with DAPI (blue)

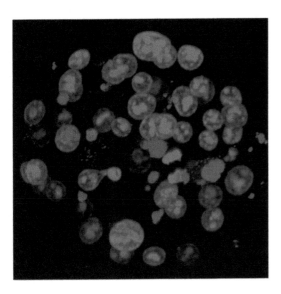

Figure 9.17 Confocal micrograph of a day-6 human blastocyst with 45 nuclei, and extensive TUNEL-labeling (pink). Nuclei with intact DNA are labeled with DAPI (blue)

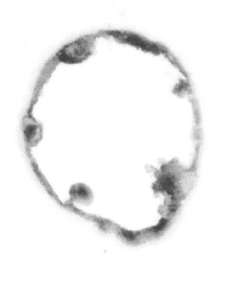

Figure 9.18 Immunohistochemical localization of bcl-2 (brown staining) in a day-5 human blastocyst of poor morphology. Reproduced with permission from Spanos S, *et al.* Caspase activity and expression of cell death genes during development of human preimplantation embryos. *Reproduction* 2002;124:353–63

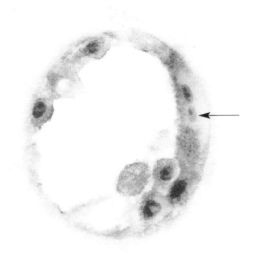

Figure 9.19 Immunohistochemical localization of bax (brown staining) in a day-5 human blastocyst of poor morphology (same blastocyst as Figure 9.18). Note low level of staining in some cells (arrow). Reproduced with permission from Spanos S, *et al.* Caspase activity and expression of cell death genes during development of human preimplantation embryos. *Reproduction* 2002;124:353–63

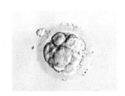

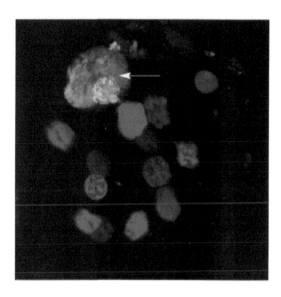

Figure 9.20 Confocal micrograph of a day-3 compacting human embryo with 15 nuclei showing one cell with active caspases present in the cytoplasm (arrowed, green). Nuclei are labeled with DAPI (red). Reproduced with permission from Spanos S, *et al*. Caspase activity and expression of cell death genes during development of human preimplantation embryos. *Reproduction* 2002;124:353–63

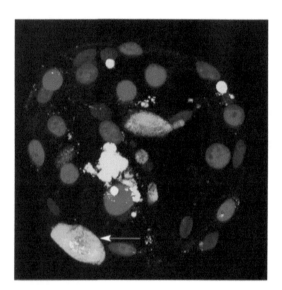

Figure 9.21 Confocal micrograph of a day-6 expanded human blastocyst with 31 nuclei. Active caspases are green. Note association of active caspases with a fragmented nucleus (arrowed). Nuclei are labeled with DAPI (red). Reproduced with permission from Spanos S, *et al*. Caspase activity and expression of cell death genes during development of human preimplantation embryos. *Reproduction* 2002;124:353–63

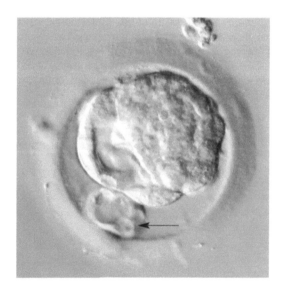

Figure 9.22 Early human blastocyst (day-6) with vacuolated excluded cell (arrowed) lying between the trophectoderm and the zona pellucida

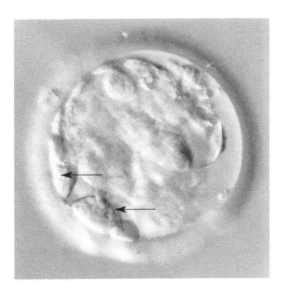

Figure 9.23 Human blastocyst of poor morphology with excluded cells (arrowed) lying between the trophectoderm and the zona pellucida

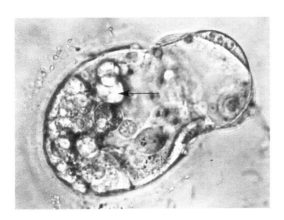

Figure 9.24 Hatching human blastocyst with excluded cells (arrowed) lying in the blastocoel cavity. Reproduced with permission from The Society for Endocrinology from Hardy K. Growth factor expression and function in the human and mouse preimplantation embryo. *J Endocrinol* 2002;172:221–36

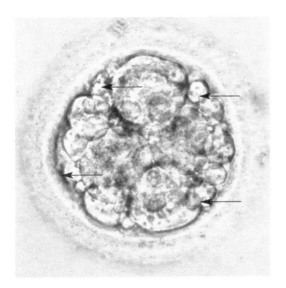

Figure 9.25 Human embryo (day 3) with extensive fragmentation (arrowed)

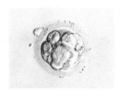

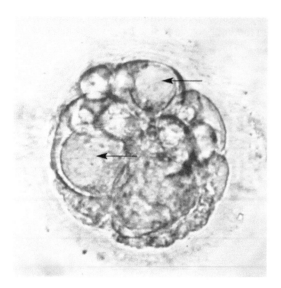

Figure 9.26 Cleavage-stage human embryo with large vacuoles in the cytoplasm

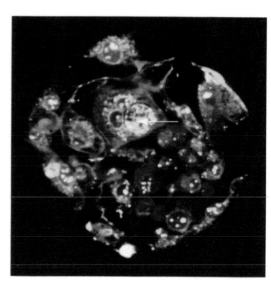

Figure 9.27 Confocal micrograph of day-5 human blastocyst showing engulfed cell (arrow). Reproduced with permission from Hardy K. Apoptosis in the human embryo. *Rev Reprod* 1999;4:125–34

10 Human implantation

Owen Davis and Zev Rosenwaks

Introduction

The process of implantation entails complex interactions between blastocyst and uterine cells (Figure 10.1). Successful implantation can only be initiated when preembryonic development is synchronized with the receptive state of the endometrium. Preparation of the endometrial bed is dependent not only on adequate hormonal stimulation, but also on a reciprocal dialog between the blastocyst and endometrium that is mediated by several factors including cytokines, growth factors and adhesion molecules, which are elaborated by the endometrium and the blastocyst. This chapter provides an overview of currently postulated mechanisms of implantation in the human.

Early embryogenesis (Figure 10.2)

Fertilization of the mature, metaphase II oocyte occurs in the ampullary region of the Fallopian tube. A combination of segmental tubal contractions and endosalpingeal ciliary activity transports the preembryo into the uterine lumen at the morula stage, within 72 h of ovulation. Further mitotic cleavage ensues over the next few days while the conceptus remains free within the uterine cavity. Requisite to the process of implantation is the differentiation of the preembryo into a blastocyst, comprising specialized extraembryonic epithelial cells (trophectoderm) and the inner cell mass. All mammalian preembryos must hatch from their zonae pellucidae prior to their initial loose attachment to the endometrial surface (apposition). The process of thinning and degradation of the zona pellucida appears to be primarily driven by the blastocyst, and permits the

initial cell membrane contact of the blastocyst polar trophectoderm with the endometrial luminal epithelium. Studies in non-human primates have shown that mononuclear cytotrophoblasts have fused into syncytia prior to attachment of these cells to the endometrial surface[1]. In the human it is the syncytial trophoblast that first adheres to the endometrial surface and subsequently invades the epithelium during the initial days of implantation (Figure 10.3). Once the blastocyst is completely embedded, cytotrophoblast columns further invade the uterine wall.

The window of implantation

Although the human blastocyst's requirements for nidation may not be rigorous, as evidenced by the occurrence of ectopic gestation, the uterus is receptive to implantation only during a discrete interval. The search for molecular markers and/or mediators of the receptive state must therefore focus on this temporal window.

In vitro fertilization (IVF) has provided investigators with a useful scientific model for studying the window of transfer (and by extrapolation, implantation) in the human. Here, preembryos of known 'age' are transferred into temporally defined endometria. With conventional IVF, however, oocytes are harvested following controlled ovarian hyperstimulation, which typically results in peak luteal phase peripheral estradiol and progesterone levels and estradiol/progesterone ratios far exceeding those seen in the natural cycle. Endometria from pharmacologically stimulated cycles typically display histological and morphological advancement[2].

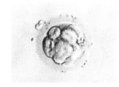

A more physiological model for study of the window of transfer is provided by oocyte donation. Preembryos of defined age, derived from *in vitro* fertilized donated oocytes, are transferred to recipients lacking endogenous ovarian function whose endometria are exposed to physiological levels of estrogen and progesterone. Steroid replacement regimens are specifically designed to mimic the normal pattern of hormone secretion observed in the natural menstrual cycle. Late secretory-phase endometrial biopsies obtained in preparatory hormone-replacement cycles typically demonstrate in-phase histology, while biopsies performed on cycle day 20–21 reveal appropriately developed stroma with lagging glandular histology (day 17–18)[3]. An analysis of the donor oocyte literature suggests that the window for transfer of 4–8-cell stage preembryos spans endometrial cycle days 16–20. Given the expected time for early cleavage-stage preembryos to develop into blastocysts, this suggests that the window of implantation in the human is approximately 4 days, commencing on cycle day 19–20 and extending to day 24.

Endometrial ultrastructure in the window of implantation

Scanning electron microscopy has revealed a striking morphological transformation of the endometrial surface in the perinidatory window. Surface microvilli and cilia are seen to regress and, under the influence of progesterone, bulbous luminal apical protrusions termed 'pinopods' develop[4] (Figure 10.4). Pinopods are seen in 78% of endometrial biopsies on postovulatory day 6, yet are scarce on postovulatory days 2 and 9. This temporal expression of pinopods suggests that they may play an as yet undetermined functional role in implantation, such as pinocytosis/endocytosis of uterine fluid and/or increasing the surface of blastocyst–epithelial contact.

Histological evaluation of secretory endometrium in the window of implantation reveals pronounced stromal edema[5]. Theoretically, this could serve to facilitate engulfment of the blastocyst. Although these various morphological changes in the endometrium may serve as markers of uterine receptivity, their functional significance remains unclear.

Cell adhesion molecules

Cell adhesion molecules are subdivided into four major subclasses: integrins, cadherins, selectins and members of the immunoglobulin superfamily. Cell adhesion molecules have been implicated in both the cyclic regeneration of the functional layer of the endometrium and blastocyst implantation.

Integrins

Integrins are ubiquitous heterodimeric transmembrane glycoproteins, comprising non-covalently bound α- and β-subunits. Integrins play a role in cell–cell binding and in cellular interactions with the extracellular matrix. The endometrium expresses both constitutive and cycle-dependent integrins. It should be noted that both endometrial epithelial estrogen and progestin receptors are down-regulated in the mid-luteal phase, during the window of implantation[6]. The decline of progesterone receptors is temporally associated with the appearance of integrin avb3 on the surface epithelium, which is expressed after day 19[7]. Additionally, αvβ3 has been found covering the preimplantation embryo[8] It is theorized that αvβ3 may offer adhesion sites for the blastocyst. Additionally, it has been suggested that αvβ3 binds and activates matrix metalloproteinases and plasminogen activators in the extracellular matrix[9], indicating that this integrin may function as both an endometrial receptor for the blastocyst and a facilitator of trophoblastic invasion.

Clinical investigation has suggested that mid-luteal αvβ3 is a marker of human uterine receptivity. A number of disorders associated with infertility have been associated with reduced expression of αvβ3, including endometriosis[10], luteal phase defect[11], idiopathic infertility[12] and the presence of hydrosalpinges[13] (which in turn have been associated with impaired implantation following IVF and embryo transfer). Although a functional role for specific integrins has not been established, further research encompassing their clinical utility as markers, or a physiological role as mediators of implantation, is warranted.

Mucins

As a class, mucins are high-molecular-weight and highly glycosylated molecules found in many secretory epithelia, and specifically on the apical aspect of endometrial epithelial cells. Various mucins may play a role in blastocyst attachment[14]. In the human, MUC-1 is up-regulated during the implantation window in endometrial samples[15]. It has been suggested that MUC-1 may regulate blastocyst adhesion, and that the blastocyst, in turn, locally modulates MUC-1 at the implantation site, focally rendering the uterine epithelium adhesive while the remainder remains non-adhesive[16]. Another mucin which has received attention as a possible marker of human endometrial receptivity is MAG (mouse ascites Golgi). MAG appears on the luminal epithelial surface of the endometrium on cycle day 18–19; abnormal expression of MAG has been cited in some patients with idiopathic infertility[17].

Attachment: the role of growth factors and cytokines

Growth factors and cytokines are ubiquitous families of peptides and proteins which variously exhibit paracrine, autocrine and endocrine activity. In the endometrium, specific growth factors, cytokines and their respective receptors and binding proteins demonstrate cycle dependence, and appear to play a role in the dialog between the preembryo and uterus.

The epidermal growth factor (EGF) family includes the polypeptides EGF, heparin-binding EGF-like growth factor (HB-EGF), transforming growth factor-α (TGF-α), amphiregulin and betacellulin; all interact with the EGF receptor (EGF-R). Studies in the murine model have demonstrated uterine epithelial expression of HB-EGF around the pre-attachment blastocyst; furthermore, HB-EGF appears to stimulate blastocyst growth and hatching *in vitro*, via EGF receptors on the blastocyst surface[18].

Colony-stimulating factor-1 (CSF-1) is a glycosylated homodimer, also referred to as macrophage CSF-1. CSF-1 is preferentially expressed in human endometrial glands during the mid-secretory phase and in first-trimester decidua[19]. Furthermore, transcripts encoding the CSF-1 receptor have been identified in the preimplantation human embryo[20], suggesting a possible role for endometrial CSF-1 in implantation.

Leukemia inhibitory factor (LIF) is a glycoprotein displaying both proliferative and differentiative effects through interaction with its receptor. The LIF receptor is composed of two subunits, the LIF receptor (LIF-R) and glycoprotein 130 (gp130). Blastocyst implantation fails to occur in knock-out mice lacking a functional LIF gene[21]. In the human, LIF is maximally expressed in mid- and late secretory-phase glandular and luminal epithelium[22]. LIF appears to regulate human cytotrophoblasts, modulating their differentiation to the anchoring phenotype[23]. *In vitro* studies have additionally indicated that LIF regulates human trophoblast differentiation along the invasive pathway, suggesting a role in the invasive phase of implantation[24]. Clinical studies have indicated that abnormal expression of endometrial LIF may be associated with human infertility. Mutations in the coding region of the LIF gene have been identified in some infertile women[25], and a greater proportion of secretory phase uterine flushings have undetectable levels of LIF in women with idiopathic infertility when compared with fertile controls[26].

The interleukin-1 (IL-1) family comprises two homologous polypeptides (IL-1α and IL-1β), their receptors (IL-1R) and the IL-1 receptor antagonist (IL-1ra). The entire IL-1 system is expressed in human endometrium; IL-1 receptors have been found to increase significantly in the mid-luteal phase[27]. Human preimplantation embryos also express IL-1, IL-1R and IL-1ra[28]. Of note, the presence of IL-1 in preembryo culture fluid is a positive predictor of implantation potential[29]. Interaction of the blastocyst with receptive endometrium elicits embryonic secretion of IL-1, which in turn effects localized changes in the endometrium prior to adhesion; the embryonic IL-1 system appears to play a role specifically in the up-regulation of endometrial β3 integrin[30].

Trophoblast invasion (Figure 10.5)

Following adhesion, the trophoblast intrudes, penetrating through the luminal epithelium, reaching and then extending through the basal lamina with subsequent invasion into the endometrial stroma, and ultimately invades the maternal vessels with establishment of the hemochorial placenta. The presence of the blastocyst initiates the decidual reaction, wherein stromal cells undergo proliferation and differentiation into specialized cells which may provide nutritional support to the preembryo and play a regulatory role in trophoblast invasion into the stroma. Of note, the decidual reaction can be experimentally induced via stimulation/trauma to the endometrium.

The attachment of the invading trophoblast to the extracellular matrix (ECM) is mediated by cell adhesion molecules. It is likely that switching of specific integrins on the trophoblast membranes is one manifestation of the transition of the cytotrophoblasts to the invasive phenotype[31]. Modulated and localized proteolysis of

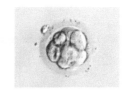

ECM is another key component of the invasive phase of implantation. First-trimester invading cytotrophoblasts express specific matrix-degrading enzymes such as the matrix metalloproteinases MMP-2 and MMP-9[32]; the latter degrades laminin/type IV collagen-rich basement membranes. Of note, IL-1β may play an autocrine role in the promotion of cytotrophoblast invasiveness via stimulation of MMP-9 production[33]. Other proteinases, such as urokinase-type plasminogen activator, may also facilitate degradation of the ECM by the invading trophoblast, either directly or via activation of pro-MMPs[34]. The activity of the various proteinases is in turn modulated by specific protease inhibitors of both decidual and trophoblastic origin. These inhibitors appear to play an important role in limiting invasion. A number of tissue inhibitors of metalloproteinases (TIMPs) have been identified. TIMP-3 is expressed in both endometrial stroma and trophoblasts, and regulates the activity of MMP-9[35]. IL-1b has been observed to inhibit the activity of TIMP-3 in human decidua, indicating that the trophoblast can promote its own invasiveness through the inhibition of maternal restraint mechanisms[36].

Specific ECM proteins also play a role in implantation. Decidualized endometrial stromal cells elaborate both laminin and fibronectin. Laminin may play a permissive role in invasion; *in vitro* studies have shown that human trophoblasts readily attach to laminin-coated surfaces[37]. Conversely, fibronectin appears to promote maternal restraint through the inhibition of cytotrophoblast invasion. Other factors have additionally been implicated in the maternal inhibition of trophoblastic invasion. Insulin growth factor binding protein-1 (IGFBP-1) is abundantly produced in secretory endometrium and decidua. IGFBP-1 has been demonstrated to bind human cytotrophoblast via α5β1 integrin in the cell membrane, and restrains cytotrophoblast invasion in endometrial stromal culture[38]. Transforming growth factor-β1 (TGF-β1) also appears to be an effector of maternal restraint on trophoblast invasion. TGF-β1 is abundantly expressed in maternal endometrium, and exerts several modulatory effects, including: inhibition of cytotrophoblast proliferation and promotion of differentiation into syncytiotrophoblasts, and induction of cytotrophoblast protease inhibitors such as TIMP-1 and plasminogen activator inhibitor (PAI)[39].

Conclusion

The successful propagation of the human species depends on reproductive efficiency. Implantation, a critical component of reproductive physiology, remains one of the most incompletely understood processes in reproductive biology. Implantation involves the introduction of a competent blastocyst into the uterine lumen during a temporally restricted interval when ovarian hormones induce a receptive uterine phase. Reciprocal signalling between the blastocyst and the endometrium is mediated in some measure by cytokines, growth factors and adhesion molecules. Successful 'cross-talk' leads to apposition and attachment of the blastocyst to the uterine wall, followed by intrusion and invasion. The process of trophoblastic invasion entails a delicate interplay between invasion facilitators and invasion inhibitors, i.e. promotion and restraint. Further elucidation of the complex mechanisms underlying the process of implantation in the human should provide clinical inroads into the diagnosis and treatment of reproductive failure.

References

1. Enders AC. Current topic: structural responses of the primate endometrium to implantation. *Placenta* 1991;12:309–25

2. Martel D, Frydman R, Sarantis L, Roihe D, Psychoyos A. Scanning electron microscopy of the uterine luminal epithelium as a marker of the implantation window. In Yoshinaga K, ed. *Blastocyst Implantation*. Boston: Serono Symposia, 1989:225–30

3. Rosenwaks Z. Donor eggs: their application in modern reproductive technologies. *Fertil Steril* 1987;47:895–909

4. Martel D, Monier MN, Roiche D, Psychoyos A. Hormonal dependence of pinopode formation at the uterine luminal surface. *Hum Reprod* 1991;6:597–603

5. Noyes RW, Hertig AT, Rock J. Dating the endometrial biopsy. *Fertil Steril* 1950;1:3–25

6. Lessey BA, Killam AP, Metzger DA, *et al.* Immunohistochemical analysis of human uterine estrogen and progesterone receptors throughout the menstrual cycle. *J Clin Endocrinol Metab* 1988;647:334–40

7. Lessey BA, Damjanovich L, Coutifaris C, *et al.* Integrin adhesion molecules in human endometrium: correlation with normal and abnormal menstrual cycles. *J Clin Invest* 1992;90:188–95

8. Campbell S, Swann HR, Seif MW, *et al.* Cell adhesion molecules on the oocyte and preimplantation human embryo. *Hum Reprod* 1995;10:1571–8

9. Brooks PC, Stromblad S, Sanders LC, *et al.* Localization of matrix metalloproteinase MMP-2 to the surface of invasive cells by interaction with integrin $\alpha v\beta 3$. *Cell* 1996;85:683–93

10. Lessey BA, Castelbaum AJ, Sawin SW, *et al.* Aberrant integrin expression in the endometrium of women with endometriosis. *J Clin Endocrinol Metab* 1994;79:643–9

11. Lessey BA, Yeh I, Castelbaum AJ, *et al.* Endometrial progesterone receptors and markers of uterine receptivity in the window of implantation. *Fertil Steril* 1996;65:477–83

12. Lessey BA, Castelbaum AJ, Sawin SW, *et al.* Integrins as markers of uterine receptivity in women with primary unexplained infertility. *Fertil Steril* 1995;63:535–42

13. Meyer WR, Castelbaum AJ, Somkuti S, *et al.* Hydrosalpinges adversely affect markers of endometrial receptivity. *Hum Reprod* 1997;12:1393–8

14. Carson DD, Rohde LH, Surveyor G. Cell surface glycoconjugates as modulators of embryo attachment to uterine epithelial cells. *Int J Biochem* 1994;26:1269–77

15. Hey NA, Graham RA, Seif MW, *et al.* The polymorphic epithelial mucin MUC 1 in human endometrium is regulated with maximal expression in the implantation phase. *J Clin Endocrinol Metab* 1994;78:337–42

16. Meseguer M, Aplin JD, Caballero-Campo P, *et al.* Human endometrial mucin MUC1 is up-regulated by progesterone and down-regulated *in vitro* by the human blastocyst. *Biol Reprod* 2001;64:590–601

17. Kliman HJ, Feinberg RJ, Schwartz LB, *et al.* A mucin-like glycoprotein identified by MAG (mouse ascites Golgi) antibodies. Menstrual cycle-dependent localization in human endometrium. *Am J Pathol* 1995;146:166–81

18. Das SK, Wang X, Paria BC, *et al.* Heparin-binding EGF-like growth factor gene is induced in the mouse uterus temporally by the blastocyst solely at the site of its apposition: a possible ligand for interaction with blastocyst EGF-receptor in implantation. *Development* 1994;120:1071–83

19. Bartocci A, Pollard JW, Stanley ER. Regulation of CSF-1 during pregnancy. *J Exp Med* 1986;164:956–61

20. Sharkey AM, Dellow K, Blayney M, *et al.* Stage-specific expression of cytokine and receptor messenger ribonucleic acids in human preimplantation embryos. *Biol Reprod* 1995;53:974–81

21. Stewart CL, Kaspar P, Brunet LJ, *et al.* Blastocyst implantation depends on maternal expression of leukaemia inhibitory factor. *Nature (London)* 1992;359:76–9

22. Charnock-Jones DS, Sharkey AM, Fenwick P, *et al.* Leukaemia inhibitory factor mRNA concentration peaks in human endometrium at the time of implantation and the blastocyst contains mRNA for the receptor at this time. *J Reprod Fertil* 1994;101:421–6

23. Nachtigall MJ, Kliman HJ, Feinberg RF, *et al.* The effect of leukemia inhibitory factor (LIF) on trophoblast differentiation: a potential role in human implantation. *J Clin Endocrinol Metab* 1996;81:801–6

24. Bischof P, Haenggeli L, Campana A. Effect of leukemia inhibitory factor on human cytotrophoblast differentiation along the invasive pathway. *Am J Reprod Immunol* 1995;34:225–30

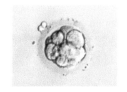

25. Giess R, Tanasescu I, Steck T, et al. Leukaemia inhibitory factor gene mutations in infertile women. Mol Hum Reprod 1999;5:581–6

26. Laird SM, Tuckerman EM, Dalton CF, et al. The production of leukaemia inhibitory factor by human endometrium: presence in uterine flushings and production by cells in culture. Hum Reprod 1997;12:569–74

27. Simon C, Piquette GN, Frances A, et al. Localization of interleukin-1 type-1 receptor and interleukin-1β in human endometrium throughout the menstrual cycle. J Clin Endocrinol Metab 1993;77:549–55

28. Krussel JS, Simon C, Rubio MC, et al. Expression of interleukin-1 system mRNA in single blastomeres from human preimplantation embryos. Hum Reprod 1998;13:2206–11

29. Sheth KV, Roca GL, al-Sedairy ST, et al. Prediction of successful embryo implantation by measuring interleukin 1α and immunosuppressive factor(s) in preimplantation embryo culture fluid. Fertil Steril 1991;55:952–7

30. Simon C, Gimeno MJ, Mercader A, et al. Embryonic regulation of integrins β3, α4 and α1 in human endometrial epithelial cells in vitro. J Clin Endocrinol Metab 1997;82:2607–16

31. Damsky CH, Librach C, Lim KH, et al. Integrin switching regulates normal trophoblast invasion. Development 1994;120:3657–66

32. Bischof P, Friedli E, Martelli M, et al. Expression of xtracellular matrix-degrading metalloptroteinases by cultured human cytotrophoblast cells: effects of cell adhesion and immuno-purification. Am J Obstet Gynecol 1991;165:1791–801

33. Librach CL, Feigenbaum SL, Bass KE, et al. Interleukin-1β regulates human cytotrophoblast metalloproteinase activity and invasiveness in vitro. J Biol Chem 1994;269:17125–31

34. Queenan JT Jr, Kao LC, Arboleda A, et al. Regulation of urokinase-type plasminogen activator production by cultured human cytotrophoblasts. J Biol Chem 1987;262:10903–6

35. Higuchi T, Kanzaki H, Nakayama H, et al. Induction of tissue inhibitor of metalloproteinase 3 gene during in vitro decidualization of human endometrial stromal cells. Endocrinology 1995;136:4973–81

36. Huang HY, Wen Y, Irwin JC, et al. Cytokine mediated regulation of tissue inhibitor of metalloproteinase-1 (TIMP-1), TIMP-3, and 92-kDa type IV collagenase mRNA expression in human endometrial stromal cells. J Clin Endocrinol Metab 1998;83:1721–9

37. Loke YW, Gardner L, Burland K, et al. Laminin in human trophoblast–decidua interaction. Hum Reprod 1989;4:457–63

38. Irwin JC, Giudice LC. IGFBP-1 binds to the α5b1 integrin in human cytotrophoblasts and inhibits their invasion into decidualized endometrial stromal cells in vitro. Growth Horm IGF Res 1998;8:21–31

39. Graham CH, McCrae KR, Lala PK. Molecular mechanisms of controlling trophoblast invasion of the uterus. Trophoblast Res 1993;7:237–50

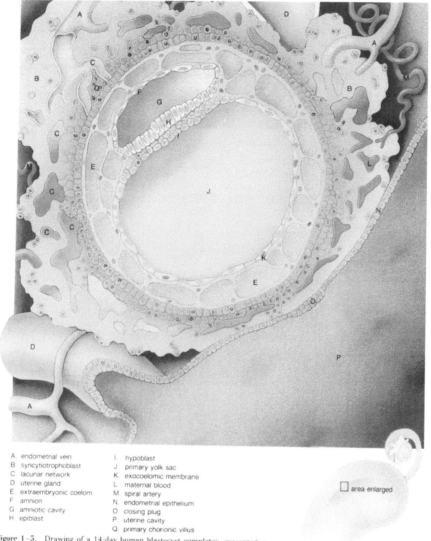

A. endometrial vein	I. hypoblast
B. syncytiotrophoblast	J. primary yolk sac
C. lacunar network	K. exocoelomic membrane
D. uterine gland	L. maternal blood
E. extraembryonic coelom	M. spiral artery
F. amnion	N. endometrial epithelium
G. amniotic cavity	O. closing plug
H. epiblast	P. uterine cavity
	Q. primary chorionic villus

☐ area enlarged

Figure 1-5. Drawing of a 14-day human blastocyst completely implanted in the endometrium. Lacunar networks (C) have developed in the external layer of the trophoblast known as the syncytiotrophoblast (B). Observe that maternal blood is entering the deepest lacunar network (*top left*). The embryo appears as the bilaminar embryonic disc. Observe that coelomic spaces appear in the extraembryonic mesoderm (E). These spaces will fuse to form the extraembryonic coelom (primordium of the chorionic cavity.)

Figure 10.1 Implantation involves complex interactions between blastocyst and uterine cells. Reprinted with permission from Moore KL, Persaud TVN, Shiota K, eds. *Color Atlas of Clinical Embryology.* Philadelphia: WB Saunders, 1994:5

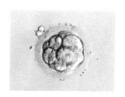

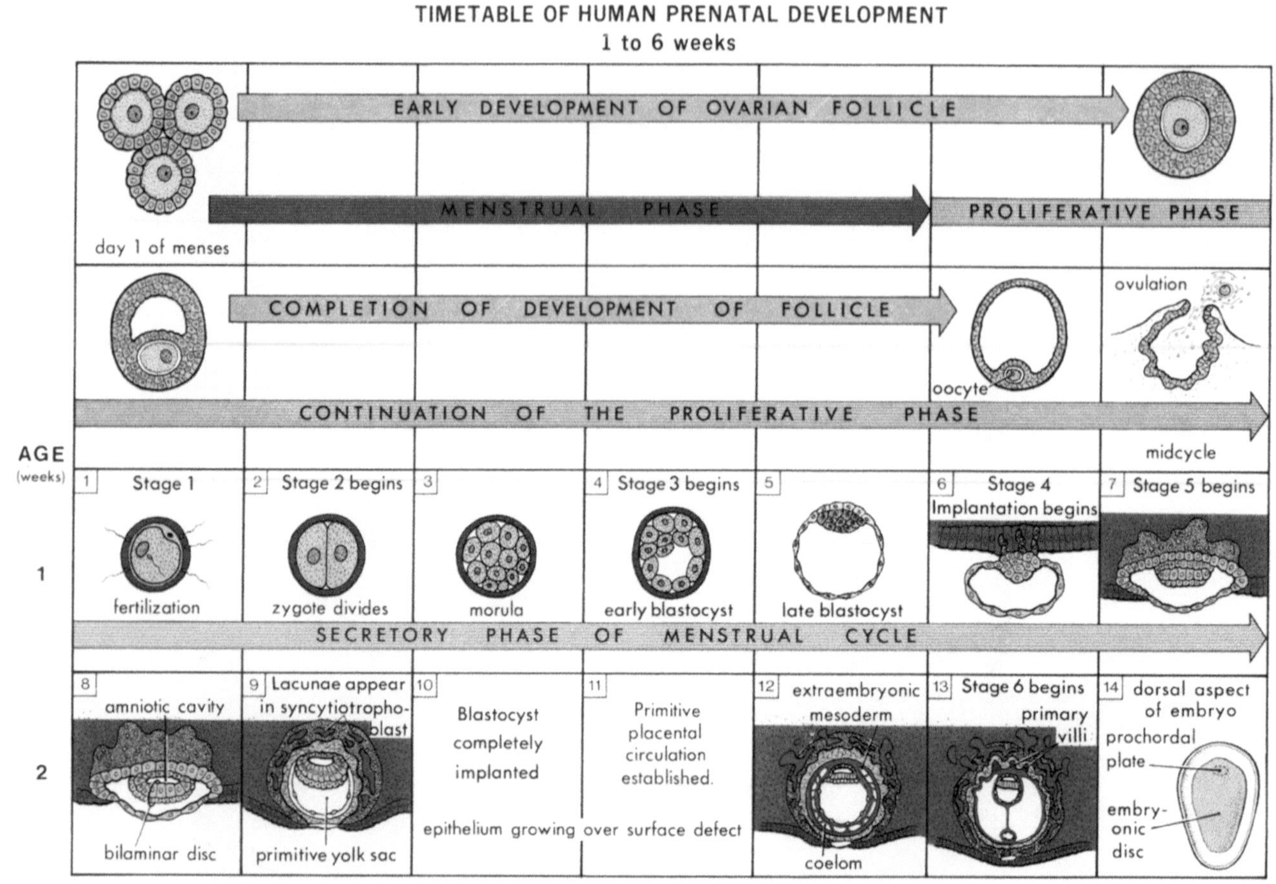

Figure 10.2 Timetable of early embryogenesis. Schematic courtesy of Keith L. Moore, *The Developing Human: Clinically Oriented Embryology,* 3rd edn. Philadelphia: WB Saunders, 1982

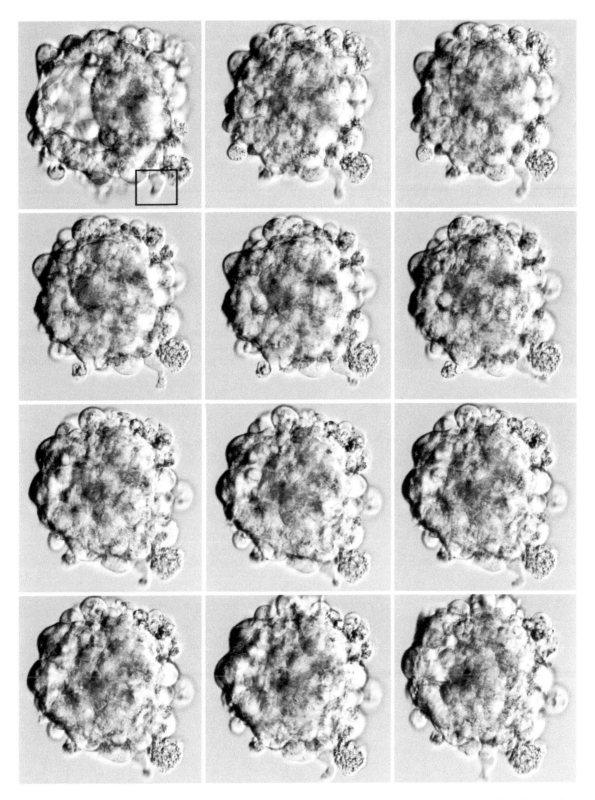

Figure 10.3 Trophoblastic projections. As observed in this sequence of time-lapse photographs, the hatched human blastocyst produces small projections that exhibit amoeboid movement, appear fimbriated and move in a fashion that suggests they seek an implantation site. Sequence courtesy of L. Veeck

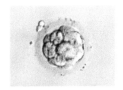

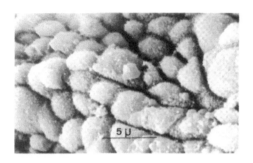

Figure 10.4 Pinopods. Luminal epithelium of the human uterus on day 6 after ovulation during spontaneous menstrual cycle. Courtesy of D. Martel[2]. In Koji Yoshinaga, ed. *Blastocyst Implantation*. Boston: Serono Symposia, 1989:228

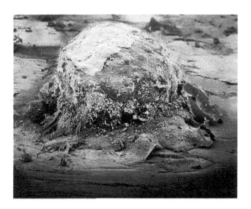

Figure 10.5 Implanting human blastocyst. The blastocyst securely anchors itself in the endometrium; to the right, veritable cables are visible. Courtesy of Lennart Nilsson/Albert Bonniers Forlag AB, *A Child is Born,* Dell Publishing Company

11 Human embryonic stem cells

Michal Amit and Joseph Itskovitz-Eldor

Introduction

Embryonic stem (ES) cells are continuously growing cell lines of embryonic origin, first isolated from the inner cell mass (ICM) of mouse blastocysts[1,2]. These unique cells are characterized by the following features:

(1) They are derived from preimplantation embryos;

(2) In culture, they indefinitely maintain uniform colonies of undifferentiated morphology, i.e. high nucleus/cytoplasm ratio and the presence of two to four nucleoli;

(3) They form teratomas after injection into SCID (severe combined immunodeficiency) mice, proving their potential to form all three embryonic germ layers;

(4) They maintain normal karyotype after continuous culture. These features are summarized in Table 11.1.

Given their ability to differentiate into any cell type of the adult body, it is not surprising that much effort was invested in the development of human ES cell lines. Since the first publication on the derivation of human pluripotent cell lines[3], additional lines have been reported that meet the ES cell criteria[4-6]. According to a list published by the National Institutes of Health (NIH, www.nih.gov/news/stemcell/index.htm), there are more than 70 human ES cell lines in several laboratories around the world that fulfil the listed features (Table 11.1) of ES cells. The availability of dozens of cell lines suggests that the derivation of these lines is a reproducible procedure with reasonable success rates.

Derivation of human ES cell lines

Human ES cell lines may be derived using two alternative methods, namely immunosurgical or mechanical isolation of the ICM. In both cases, surplus blastocysts donated by couples undergoing *in vitro*

Table 11.1 Main features of embryonic stem (ES) cells

---

(1) Derived from preimplantation embryos

(2) Pluripotent, capable of differentiating into representative cells from all three germ layers of the embryo

(3) Immortal, with long-term proliferative ability at the undifferentiated stage (self-maintenance) and high telomerase activity

(4) Express unique markers typical of cells at the undifferentiated stage, such as transcription factor Oct-4, or cell surface markers such as stage-specific embryonic antigen-3 (SSEA3), SSEA4 and tumor-rejecting antigen-60 (TRA-1-60), TRA1-81

(5) Maintain normal karyotype after prolonged culture

(6) Clonogenic, i.e. each individual cell possesses these characteristics

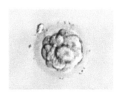

fertilization (IVF) treatments are grown *in vitro* to the blastocyst stage (Figure 11.1). The first method was developed in the early 1970s by Solter and Knowles, to derive embryonic teratocarcinoma (EC) lines and for early embryonic development research[7]. During immunosurgery, the outer layer of the trophectoderm is selectively removed, leaving an intact ICM. Initially, the zona pellucida of the embryo is removed using ether Tyrode's solution or pronase, after which the embryo is exposed to anti-human whole antiserum (Figure 11.2a). These antibodies recognize and attach to any human cell, thereby marking all trophoblast cells. As cell–cell connections between the trophoblast cells prevent antibody penetration into the embryo, the ICM of the embryo remains intact. The next stage includes exposure of the embryo to guinea-pig complement, which lyses all cells marked with the antibody, i.e. the trophectoderm cells (Figure 11.2b). The intact ICM is further cultured on a mitotically inactivated mouse embryonic fibroblast (MEF) feeder layer (Figure 11.2c).

Human ES cell lines may also be derived using mechanical separation of the trophectoderm and from ICM. The latter may be conducted by either removing the trophectoderm using 27-gauge needles followed by plating the ICM on MEFs, or plating an intact blastocyst on MEFs, culturing until the ICM cells expand and then mechanically removing the ICM cells into a fresh culture plate.

MEF feeder layers perform a dual role: they support ES cell growth and prevent their spontaneous differentiation during culture. The mechanism by which MEFs prevent differentiation is still not completely understood.

Six human ES cell lines (I-3, I-4, I-6, I-8, J-6 and J-3) have been derived in our laboratory that fulfil the characteristics of existing human pluripotent cell lines. These lines demonstrate typical morphology of human ES cell colonies (illustrated in Figure 11.3) and single cells, i.e. high nucleus/cytoplasm ratio and the presence of at least two nucleoli (shown in Figure 11.4). In addition, scanning electron microscopy reveals the existence of cytoplasmic connections between human ES cells and MEF (Figure 11.5).

Compared with mouse ES cells, primate ES cells have been found to express different surface markers, specific to undifferentiated cells. While mouse ES cells highly express surface marker stage-specific embryonic antigen-1 (SSEA1), and do not express SSEA3, SSEA4, tumor-rejecting antigen-60 (TRA-1-60) and TRA-1-81,

non-human primate ES cells and human ES cells strongly express SSEA4, TRA-1-60 and TRA-1-81, weakly express SSEA3 and do not express SSEA1[3,4]. The typical antibody expression of human ES cells is demonstrated in Figure 11.6.

Human ES cell culture

At first, human ES cells required an MEF feeder layer to grow continuously at the undifferentiated stage. Mouse ES cells can be grown as undifferentiated cells directly on gelatin-coated plates with the addition of leukemia inhibitory factor (LIF). Unfortunately, LIF does not have the same effect on human ES cells[3,4].

Three major improvements in the basic culture methods of human ES cells have been developed since their original derivation on an MEF feeder layer:

(1) The use of serum-free medium, which provides better defined culture conditions[8];

(2) The ability to grow and derive human ES cells with human feeder layer[9];

(3) The ability of human ES cells to grow under feeder-free culture conditions[10].

Human ES cells can be grown as undifferentiated cells using serum replacement supplemented with 4 ng/ml basic fibroblast growth factor (bFGF) while maintaining all ES cell features[8]. Under these culture conditions, the morphology of human ES cell colonies is slightly different: the cells are organized in more than one layer, while in fetal bovine serum (FBS) the colonies consist of a monolayer of ES cells. Representative examples of colonies in these two conditions are illustrated in Figure 11.7. The serum-free growth of human ES cells leads to better-defined culture conditions for the growth and manipulation of these cells.

Another advantage of the serum-free condition is that it has been found to be suitable for the derivation of single-cell human ES cell clones[8]. As mentioned above, human ES cell lines are derived from the ICM. The ICM cells may not represent a homologous cell population; therefore, it is possible that the pluripotency of human ES cells reflects the combined developmental potential of this cell population. However, the ability of single-cell clones to differentiate into representative tissues of the three embryonic germ layers eliminates this possibility. To date, nine single-cell clones from six various parental ES cell lines have been derived in our laboratory using serum-free conditions. A clonally derived human ES cell line in a 96-well plate is shown in Figure 11.8.

Human ES cells have also been reported to grow in an animal-free system[9]. The suggested animal-free culture system for human ES cells consists of coculture with human fetal-derived feeder layers or human adult Fallopian tube epithelial feeder layers, using medium supplemented with human serum. These conditions are suitable both for the maintenance of their characteristics during prolonged culture and for the derivation of new human ES cell lines. We have demonstrated that foreskin feeder layers support the growth of human ES cells in the above serum-free conditions[11]. After more than 70 passages, human ES cell lines grown on foreskin feeders exhibited all human ES cell features, including teratoma and embryoid body (EB) formation, expression of surface markers typical of undifferentiated cells and preservation of normal karyotypes. The morphology of a human ES cell colony grown on a foreskin line varies from that of a colony grown on MEF in the tendency of the cells to organize in an elliptical manner (demonstrated in Figure 11.9). Unlike fetal fibroblasts, which can grow to reach a certain limited passage, foreskin fibroblasts can grow to reach passage 42. Therefore, foreskin lines have an advantage when large-scale growth of human ES cells is concerned.

Lastly, a suggested culture system in which human ES cells are grown on matrigel, laminin or fibronectin, using 100% MEF-conditioned medium supplemented with serum replacement and bFGF, has been reported[10]. Examples of human ES cells grown using this system for 12 passages are illustrated in Figure 11.10. Since human ES cells may still be exposed to animal pathogens through the conditioned medium, and there is still a requirement for simultaneous massive growth of MEFs for the production of conditioned medium, the quest for the ideal animal- and feeder layer-free culture system for human ES cells is still taking place.

Human ES cell differentiation

As long as human ES cells are grown on an MEF feeder layer and passaged routinely every 4–6 days, they will maintain their pluripotency and remain at the undifferentiated stage. They differentiate spontaneously when grown to confluency on MEFs or removed from the MEF feeder layer, and, when plated as crowded cultures on gelatin, they differentiate rapidly and form visible structures (Figure 11.11). Another way to

encourage spontaneous differentiation of human ES cells is by inducing the formation of EBs. Human ES cells, like mouse ES cells, spontaneously create EBs when cultured in suspension[12]. Initially, after 24 h in suspension, they spontaneously form small cell aggregates (Figure 11.12a). These aggregates tend to organize into a special structure consisting of an internal ectoderm layer and an external endoderm layer (Figure 11.12b). Later on, some of the EBs form cysts (Figure 11.12c and d) and visible structures (Figure 11.12e and f). These EBs contain derivatives of the three embryonic germ layers[12]. Examples of different cell types resulted in differentiating ES cells in EBs are shown in Figure 11.13. It seems that the formation of EBs encourages ES cells to differentiate and consequently increase the rate and efficiency of differentiation. Human ES cells can create EBs with the same efficiency as mouse ES cells, although EBs formed from human ES cells have been found to be somewhat less organized than those derived from mouse ES cells[12].

The simplest and most convincing way to examine ES cell pluripotency is to look for teratoma formation. Following injection into the hind leg muscle of SCID mice, ES cells spontaneously create teratomas, in which they differentiate into representative tissues of the three embryonic germ layers. Several examples of resultant teratomas formed by lines I-3 and I-6 are illustrated in Figure 11.14: from endodermal-origin columnar epithelium, and tubules interspersed with structures resembling fetal glomeruli, from mesodermal-origin mesenchymal tissue, and hyaline cartilage, and from ectodermal-origin epithelium containing melanin-producing cells and nerve tissues.

While in EBs, ES cells differentiate mainly into simple structures or unorganized groups of cells. In teratomas, however, human ES cells can also create more complex and well-organized organ-like structures. Examples of such organs are illustrated in Figure 11.15, which shows a group of hair follicles, a salivary gland and skin tissue.

In their 4 years of existence, human ES cells have been shown to differentiate into specific cell types representative of the three embryonic germ layers in both spontaneous and directed-differentiation models. These differentiation models are summarized in Table 11.2. Overall, the reports on human ES cell differentiation models support the possibility of creating a well-developed model of differentiation for human ES cells, which would resemble the existing mouse ES cell differentiation models.

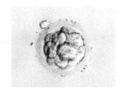

Table 11.2 Cell types formed by spontaneous and induced human ES cell differentiation

Cell types	Reference
Spontaneous differentiation	
Cardiomyocytes	Kehat et al.[13] (2001),
Endothelial cells	Levenberg et al.[14] (2002)
Insulin-secreting cells	Assady et al.[15] (2001)
Directed differentiation	
Neuronal cells	Carpenter et al.[16] (2001)
	Reubinoff et al.[17] (2001)
	Zhang et al.[18] (2001)
	Schuldiner et al.[19] (2002)
Trophoblast cells	Xu et al.[20] (2002)
Cardiomyocytes	Xu et al.[21] (2002)

Acknowledgements

The authors wish to thank Mrs Hadas O'Neill for editing the manuscript, Mrs Ruth Tal for editing the figures, Mrs Kohava Shariki and Mrs Victoria Marguletz for technical assistance, and Dr D. Levanon and Mrs Zelda Weinberg for their assistance with the electron microscopy work.

The antibodies used for the surface marker analysis (Figure 11.6) were generously provided by Professor P.W. Andrews from the University of Sheffield. The research performed in our laboratory was partly supported by the Fund for Medical Research and Development, Rambam Medical Center, and Technion Research and Development Fund, Haifa, Israel.

References

1. Evans MJ, Kaufman MH. Establishment in culture of pluripotential cells from mouse embryos. *Nature (London)* 1981;292:154–6

2. Martin GR. Isolation of a pluripotent cell line from early mouse embryos cultured in medium conditioned by teratocarcinoma stem cells. *Proc Natl Acad Sci USA* 1981;78:7634–8

3. Thomson JA, Itskovitz-Eldor J, Shapiro SS, *et al.* Embryonic stem cell lines derived from human blastocysts. *Science* 1998;282:1145–7 (erratum in *Science* 1998;282:1827)

4. Reubinoff BE, Pera MF, Fong C, Trounson A, Bongso A. Embryonic stem cell lines from human blastocysts: somatic differentiation *in vitro. Nat Biotechnol* 2000;18:399–404

5. Lanzendorf SE, Boyd CA, Wright DL, Muasher S, Oehninger S, Hodgen GD. Use of human gametes obtained from anonymous donors for the production of human embryonic stem cell lines. *Fertil Steril* 2001;76:132–7

6. Amit M, Itskovitz-Eldor J. Derivation and spontaneous differentiation of human embryonic stem cells. *J Anat* 2002;200:225–32

7. Solter D, Knowles BB. Immunosurgery of mouse blastocyst. *Proc Natl Acad Sci USA* 1975;72:5099–102

8. Amit M, Carpenter MK, Inokuma MS, *et al.* Clonally derived human embryonic stem cell lines maintain pluripotency and proliferative potential for prolonged periods of culture. *Dev Biol* 2000;227:271–8

9. Richards M, Fong CY, Chan WK, Wong PC, Bongso A. Human feeders support prolonged undifferentiated growth of human inner cell masses and embryonic stem cells. *Nat Biotechnol* 2002;20:933–6

10. Xu C, Inokuma MS, Denham J, *et al.* Feeder-free growth of undifferentiated human embryonic stem cells. *Nat Biotechnol* 2001;19:971–4

11. Amit M, Margulets V, Segev H, *et al.* Human feeder layers for human embryonic stem cells. *Biol Reprod* 2003;10:1095

12. Itskovitz-Eldor J, Schuldiner M, Karsenti D, *et al.* Differentiation of human embryonic stem cells into embryoid bodies comprising the three embryonic germ layers. *Mol Med* 2000;6:88–95

13. Kehat I, Kenyagin-Karsenti D, Snir M, *et al.* Human embryonic stem cells can differentiate into myocytes with structural and functional properties of cardiomyocytes. *J Clin Invest* 2001;108:407–14

14. Levenberg S, Golub JS, Amit M, Itskovitz-Eldor J, Langer R. Endothelial cells derived from human embryonic stem cells. *Proc Natl Acad Sci USA* 2002;99:4391–6

15. Assady S, Maor G, Amit M, Itskovitz-Eldor J, Skorecki KL, Tzukerman M. Insulin production by human embryonic stem cells. *Diabetes* 2001;50:1691–7

16. Carpenter MK, Inokuma MS, Denham J, Mujtaba T, Chiu CP, Rao MS. Enrichment of neurons and neural precursors from human embryonic stem cells. *Exp Neurol* 2001;172:383–97

17. Reubinoff BE, Itsykson P, Turetsky T, *et al.* Neural progenitors from human embryonic stem cells. *Nat Biotechnol* 2001;19:1134–40

18. Zhang S-C, Wernig M, Duncan ID, Brüstle O, Thomson JA. *In vitro* differentiation of transplantable neural precursors from human embryonic stem cells. *Nat Biotechnol* 2001;19:1129–33

19. Schuldiner M, Elges R, Eden A, Yanuka O, Itskovitz-Eldor J, Goldstein RS, Benvisty N. Induced neuronal differentiation of human embryonic stem cells. *Brain Res* 2001;913:201–5

20. Xu RH, Chen X, Li DS, *et al.* BMP4 initiates human embryonic stem cell differentiation to trophoblast. *Nat Biotechnol* 2002;online 11 November

21. Xu C, Police S, Rao N, Carpenter MK. Characterization and enrichment of cardiomyocytes derived from human embryonic stem cells. *Circulation Res* 2002;91:501–8

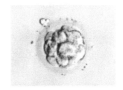

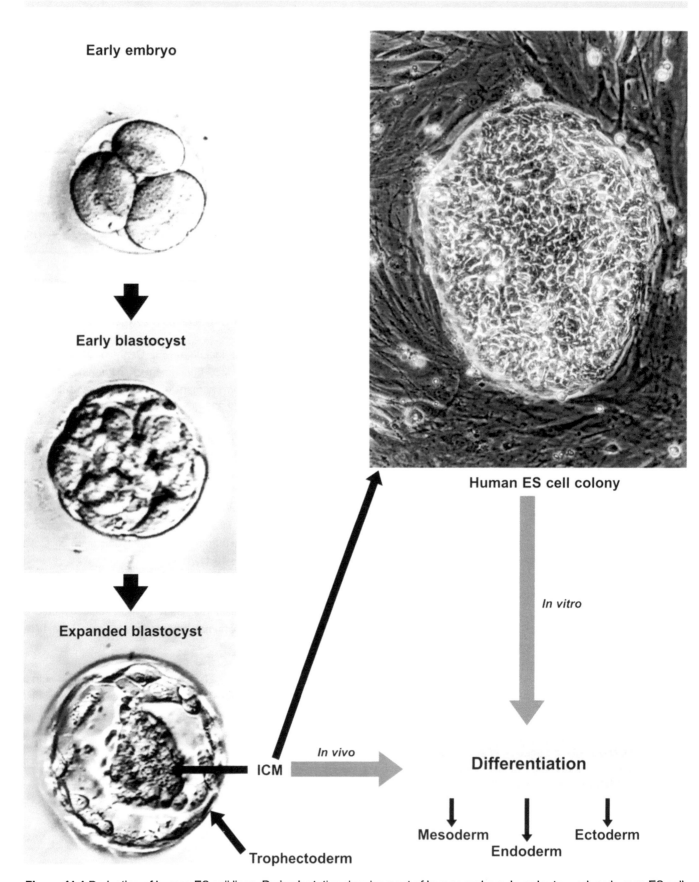

Figure 11.1 Derivation of human ES cell lines. Preimplantation development of human embryo. In order to produce human ES cell lines, surplus donated human embryos are grown *in vitro* from early embryos to the blastocyst stage. The ICM is selectively removed and further cultured on mitotically inactivated MEF. The resulting ES cells may differentiate into representative tissues of the three embryonic germ layers

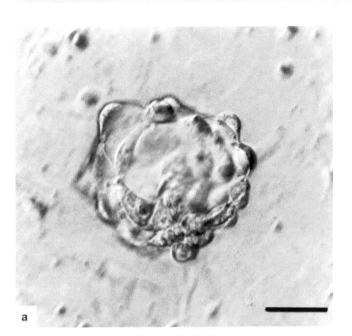

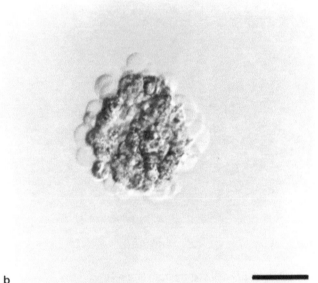

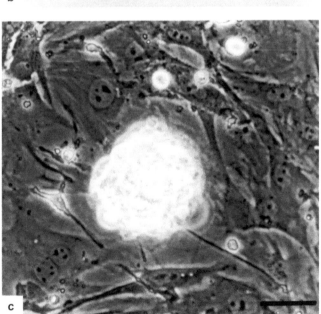

Figure 11.2 Derivation of human ES cell lines. Immunosurgery of human blastocyst for the derivation of human ES cell lines. (a) Human blastocyst after zona pellucida removal by Tyrode's solution, during exposure to rabbit anti-human whole anti-serum; (b) embryo after exposure to guinea pig complement; (c) intact inner cell mass immediately after immunosurgery on mitotically inactivated mouse embryonic fibroblast feeder layer. Bar 50 μm. From Amit and Itskovitz-Eldor, *J Anat* 2002;200:225–32

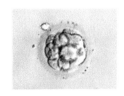

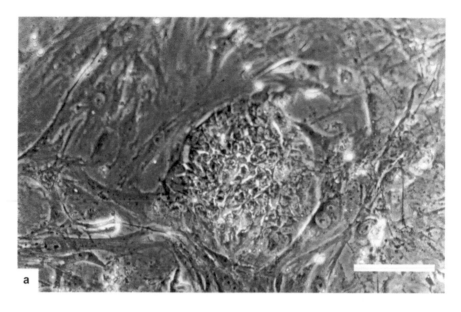

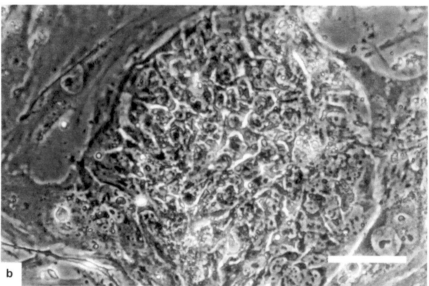

Figure 11.3 Characterization of human ES cells. Human ES cell colony from line I-4 grown for 47 passages on mitotically inactivated MEF. (a) Using low magnification: note the round shape of the colony, typical of human ES cells grown on mitotically inactivated MEF. Bar 100 µm. (b) Using high magnification: typical spaces between the ES cells and high nucleus-to-cytoplasm ratio. Bar 50 µm

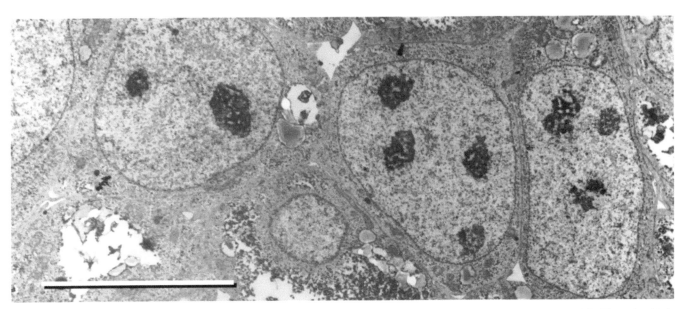

Figure 11.4 Characterization of human ES cells. Electron microscopy of single human ES cells from line H-9. Note the high nucleus-to-cytoplasm ratio and the presence of at least two nucleoli. Bar 8 μm

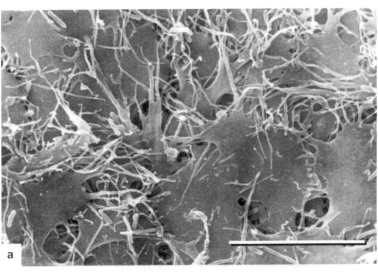

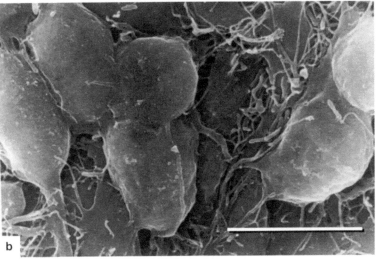

Figure 11.5 Characterization of human ES cells. Scanning electron microscopy of (a) MEF feeder layer. Note the cytoplasmatic extensions between the cells; (b) H-9.2 cells grown on MEF. Note the cytoplasmatic extension generated by both the ES cells and the MEF. Bar 10 μm

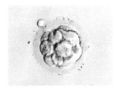

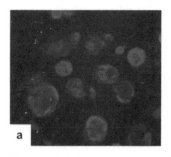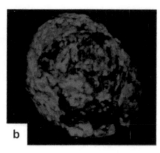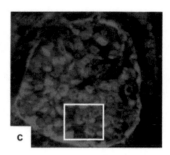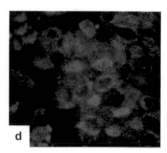

Figure 11.6 Characterization of human ES cells. Fluorescent immunostaining of human ES cells. (a) Immunostaining of human ES cell colonies I-3 with anti-TRA-1-60 (tumor-rejecting antigen-60) antibodies (× 5); (b) immunostaining of human ES cell colony I-6 with anti-SSEA4 (stage-specific embryonic antigen-4) antibodies (× 20); (c) immunostaining of human ES cell colony I-6 with anti-TRA-1-81 (× 20); (d) high-power picture from the marked area in (c) (× 63). From Amit and Itskovitz-Eldor, *J Anat* 2002;200:225–32

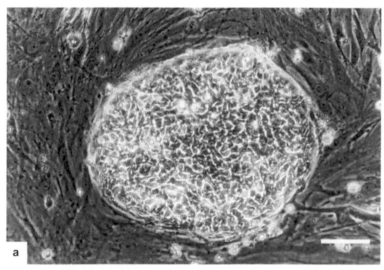

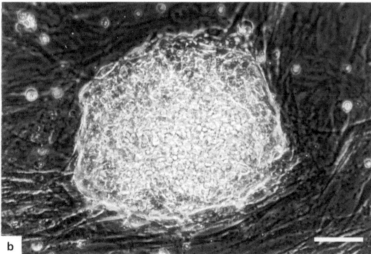

Figure 11.7 Human ES cell culture. Typical morphology of ES cell colonies of clone H-9.2 in different types of medium. (a) Medium supplemented with FBS; (b) medium supplemented with serum replacement and bFGF. Bar 50 μm

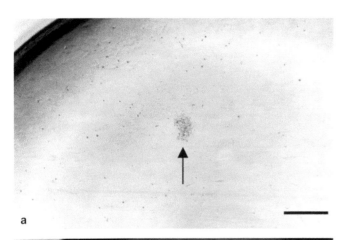

a

b

Figure 11.8 Human ES cell culture. A clonally derived human ES cell line in a 96-well plate. (a) Colony of single-cell clone I-3.3 7 days post-cloning; (b) the same colony at day 12 post-cloning. Bar 38 μm

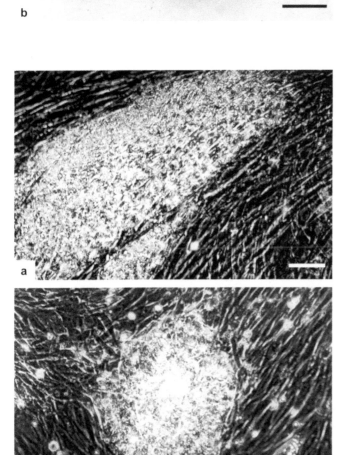

a

b

Figure 11.9 Human ES cell culture. Typical morphology of ES cell colony grown on human foreskin feeder layer. (a) The common morphology: elliptic-like colony of line I-6 after 57 passages on the human feeders, and (b) a rare morphology, irregular shape of line I-3 after 21 passages on the human feeders. Bar 50 μm

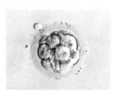

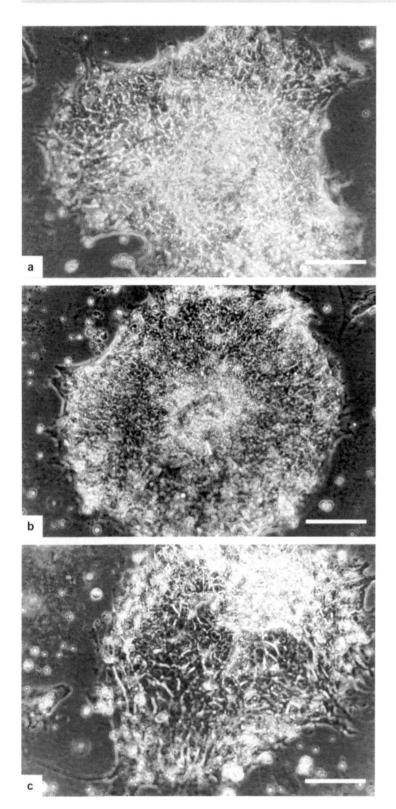

Figure 11.10 Human ES cell culture. Three examples of the colonial morphology of undifferentiated ES cells from clone I-3.2, grown for 12 passages on Matrigel® (BD Biosciences, Bedford, MA, USA) matrix using MEF-conditioned medium. Note the typical spaces between the ES cells and the high nucleus-to-cytoplasm ratio ((a) and (c)), and small and dense cells in (b) typical of dividing cells. Bar 50 μm

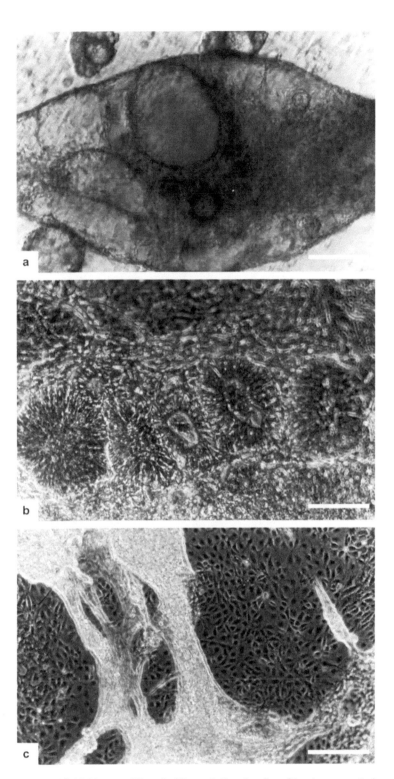

Figure 11.11 Human ES cell differentiation *in vitro*. Structure created by human ES cells H-9 at passage 33, grown to confluency on gelatin (a) for 9 days: note the cyst created by the differentiating ES cells, whose structure resembles that of an embryoid body (EB), bar 100 μm; (b) for 10 days: rosettes of neural epithelium-like structures have been formed, bar 75 μm; (c) for 13 days, bar 100 μm

225

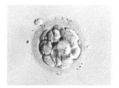

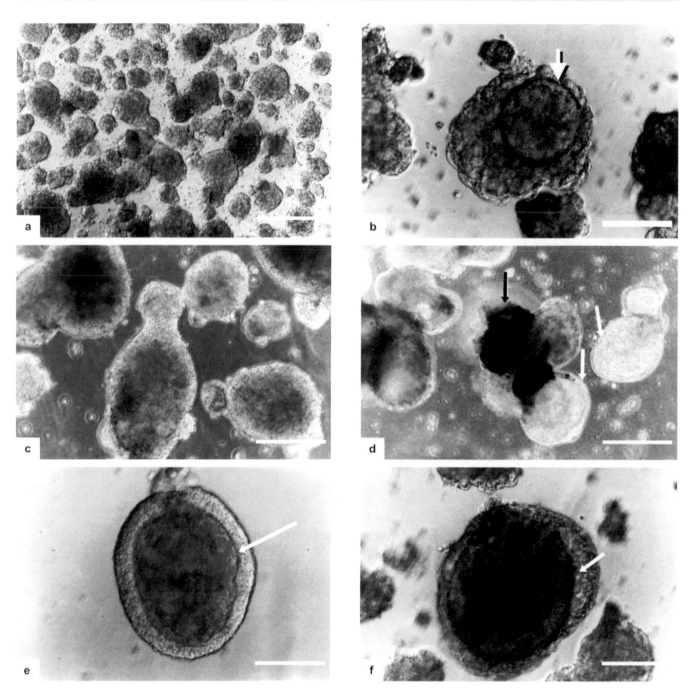

Figure 11.12 Human ES cell differentiation *in vitro*. Embryoid body (EB) development. (a) EB formed by cells H-9 after 24 h in suspension. Bar 100 μm; (b) EB from line I-6 after 48 h in suspension. Note the ectoderm layer (arrow) surrounding the EB. Bar 75 μm; (c) EB formed by line H-9 starts to create a cyst after 4 days in suspension. Bar 50 μm; (d) EB formed by line H-9 after 6 days in suspension. Note the well-developed cyst (white arrows) and some melanin-containing cells (black arrow). Bar 75 μm; (e) and (f) 1-month-old EB from single-cell clones H-9.2 and H-9.2.4, respectively, containing notable structures (white arrows). Bar 50 μm

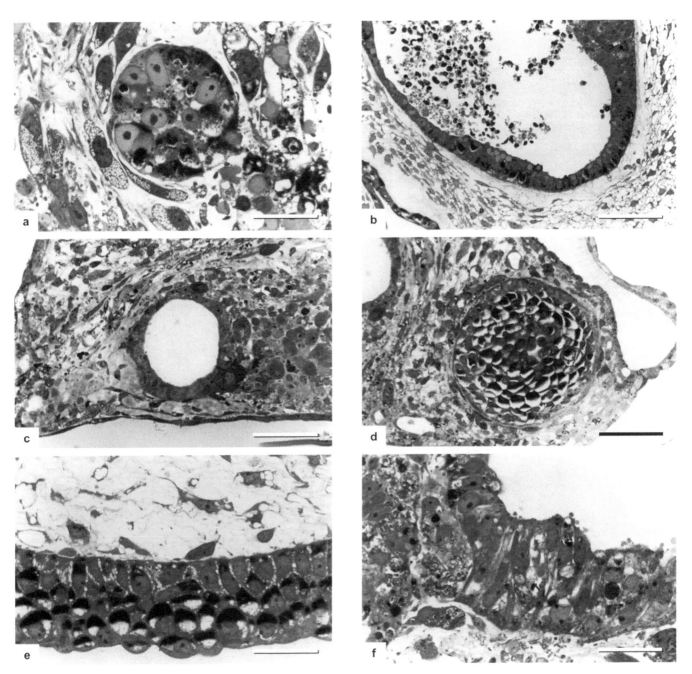

Figure 11.13 Human ES cells differentiation *in vitro*. Examples of 1-μm epon sections of 1-month-old EB from single-cell clone H-9.2 stained in alkaline toluidine blue. (a) Ball of epithelial-like cells with large regular nuclei and very pronounced nucleoli, which indicate intense synthetic activities. Isolated cells are seen with many cytoplasmic lipid droplets. Bar 10 μm; (b) stratified epithelium lining a tube-like structure in which aggregates of unidentified cells can be observed. Bar 25 μm; (c) differentiation of epithelial cells lining a tube-like structure. The surrounding cells are quite varied and probably develop connective tissue cells and intracellular matrices. Bar 25 μm; (d) epithelial-like cells arranged in a solid ball. The cells contain cytoplasmic granular material, which is stained with a deep purple color. Bar 25 μm; (e) stratified epithelium at the periphery of an EB and underlying mesenchymal-like cells of developing connective tissue. Bar 10 μm; (f) development of columnar epithelium seen in a differentiating structure within an EB. Bar 10 μm

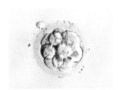

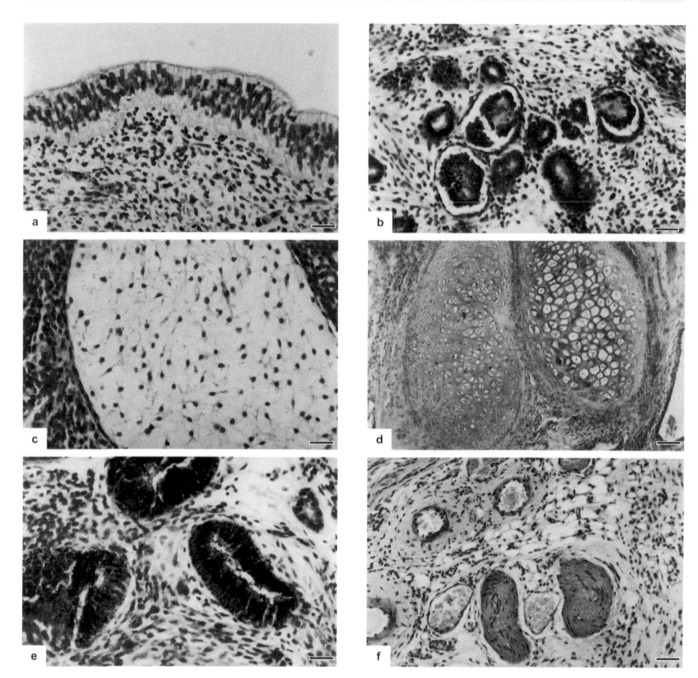

Figure 11.14 Human ES cells differentiation *in vivo*. Differentiated human ES cells from lines I-3 and I-6 in teratomas. (a) Columnar-epithelium, I-3 (H&E) Bar 25 μm; (b) tubules interspersed with structures resembling fetal glomeruli, I-6 (H&E) Bar 25 μm; (c) mesenchymal tissue, I-6 (H&E) Bar 25 μm; (d) hyalinic cartilage, I-3 (H&E) Bar 100 μm; (e) epithelium containing melanin-producing cells, I-6 (H&E) Bar 25 μm; (f) nerve tissue and blood vessels, I-6 (H&E). Bar 50 μm

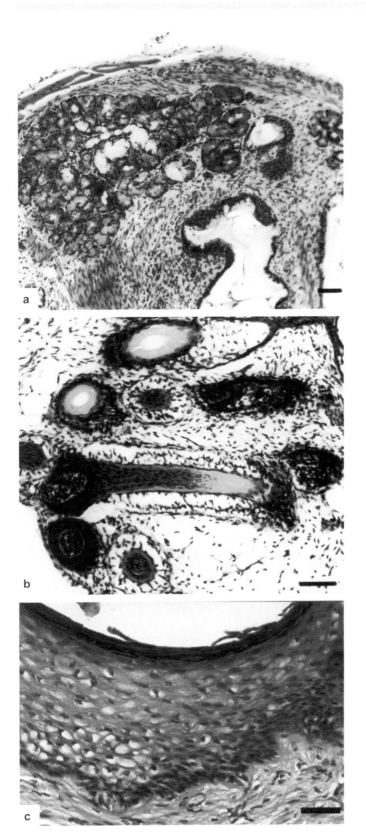

Figure 11.15 Differentiated human ES cells from subclone H-9.2.4 in teratomas. (a) Mixed salivary gland with serous and mucous secretory cells (H&E); (b) group of developing hair follicles (H&E); (c) complete skin tissue formed by line J-3. Keratin-containing cells facing a large lumen. Bar 50 μm. (a) and (b) taken from reference 6, with permission

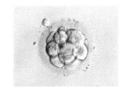

12 The mammalian blastocyst as an experimental model

Shoukhrat M. Mitalipov, Hung-Chih Kuo and Don P. Wolf

Introduction

In the development and application of assisted reproductive technology (ART), clinical experience in the human has often led the way. However, when invasive experimentation is required, the rodent or non-human primate may be the only suitable model. Furthermore, it can be argued that all ART applications should ideally be first applied in animals. Recent advances in non-human primate ART, with emphasis on experiments that cannot be conducted in humans for ethical reasons, are highlighted here.

Preimplantation development of the mammalian embryo incorporates explicit developmental stages from the formation of the zygote after fertilization to cleavage, morula formation, compaction and, finally, cavitation with the formation of the blastocyst (Figure 12.1). *In vitro*, in the rhesus monkey, preimplantation development is slower than in the human, with early blastocysts containing 100 or so cells seen on day 6–7 instead of day 5. Admittedly, *in vivo* rates are probably somewhat faster than *in vitro*, which may reflect suboptimal culture conditions.

During preimplantation development there is little or no growth in embryo volume, rather the large oocyte simply cleaves into smaller and smaller cells until blastulation. After fertilization, the embryonic genome is transcriptionally inactive and the first divisions of the embryo are supported primarily by maternally inherited proteins and mRNAs present in the cytoplasm of the unfertilized oocyte. The onset of embryonic transcription at the maternal–embryonic transition is species-dependent, starting as early as the 1–2-cell stage in the mouse[1] and the 4–8-cell stage in the rhesus monkey and humans[2-4]. Cavitation (early blastocyst formation) is driven by the expression of specific sets of gene products, including critical gene families: the E-cadherin–catenin cell adhesion family, the tight junction gene family, the Na/K-adenosine triphosphatase (ATPase) gene family and perhaps the aquaporin gene family[5]. During early preimplantation development, individual blastomeres are totipotent, that is, each blastomere is capable of supporting a pregnancy and the development of a viable fetus.

Blastocyst formation marks the first obvious differentiation of the mammalian preimplantation embryo when two distinctive cell types are present: the inner cell mass (ICM) and the trophectoderm. The trophectoderm comprises a sphere of single-layered flat epithelial cells surrounding a fluid-filled cavity, the blastocoel. A compact group of cells within the sphere represents the ICM, whose formation is dependent upon expression of the transcription factor *Oct4*. During development, trophectoderm and ICM cells contribute to distinctive embryonic lineages. Experimental studies in the mouse indicate that the ICM gives rise to the embryo proper and to several extraembryonic membranes, while the trophectoderm contributes to the trophoblast layers of the placenta[6].

Developmental competence to the blastocyst stage is often used as assessment of embryo viability in the context of infertility treatments such as *in vitro* fertilization/intracytoplasmic sperm injection (IVF/ICSI), or in the creation of reconstructed embryos by nuclear transfer. To be sure, however, *in vitro* development to the blastocyst stage does not ensure

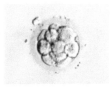

full-term development, since all blastocysts are not the same. For instance, parthenotes reach the blastocyst stage but do not develop beyond the 25-somite stage[7]. Even after fertilization, significant differences in blastocyst quality have been observed, and it is recognized that morphological assessment alone is not an absolute measure of viability[8]. The ultimate measure of embryo quality is unquestionably the ability to support full-term pregnancy following transfer to a recipient. Unfortunately, it is often impractical to use term birth as the outcome measure because of time and resource considerations. On the other hand, the embryo's ability to grow to the blastocyst stage is a significant accomplishment, as progression beyond the maternal–embryonic transition point and embryonic genome activation occur.

Blastocyst formation is essential for further development including implantation and pregnancy. It is important to evaluate embryo quality before transfer; however, we know little about the preimplantation stage embryo apart from gross morphological descriptions, cleavage timing and the ploidy status of selected chromosomes. Current studies on cellular composition and gene expression profiles in primate blastocysts require invasive techniques, but are critical to our long-term objectives of understanding and improving embryonic development. Such studies in the human are impacted upon by the scarcity of embryos available for research and by associated ethical concerns. However, because of the close physiological and genetic similarities between primates, the rhesus monkey is an excellent animal model for biomedical research on primate embryonic development. This animal model can also be used as an important experimental tool in the development and evaluation of novel technologies such as embryonic stem (ES) cell-based therapy. We believe that, in this case, translational research in a monkey model is absolutely essential before human clinical use, not only to demonstrate therapeutic efficacy, but also to allay safety concerns.

Oct4 expression in mammalian blastocysts

Although molecular mechanisms underlying the separation of ICM and trophectoderm cell lineages are still poorly understood, it is known that the transcription factor Oct4 is essential for ICM development. Oct4, also named Oct3, belongs to the Pou (Pit, Oct, Unc) family of domain transcription factors. Expression of Oct4 is

detectable throughout oogenesis and preimplantation development. However, in the mouse, Oct4 expression at the blastocyst stage is restricted to the ICM only, and later to the early epiblast, and finally confined to the developing germ cells[6,9,10]. The role of Oct4 has been elegantly demonstrated in mutant mice. Oct4 mutant mouse embryos develop into blastocyst-like structures containing trophectoderm but no ICM. Thus, Oct4 is essential for ICM development and has been used as a key marker for pluripotent cells such as embryonic stem (ES) or embryonic germ (EG) cells.

In the mouse, the two cell populations responsible for the ICM and trophectoderm can be identified at the morula stage. According to the inside–outside hypothesis, the inner and outer cell layers in the morula develop into ICM and trophectoderm, respectively[11]. Conversely, in porcine and bovine embryos, compaction and cell allocation into ICM and trophectoderm seems to be an independent and random process[12]. Mouse embryos form an egg cylinder stage, and hatching and implantation occur almost simultaneously, whereas in farm animals blastulation is followed by the germinal disc stage and implantation is delayed following hatching[13,14]. These differences in the timing of genetic and morphological transitions may relate to differences in Oct4 expression. The protein produced by Oct4 expression has been detected in the ICM and the trophectoderm of cattle and porcine expanded blastocysts.

We have been particularly interested in the pattern of Oct4 expression in primate embryos. Immunohistochemical examination of whole-mounted expanded rhesus monkey blastocysts reveals expression of Oct4 in the ICM as well as in trophectoderm. Oct4 protein is present in the nuclei of ICM cells, whereas a diffuse distribution of the signal, primarily in the cytoplasm of trophectoderm cells, is observed (Figure 12.2). Hatched blastocysts, however, show strong Oct4 expression in the ICM, with no detectable signal in the TE (Figure 12.2(d)). An Oct4 expression level was also studied in human blastocysts by reverse transcriptase-polymerase chain reaction (RT-PCR), and the mean Oct4 expression was 31 times higher in the ICM than in trophectoderm[10]. Interestingly, Oct4 was not detected in an 'empty blastocyst' lacking an ICM. This may suggest that Oct4 plays a similar role in maintaining pluripotency in humans and non-human primates as it does in mice. Mouse, human and monkey ES cells also express Oct4, and differentiation of these pluripotent cells is associated with loss of Oct4 signal. Thus, Oct4 is a candidate regulator in pluripotent and germ-line cells and is essential for the initial formation of a pluripotent founder population in the mammalian embryo. From a practical perspective, *Oct4* expression can be used as a suitable marker to establish and maintain primate ES cell lines.

Cloning by nuclear transfer and embryo twinning

In the past decade, tremendous progress has been made in the development of nuclear transfer (NT) technology. Live offspring have been produced in sheep, cattle, mouse, goat, pig and rabbit by nuclear transfer from differentiated somatic cells[15–22]. The possibility of cloning non-human mammals from somatic cells carries potential applications in a basic research context as well as at the applied level. Understanding the mechanisms of nuclear reprogramming after somatic cell nuclear transfer not only could lead to improving the efficiency of routine NT protocols but also could enhance our knowledge of early mammalian development. Improved efficiencies in producing healthy offspring by somatic cell nuclear transfer will allow its commercial use in agriculture and pharmaceutics. Coupling gene targeting with NT technology extends the possibility of producing transgenic and knock-out animals in species where it has not heretofore been possible[23–25].

The first requirement for cloning protocols is a reliable source of high-quality oocytes matured *in vitro* or *in vivo* following ovarian stimulation. Mature metaphase II (MII) oocytes are then enucleated using micromanipulation (Figure 12.3). Confirmation of metaphase spindle removal by staining with DNA-specific fluorochromes and epifluorescence is important, since artificial activation may induce parthenogenetic development of non-enucleated oocytes and developmental chaos after NT. The absence of a nuclear membrane makes it almost impossible to visualize the MII oocyte's spindle under conventional microscopy. Blind enucleation based on removal of the first polar body and adjacent cytoplasm may ensure a high degree of complete enucleation in freshly matured MII oocytes. However, within 2–3 h of first polar body extrusion, polar body movement within the perivitelline space makes blind enucleation impractical and inefficient.

The next step in NT is introducing the donor DNA (nucleus), from cultured or freshly isolated cells, into the enucleated oocyte (cytoplast). Conventionally, this is achieved by placing an isolated intact donor cell into the perivitelline space of the cytoplast followed by electrofusion. Alternatively, an isolated nucleus is injected directly into the cytoplast, similar to sperm transfer in the ICSI procedure (Figure 12.4). Synchrony between the nuclear donor cell and the cytoplast is important for maintaining the correct ploidy in the resulting reconstructed embryo. When a donor nucleus is transferred into an MII cytoplast prior to activation, high levels of maturation/meiosis/mitosis-promoting factor (MPF) induce rapid donor nucleus envelope-breakdown followed by premature chromosome condensation (Figure 12.5). This is the 'normal' response observed in many species, and may presage the reprogramming process necessary for successful full-term development. Of course, somatic cell nuclear transfer protocols bypass sperm-induced oocyte activation. Instead, artificial activation strategies designed to initiate cleavage and development are employed. The prerequisite oscillation in intracellular calcium concentrations followed by MPF inactivation can be accomplished, more or less, by exposure to ionophores and general protein synthesis or phosphorylation inhibitors. Cytoplast activation is followed by pronuclear formation and cleavage of the reconstructed embryo (Figure 12.6). For normal full term development of embryos created by NT from somatic cells, genes normally expressed during embryogenesis, but silent in the somatic donor cell, must be reactivated in an appropriate temporal and spatial manner. The genetic reprogramming required to reverse many, if not all, of these epigenetic changes in the somatic nucleus after NT is radically different from the process that occurs during natural gametogenesis, and must take place within the short interval between NT and the time of embryonic genome activation.

While the production of NT embryos is now relatively routine in several species, the establishment of viable pregnancies and live offspring following transfer into recipients remains challenging, owing to high fetal and neonatal losses. These low success rates most likely reflect poor or incomplete genetic reprogramming of the donor nucleus followed by improper gene expression. DNA methylation is one of the epigenetic modifications controlling gene expression, and global methylation patterns are dynamic during preimplantation development and dramatically different from those seen in somatic nuclei. In several mammalian species studied including mice, rats, pigs and cattle, preimplantation embryos undergo genome-wide demethylation after fertilization followed by remethylation[26]. Somatic cell

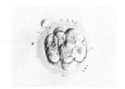

NT embryos showed a slight reduction in methylation consistent with active demethylation, but demethylation was subnormal. *De novo* methylation, resembling the methylation patterns of somatic cells, occurred precociously in many NT embryos[26]. This indicates that low efficiencies in somatic cell NT may to some degree be due to improper reprogramming as reflected by methylation levels.

The advantage of producing identical animals for biomedical research is that, in general, a substantial reduction in animal number requirements can be realized[27]. Additionally, genetically identical animals are absolute requirements for some experimentation, for instance when immune system function is under study. Somatic cell NT may eventually provide a solution, given marked improvements in fetal and neonatal outcomes, although true clones or animals that are 100% genetically identical will not result, because of differences in the source of nuclear and mitochondrial DNA. The production of monozygotic offspring by manipulation of the preimplantation embryo remains an important alternative. Two approaches have been established in several mammalian species: blastomere separation at cleavage stages and blastocyst bisection.

The ability of isolated blastomeres, either singly or in pairs, from 2-, 4- and 8-cell stage embryos to support term pregnancies and to produce genetically identical animals has been described in the mouse[28], rat[29], goat[30], horse[31] and, on repeated occasions, in cattle[32,33]. Although the usual outcome in producing monozygotic offspring is a singleton pregnancy, twins, triplets and even quadruplets have been reported upon transfer of one-quarter embryos in cattle[34,35]. On average, 25–40% of live offspring resulted after transfer of in vivo-produced and -twinned cattle and sheep embryos as identical sets. However, in the mouse, rabbit and pig, the incidence of monozygotic twinning among offspring reached only 2–5%[36]. For blastomere separation, zonae pellucidae of 2–4-cell stage embryos are enzymatically removed and then individual (from 2-cell embryos) or paired (from 4-cell embryos) blastomeres are separated mechanically, aspirated into a micropipette and transferred into surrogate zonae pellucidae immobilized on a holding pipette (Figure 12.7). A convenient measure of the resulting demi-embryo viability is growth to the blastocyst stage *in vitro* compared with intact, or IVF- or ICSI-produced controls.

The splitting of uterine stage embryos (morulae/-blastocysts) has also led to the production of monozygotic offspring. Embryos can be recovered non-surgically by flushing the uterus of mated animals or by application of the assisted reproductive technologies. For bisection, the blastocyst is immobilized with a holding pipette, positioned across from the ICM, in a micromanipulation chamber on the stage of an inverted microscope. A surgical microblade attached to a micromanipulator is used to split the embryo, with even distribution of ICM and trophectoderm into each demi-embryo (Figure 12.8). The zone-free demi-embryos produced by bisection are placed in culture and monitored for re-expansion.

The number of identical animals that can be produced by blastomere separation or blastocyst bisection is realistically limited to twins or triplets, as the developmental potential of one-quarter embryos and less is poor, secondary to inadequate cell numbers to support the allocation of cells required during blastulation, as evidenced by extensive experience in agricultural species[37]. Thus, there may be insufficient embryonic mass for normal development or for the appropriate signalling that must occur between embryo and host. Demi-embryos separated at the 2- or 4-cell stage grow to the blastocyst stage at the same rate as intact controls, and contain, as evidenced by differential staining and confocal microscopy, half the number of cells[38]. Demi-blastocysts, when compared as averaged values and independent of the twinning method, also maintain allocations of ICM and trophectoderm cells with ICM/trophectoderm or ICM/total cell ratios the same as those of intact controls. Our preliminary results[38] suggest that, for specific biomedical and genetic purposes, pairs of monozygotic monkeys can be produced by either embryo twinning technique, although we have yet to realize a monozygotic twin pregnancy to term.

While spontaneous monozygotic twinning has been reported following blastocyst transfer in women[39], it seems unlikely that the twinning approaches described here in monkeys will be used clinically, at least in the near future.

Blastocyst evaluation by differential staining

As noted above, the embryo at the blastocyst stage comprises a morphologically distinct ICM and trophectoderm. Clearly, both of these cellular types are required for normal implantation and pregnancy to ensue. The possibility that differences in cell allocation and count could impact upon viability has led to the development of specialized techniques for quantifying these cells. Such examinations are most commonly performed by differential staining (*see* reference 40 for review). One procedure is based on partial lysis of trophectodermal cells with complement, following labelling with species-specific antibody[41]. The ICM, however, is protected from antibody exposure by the selective permeability of the outer trophoblast layer. The embryo is stained with the DNA-specific dye, propidium iodide, which does not penetrate intact membranes and stains only partially lysed trophectodermal cell nuclei. The embryo is then counter-stained with a different DNA-specific dye, bisbenzimide (Hoechst 33342), which penetrates the membranes and labels the ICM.

A modification of this technique has been developed that avoids the need for species-specific antibodies[42]. In this case, trophoblastic cell surface proteins are first labelled with trinitrobenzenesulfonic acid (TNBS) and subsequently recognized by a universal TNBS-specific antibody. The advantage of this approach is that all reagents are commercially available and suitable for any species. In yet another approach, the trophectodermal layer can be permeabilized by treatment with calcium ionophore combined with propidium iodide[43]. Calcium ionophore treatment triggers an osmotic response and formation of cell membrane vesicles, leading to permeation of trophectoderm cells exclusively. The ICM cells remain intact, and can be differentially counterstained with bisbenzimide.

The final examination of whole mounted specimens is carried out under a fluorescence microscope, equipped with excitation and emission filters appropriate for the fluorochromes in use. ICM nuclei labelled with bisbenzimide appear blue, while trophectoderm nuclei labelled with both bisbenzimide and propidium iodide appear pink or red (Figure 12.9). The numbers of ICM and trophectoderm nuclei can be counted directly under the microscope. More precise imaging can be performed using confocal microscopy, where different lasers can be used to excite bisbenzimide and propidium iodide. Fluorescent light in the specific spectral range is detected simultaneously in separate channels for either the propidium iodide or the Hoechst stain. Following this, optical sections approximately 0.5 µm in thickness can be sampled at 1–5-µm intervals throughout the entire blastocyst. Digital optical sections are analyzed by combining them into three-dimensional images using image-processing software such as MetaMorph 4.5. This approach allows automatic or semi-automatic cell counts of each section, and minimizes errors.

In experimental embryology, differential staining techniques have numerous applications, such as defining the 'normal' allocation of ICM and trophectoderm cells in blastocysts and then comparing allocations for *in vivo*-versus *in vitro*-produced blastocysts. The impact of different culture media or embryo manipulations (blastomere biopsy, twinning, NT) on development can also be assessed. In the clinical arena, the technique could help correlate cell numbers and allocations with morphological criteria of blastocyst quality. This approach would ultimately improve the non-invasive evaluation and selection of blastocysts for intrauterine transfer or cryopreservation.

Primate embryonic stem cells: pluripotency assessment

Embryonic stem (ES) cells and embryonic germ (EG) cells are pluripotent cell lines as derived initially from mouse preimplantation embryos[44,45] and primordial germ cells[46,47]. Application of mouse ES cell technology coupled with gene targeting for the production of mice carrying predetermined genetic alterations has become a revolutionary tool for the study of mammalian gene function (for review *see* reference 48). ES and EG cells are morphologically distinct, and express specific cellular markers. They remain immortal and undifferentiated under certain conditions, and their pluripotency has been demonstrated both *in vitro* and *in vivo*. In the absence of feeder layers *in vitro*, ES cells are capable of differentiating into a variety of cell types representing all three embryonic germ layers. *In vivo*, when injected into immunocompromised mice, ES cells can form teratomas also containing cells representative of all three germ layers, however, this property is shared with mouse and rat visceral endoderm (yolk sac)[49] and, therefore, may not be the most definitive measure of pluripotency. The ultimate measure perhaps, despite feasibility limitations, is the participation of ES cells in chimeric animals. Combined with host cells in a chimeric embryo, ES cells in the mouse can participate in development of all adult tissues, including germ cells[50].

Human pluripotent (ES and EG) cells have been isolated recently both from ICM cells of IVF-produced blastocysts[51] and from primordial germ cells recovered from gonadal ridges and mesenteries of 5–9-week-old

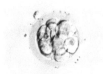

fetuses[52]. The use of such cells may eventually revolutionize the practice of medicine, with implications as far-ranging as our understanding of human embryogenesis and the development of transplantation therapies. The potency of human ES cells is important to establish as a prerequisite to clinical research that evaluates human ES cell use for cell, tissue or organ replacement/repair purposes. Pluripotency can most appropriately be established by quantitating participation of ES cell derivatives in chimeric embryos and in all cell lineages of chimeric fetuses and term infants, an undertaking that cannot be done in the human for ethical reasons. However, because of the close similarities between human and monkey ES cells, the use of rhesus monkey ES cells would serve as a valuable biomedical research model, and should catalyze progress towards clinical applications of ES cells.

Rhesus ES cells proliferate indefinitely *in vitro* as undifferentiated stem cells, and retain the potential to differentiate into derivatives of trophectoderm and all three embryonic germ layers *in vitro* or *in vivo* after injection into immunodeficient mouse[53,54]. Based on morphology and the presence of specific markers (alkaline phosphatase activity, *Oct4*, cell-surface markers stage-specific embryonic antigen-3 (SSEA-3), SSEA-4, TRA-1-60 and TRA-1-81) (the high-molecular-weight glycoproteins), rhesus ES cells resemble early totipotent embryonic and human embryonic carcinoma (EC) cells[54].

Presumptive ES cell lines with *in vitro* pluripotent characteristics similar to mouse ES cells have been established in several mammalian species, but only a few of them are able to generate chimeras: rat[55], rabbit[56], pig[57] and cow[58]. Although the precise requirements for maintaining pluripotency in such cell lines are unknown, the rigorous application of specialized culturing techniques as well as the use of early passage cells significantly increases the chances of obtaining highly chimeric animals.

The methods of production of ES cell–embryo chimeras currently fall into three groups: microinjection, aggregation and coculture. The predominant method used so far has been injection of 10–15 ES cells into the blastocoel cavity of blastocysts, followed by embryo transfer into pseudopregnant recipients[50]. Simplified techniques have been developed, based on the ability of ES cells to aggregate readily with cleavage stage embryos. For example, ES cell clumps aggregated with 4–8-cell stage zona pellucida-free mouse embryos or were sandwiched between two tetraploid embryos[59]. The use of tetraploid embryos is predicated on the observation that tetraploid host embryonic cells are effectively selected against in the developing chimeric embryo, producing 100% ES cell-derived mice; the tetraploid cells are well represented in the extraembryonic membranes and tissues. The third alternative employs simple short-term coculture of 8-cell stage, zona-free embryos on a 'lawn' of disaggregated ES cells[60] with the chimeric embryos cultured overnight to the blastocyst stage before transfer into recipients. The aggregation and coculture approaches involving zona-free embryos may not be an option for chimera production in mammalian species that require the presence of a zona pellucida during preimplantation development. A variation on the blastocyst injection and aggregation technique, which seems to be more efficient, involves injection of ES cells into cleavage stage embryos, where 10–15 ES cells are injected into the perivitelline space[61-64]. A similar approach has been successfully used to generate bovine ES cell-derived chimeras after injecting ES-like cells into 8-cell stage embryos[58]. Injection of ES cells into 4–8-cell stage host embryos has been shown to be more efficient than blastocyst injection in terms of ES cell contribution to somatic and germ line tissue in the resultant chimeras. This approach also carries the possibility of confirming ES cell participation in chimeric blastocysts *in vitro* before further *in vivo* studies are undertaken.

While phenotypic markers are readily available in mice, cellular markers are also important in assessing the extent of ES colonization of chimeric blastocysts. The *lac*-Z reporter gene, coding for β-galactosidase whose activity can be followed *in situ* directly on whole-mounted embryos, has been used for this purpose in the mouse[61,63]. The presence of bovine ES-like cell derivatives, transgenic for *lac*-Z in multiple tissues of 5-month-old chimeric animals, was identified and quantified by Southern blot analysis and fluorescence *in situ* hybridization (FISH) owing to the presence of the *lac*-Z reporter gene[58]. Thus, transfection of rhesus monkey ES cells with a *lac*-Z or green fluorescence protein (GFP) construct is of considerable importance to success in the identification of ES cell derivatives in chimeric fetuses and offspring. Unfortunately, we have not yet succeeded in producing *GFP*-positive monkey ES cells. In an alternative approach, PKH-26, a red fluorescent cell linker was used, based on its established application in cell labelling and short-term tracking. PKH-26 labelling has also shown low toxicity, with no cross-contamination of the label to neighboring cells.

Rhesus monkey ES cells were dispersed into single cells or small clusters of 2–3 cells each and labelled with PKH-26. A total of 10–15 labelled cells were then injected into embryos at the 4–8-cell stage (Figure 12.10a and b), and the incorporation of cells into the chimeric embryos was monitored under epifluorescent microscopy throughout preimplantation development. Monitoring labelled, injected cells provides valuable insights into the proliferative activities and localization of ES cells in morulae and blastocysts. Images taken from live embryos (Figure 12.10) clearly demonstrate ES cell colonization of both the ICM and trophectoderm. These chimeric blastocysts can be further analyzed by differential staining, followed by confocal microscopy and quantitation of ES derivatives in the ICM and trophectoderm.

In summary, clear evidence of ES cell proliferation in early preimplantation development was obtained in monkey embryos with distribution into both the trophectoderm and ICM. These results demonstrate that chimeric embryos can be produced readily in the rhesus monkey by ES cell injection, and set the stage for potency determination in chimeric fetuses or offspring when permanently labelled ES cells become available.

Preimplantation genetic diagnosis

Preimplantation genetic diagnosis (PGD) allows embryos to be screened for genetic disorders, followed by the selection of unaffected embryos for transfer before the establishment of pregnancy. Basically, the procedure of PGD involves two major steps, collecting diagnostic material via polar body or embryo biopsy, and genetic testing for a specific genetic disorder by molecular or molecular–cytogenetic approaches. Couples either affected by or carriers of a specific genetic disorder can create embryos by IVF and have one or two blastomeres aspirated from the 6–8-cell stage embryo, or polar bodies can be removed from the oocyte or zygote. In the latter case, genetic analysis can detect a disorder if it is of maternal origin. The collected materials are then processed for genetic diagnosis. There are two major methods currently used for PGD testing, polymerase chain reaction (PCR) and FISH. PCR-based methodologies are mainly used to diagnose single-gene disorders, while FISH-based methodologies are used to detect numerical and structural chromosomal abnormalities.

Although PGD has now been practiced for more than 10 years, there are still few centers worldwide that can effectively offer these clinical services to patients. As there are several cases of misdiagnosis reported[65,66], concerns of accuracy along with substantial technical demands impact upon the widespread application of PGD. Misdiagnosis in PGD may reflect biological or technical factors. Biological factors indicate abnormalities inherent to the embryo(s) or blastomere(s) taken for genetic analysis, such as chromosome mosaicisms or nuclear abnormalities. The high rate of chromosome mosaicism detected in cleavage stage embryos[67–69] has been regarded as a potential problem for the accuracy of single-cell PCR diagnosis for single gene defects or FISH diagnosis for chromosomal abnormalities or gender selection[70,71]. Technical factors include improper processing of diagnostic materials, contamination by exogenous genetic materials, amplification failure or inaccurate signal detection.

As described above, many factors impact upon PGD when single cells are used; however, improved protocols will undoubtedly further reduce the misdiagnosis rate due to technical limitations[72]. Errors secondary to genetic diagnostic attempts involving only one or two cells remain. The biopsy of trophectoderm cells of blastocysts may provide a way of obtaining more diagnostic material for PGD testing, as 2–30 cells can be obtained from human blastocysts with various biopsy strategies[73–75].

Blastocyst biopsy has several potential advantages over cleavage stage or polar body biopsy. First, since blastocyst biopsy involves removal of cells from the trophectoderm, an exclusively extraembryonic lineage, the ICM, or cells that contribute to the embryo proper, should remain unperturbed. Second, as noted above, many more cells can be removed from the trophectoderm, providing the basis for more reliable genetic testing. Third, embryos that reach the blastocyst stage in culture may have an increased implantation potential, ensuring a higher overall success rate for PGD, when carried out at this stage.

The feasibility of trophectoderm biopsy has been demonstrated in various species (rabbit[76], mouse[77,78], cattle[79], marmoset[80], human[73]) with several biopsy strategies including: trophectoderm incision, where a microblade inserted through a small hole made in the zona pellucida is used to excise trophectoderm cells; and zona drilling and excision, drilling with acidified Tyrode's solution (Figure 12.11a) away from the ICM and dissecting trophectoderm after partial hatching with a microblade (Figure 12.11b and c). A laser-mediated approach has been used to perform zona drilling and

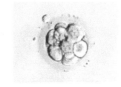

subsequent trophectoderm biopsy on human blastocysts[75]. Development of biopsied blastocysts seems unimpaired, as it has been shown that more than 40% of manipulated human blastocysts reach the hatching stage after biopsy[73]. In addition, birth of normal offspring after trophectoderm biopsy has been reported in the mouse[81] and marmoset[80].

Although trophectoderm biopsy has been performed on human blastocysts for research purposes for many years, this technique has not been widely applied in clinical PGD. A main concern has been the inefficient development of embryos to the blastocyst stage. Furthermore, only limited data are available in the human on the effects of trophectoderm biopsy on implantation, pregnancy rate and postimplantation embryonic development. With improvements in culture conditions, high blastocyst rates are now routinely achieved in vitro[82,83]. This should encourage further interest in blastocyst biopsy; however, a greater understanding of implantation and postimplantation development of biopsied blastocysts is still needed. This knowledge base should ideally be preceded by safety and efficiency assessments in animal models such as the monkey.

In conclusion, the potential applications of PGD expand as our knowledge of the human genome increases. This technology will significantly impact upon the future of human assisted reproductive technologies, and could lead to use in fertile patients at genetic risk. Additionally, microarray technologies will allow the determination of gene expression patterns or the ability to analyze the genetic polymorphism within individual embryos, and, therefore, provide an opportunity to identify embryonic viability markers or specific genetic disorders. Clearly, these objectives provide incentives to overcome the current limitations of PDG, namely the limited genetic material available for diagnosis. Translational research in animal models, including the non-human primate, we believe will contribute significantly to the further development of PGD.

References

1. Bolton VN, Oades PJ, Johnson MH. The relationship between cleavage, DNA replication, and gene expression in the mouse 2-cell embryo. *J Embryol Exp Morphol* 1984;79:139–63

2. Braude P, Bolton V, Moore S. Human gene expression first occurs between the four- and eight-cell stages of preimplantation development. *Nature (London)* 1988;332:459–61

3. Weston AM, Wolf DP. Timing of the maternal to embryonic transition in rhesus monkey embryos. Presented at the *27th Annual Meeting, Society for the Study of Reproduction*. Ann Arbor, MI, 1994: abstr P297

4. Schramm RD, Bavister BD. Onset of nucleolar and extranucleolar transcription and expression of fibrillarin in macaque embryos developing *in vitro*. *Biol Reprod* 1999;60:721–8

5. Watson AJ, Barcroft LC. Regulation of blastocyst formation. *Front Biosci* 2001;6:D708–30

6. Rossant J. Stem cells from the mammalian blastocyst. *Stem Cells* 2001;19:477–82

7. Tarkowski AK, Witkowska A, Nowicka J. Experimental partheonogenesis in the mouse. *Nature (London)* 1970;226:162–5

8. Gardner DK, Schoolcraft WB. Human embryo viability: what determines developmental potential, and can it be assessed? *J Assist Reprod Genet* 1998;15:455–8

9. Palmieri SL, Peter W, Hess H, Scholer HR. *Oct-4* transcription factor is differentially expressed in the mouse embryo during establishment of the first two extraembryonic cell lineages involved in implantation. *Dev Biol* 1994;166:259–67

10. Hansis C, Grifo JA, Krey LC. Oct-4 expression in inner cell mass and trophectoderm of human blastocysts. *Mol Hum Reprod* 2000;6:999–1004

11. Johnson MH, Maro B. Time and space in the mouse early embryo: a cell biological approach to cell diversification. In Rossant J, Pedersen RA, eds. *Experimental Approaches to Mammalian Embryonic Development*. Cambridge: Cambridge University Press, 1986:35–65

12. Kirchhof N, Carnwath JW, Lemme E, Anastassiadis K, Scholer H, Niemann H. Expression pattern of *Oct-4* in preimplantation embryos of different species. *Biol Reprod* 2000;63:1698–705

13. Evans MJ, Notarianni E, Laurie S, Moor RM. Derivation and preliminary characterization of pluripotent cell lines from porcine and bovine blastocysts. *Theriogenology* 1990;33:125–8

14. Stewart CL. Prospects for the establishment of embryonic stem cells and genetic manipulation of domestic animals. In Pedersen RA, McLaren A, First NL, eds. *Animal Applications of Research in Mammalian Development*. Cold Spring Harbor, NY: Cold Spring Harbor Laboratory Press, 1991:267–284

15. Campbell KH, McWhir J, Ritchie WA, Wilmut I. Sheep cloned by nuclear transfer from a cultured cell line. *Nature (London)* 1996; 380:64–6

16. Wilmut I, Schnieke AE, McWhir J, Kind AJ, Campbell KH. Viable offspring derived from fetal and adult mammalian cells. *Nature (London)* 1997;385:810–13

17. Cibelli JB, Stice SL, Golueke PJ, *et al*. Cloned transgenic calves produced from nonquiescent fetal fibroblasts. *Science* 1998;280:1256–8

18. Wakayama T, Perry AC, Zuccotti M, Johnson KR, Yanagimachi R. Full-term development of mice from enucleated oocytes injected with cumulus cell nuclei. *Nature (London)* 1998;394:369–74

19. Baguisi A, Behboodi E, Melican DT, *et al*. Production of goats by somatic cell nuclear transfer. *Nat Biotechnol* 1999;17:456–61

20. Onishi A, Iwamoto M, Akita T, *et al*. Pig cloning by microinjection of fetal fibroblast nuclei. *Science* 2000;289:1188–90

21. Polejaeva IA, Chen SH, Vaught TD, *et al*. Cloned pigs produced by nuclear transfer from adult somatic cells. *Nature (London)* 2000;407:86–90

22. Chesne P, Adenot PG, Viglietta C, Baratte M, Boulanger L, Renard JP. Cloned rabbits produced by nuclear transfer from adult somatic cells. *Nat Biotechnol* 2002;20:366–9

23. McCreath KJ, Howcroft J, Campbell KH, Colman A, Schnieke AE, Kind AJ. Production of gene-targeted sheep by nuclear transfer from cultured somatic cells. *Nature (London)* 2000;405:1066–9

24. Lai L, Kolber-Simonds D, Park KW, *et al*. Production of a-1,3-galactosyltransferase knockout pigs by nuclear transfer cloning. *Science* 2002;295:1089–92

25. Dai Y, Vaught TD, Boone J, *et al*. Targeted disruption of the a1,3-galactosyltransferase gene in cloned pigs. *Nat Biotechnol* 2002;20:251–5

26. Dean W, Santos F, Stojkovic M, *et al*. Conservation of methylation reprogramming in mammalian development: aberrant reprogramming in cloned embryos. *Proc Natl Acad Sci USA* 2001;98:13734–8

27. Biggers JD. The potential use of artificially produced monozygotic twins for comparative experiments. *Theriogenology* 1986;26:1–25

28. Papaioannou VE, Mkandawire J, Biggers JD. Development and phenotypic variability of genetically identical half mouse embryos. *Development* 1989;106:817–27

29. Matsumoto K, Miyake M, Utsumi K, Iritani A. Production of identical twins by separating two-cell rat embryos. *Gamete Res* 1989;22:257–263

30. Tsunoda Y, Uasui T, Sugie T. Production of monozygotic twins following transfer of separated half embryos in the goat. *Jpn J Zootech Sci* 1984;55:643–7

31. Allen WR, Pashen RL. Production of monozygotic (identical) horse twins by embryo micromanipulation. *J Reprod Fertil* 1984;71:607–13

32. Willadsen SM, Lehn-Jensen H, Fehily CB, Newcomb R. The production of monozygotic twins of preselected parentage by micromanipulation of non-surgically collected cow embryos. *Theriogenology* 1981;15:23–9

33. Ozil JP, Heyman Y, Renard JP. Production of monozygotic twins by micromanipulation and cervical transfer in the cow. *Vet Rec* 1982;110:126–7

34. Willadsen SM, Polge C. Attempts to produce monozygotic quadruplets in cattle by blastomere separation. *Vet Rec* 1981;108:211–13

35. Johnson WH, Loskutoff NM, Plante Y, Betteridge KJ. Production of four identical calves by the separation of blastomeres from an *in vitro* derived four-cell embryo. *Vet Rec* 1995;137:15–16

36. Niemann H, Rath D. Progress in reproductive biotechnology in swine. *Theriogenology* 2001;56:1291–304

37. Eckert J, Tao T, Niemann H. Ratio of inner cell mass and trophoblastic cells in blastocysts derived from porcine 4- and 8-cell embryos and isolated blastomeres cultured *in vitro* in the presence or absence of protein and human leukemia inhibitory factor. *Biol Reprod* 1997;57:552–60

38. Mitalipov SM, Yeoman RR, Kuo HC, Wolf DP. Monozygotic twinning in rhesus monkeys by manipulation of *in vitro*-derived embryos. *Biol Reprod* 2002;66:1449–55

39. da Costa AL, Abdelmassih S, de Oliveira FG, *et al.* Monozygotic twins and transfer at the blastocyst stage after ICSI. *Hum Reprod* 2001;16:333–6

40. Van Soom A, Vanroose G, de Kruif A. Blastocyst evaluation by means of differential staining: a practical approach. *Reprod Domest Anim* 2001;36:29–35

41. Handyside AH, Hunter S. A rapid procedure for visualising the inner cell mass and trophectoderm nuclei of mouse blastocysts *in situ* using polynucleotide-specific fluorochromes. *J Exp Zool* 1984;231:429–34

42. Hardy K, Handyside AH, Winston RM. The human blastocyst: cell number, death and allocation during late preimplantation development *in vitro*. *Development* 1989;107:597–604

43. de la Fuente R, King WA. Use of a chemically defined system for the direct comparison of inner cell mass and trophectoderm distribution in murine, porcine and bovine embryos. *Zygote* 1997;5:309–20

44. Evans MJ, Kaufman MH. Establishment in culture of pluripotent stem cells from mouse embryos. *Nature (London)* 1981;292:154–6

45. Martin GR. Isolation of a pluripotent cell line from early mouse embryos cultured in medium conditioned by terato-carcinoma stem cells. *Proc Natl Acad Sci USA* 1981;78:7634–8

46. Matsui Y, Zsebo K, Hogan BL. Derivation of pluripotential embryonic stem cells from murine primordial germ cells in culture. *Cell* 1992;70:841–7

47. Resnick JL, Bixler LS, Cheng L, Donovan PJ. Long-term proliferation of mouse primordial germ cells in culture. *Nature (London)* 1992;359:550–1

48. Muller U. Ten years of gene targeting: targeted mouse mutants, from vector design to phenotype analysis. *Mech Dev* 1999;82:3–21

49. Sobis H, Verstuyf A, Vandeputte M. Endodermal origin of yolk-sac-derived teratomas. *Development* 1991;111:75–8

50. Bradley A, Evans M, Kaufman MH, Robertson E. Formation of germ-line chimeras from embryo derived teratocarcinoma cell lines. *Nature (London)* 1984;309:255–6

51. Thomson JA, Itskovitz-Eldor J, Shapiro SS, *et al.* Embryonic stem cell lines derived from human blastocysts. *Science* 1998;282:1145–7

52. Shamblott MJ, Axelman J, Wang S, *et al.* Derivation of pluripotent stem cells from cultured human primordial germ cells. *Proc Natl Acad Sci USA* 1998;95:13726–31

53. Kuo H-C, Pau PK-Y, Okano H, Mitalipov SM, Wolf DP. Monkey embryonic stem (ES) cell-derived embryoid bodies, neural progenitor cells and neural phenotypes. Presented at the *35th Annual Meeting, Society for the Study of Reproduction*. Baltimore, MD, 2002: July Abstr 22

54. Thomson JA, Kalishman J, Golos TG, *et al.* Isolation of a primate embryonic stem cell line. *Proc Natl Acad Sci USA* 1995;92:7844–8

55. Iannaccone PM, Taborn GU, Garton RL, Caplice MD, Brenin DR. Pluripotent embryonic stem cells from the rat are capable of producing chimeras. *Dev Biol* 1994;163:288–92

56. Schoonjans L, Albright GM, Li JL, Collen D, Moreadith RW. Pluripotential rabbit embryonic stem (ES) cells are capable of forming overt coat color chimeras following injection into blastocysts. *Mol Reprod Dev* 1996;45:439–43

57. Piedrahita JA, Moore K, Oetama B, et al. Generation of transgenic porcine chimeras using primordial germ cell-derived colonies. *Biol Reprod* 1998;58:1321–9

58. Cibelli JB, Stice SL, Golueke PJ, *et al.* Transgenic bovine chimeric offspring produced from somatic cell-derived stem-like cells. *Nat Biotechnol* 1998;16:642–6

59. Nagy A, Rossant J, Nagy R, Abramow-Newerly W, Roder JC. Derivation of completely cell culture-derived mice from early-passage embryonic stem cells. *Proc Natl Acad Sci USA* 1993;90:8424–8

60. Wood SA, Pascoe WS, Schmidt C, Kemler R, Evans MJ, Allen ND. Simple and efficient production of embryonic stem cell–embryo chimeras by coculture. *Proc Natl Acad Sci USA* 1993;90:4582–5

61. Lallemand Y, Brulet P. An *in situ* assessment of the routes and extents of colonisation of the mouse embryo by

embryonic stem cells and their descendants. *Development* 1990;110:1241–8

62. Tokunaga T, Tsunoda Y. Efficacious production of viable germ-line chimeras between embryonic stem (ES) cells and 8-cell stage embryos. *Dev Growth Differ* 1992;34:561–6

63. Yagi T, Tokunaga T, Furuta Y, *et al.* A novel ES cell line, TT2, with high germline-differentiating potency. *Anal Biochem* 1993;214:70–6

64. Wolf DP, Kuo H-C, Mitalipov SM. Participation of rhesus monkey embryonic stem (ES) cells in the preimplantation development of chimeric embryos *in vitro*. Presented at the *35th Annual Meeting, Society for the Study of Reproduction*. Baltimore, MD, July 2002:abstr 21

65. Geraedts J, Handyside A, Harper J, *et al.* European Society of Human Reproduction and Embryology Preimplantation Genetic Diagnosis Consortium. Preliminary assessment of data from January 1997 to September 1998. ESHRE PGD Consortium Steering Committee. *Hum Reprod* 1999;14:3138–48

66. Lewis CM, Pinel T, Whittaker JC, Handyside AH. Controlling misdiagnosis errors in preimplantation genetic diagnosis: a comprehensive model encompassing extrinsic and intrinsic sources of error. *Hum Reprod* 2001;16:43–50

67. Munne S, Sultan KM, Weier HU, Grifo JA, Cohen J, Rosenwaks Z. Assessment of numeric abnormalities of X, Y, 18, and 16 chromosomes in preimplantation human embryos before transfer. *Am J Obstet Gynecol* 1995;172:1191–9, discussion 1199–201

68. Delhanty JD, Harper JC, Ao A, Handyside AH, Winston RM. Multicolor FISH detects frequent chromosomal mosaicism and chaotic division in normal preimplantation embryos from fertile patients. *Hum Genet* 1997;99:755–60

69. Kuo HC, Ogilvie CM, Handyside AH. Chromosomal mosaicism in cleavage-stage human embryos and the accuracy of single-cell genetic analysis. *J Assist Reprod Genet* 1998;15:276–80

70. Harper JC, Coonen E, Ramaekers FC, *et al.* Identification of the sex of human preimplantation embryos in two hours using an improved spreading method and fluorescent *in-situ* hybridization (FISH) using directly labelled probes. *Hum Reprod* 1994;9:721–4

71. Delhanty JD, Wells D, Harper JC. Genetic diagnosis before implantation. *Br Med J* 1997;315:828–9

72. Munne S, Marquez C, Magli C, Morton P, Morrison L. Scoring criteria for preimplantation genetic diagnosis of numerical abnormalities for chromosomes X, Y, 13, 16, 18 and 21. *Mol Hum Reprod* 1998.4:863–70

73. Dokras A, Sargent IL, Ross C, Gardner RL, Barlow DH. Trophectoderm biopsy in human blastocysts. *Hum Reprod* 1990;5:821–5

74. Muggleton-Harris AL, Braude PR. Preimplantation diagnosis of genetic disease. *Curr Opin Obstet Gynecol* 1993;5:600–5

75. Veiga A, Sandalinas M, Benkhalifa M, *et al.* Laser blastocyst biopsy for preimplantation diagnosis in the human. *Zygote* 1997;5:351–4

76. Gardner RL, Edwards RG. Control of the sex ratio at full term in the rabbit by transferring sexed blastocysts. *Nature (London)* 1968;218:346–8

77. Gardner RL. Manipulation on the blastocyst. *Adv Biosci* 1971;6:279–96

78. Monk M, Muggleton-Harris AL, Rawlings E, Whittingham DG. Pre-implantation diagnosis of HPRT-deficient male and carrier female mouse embryos by trophectoderm biopsy. *Hum Reprod* 1988;3:377–81

79. Betteridge KJ, Hare WCD, Singh EL. Approaches to sex selection in farm animals. In Brackett BG, Seidel GE, Seidel SM, eds. *New Technologies in Animal Breeding*. New York: Academic Press, 1981:109–25

80. Summers PM, Campbell JM, Miller MW. Normal *in-vivo* development of marmoset monkey embryos after trophectoderm biopsy. *Hum Reprod* 1988;3:389–93

81. Gentry WL, Critser ES. Growth of mouse pups derived from biopsied blastocysts. *Obstet Gynecol* 1995;85:1003–6

82. Gardner DK. Development of serum-free media for the culture and transfer of human blastocysts. *Hum Reprod* 1998;13(Suppl 4):218–25

83. Gardner DK. Schoolcraft WB. Culture and transfer of human blastocysts. *Curr Opin Obstet Gynecol* 1999;11:307–11

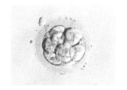

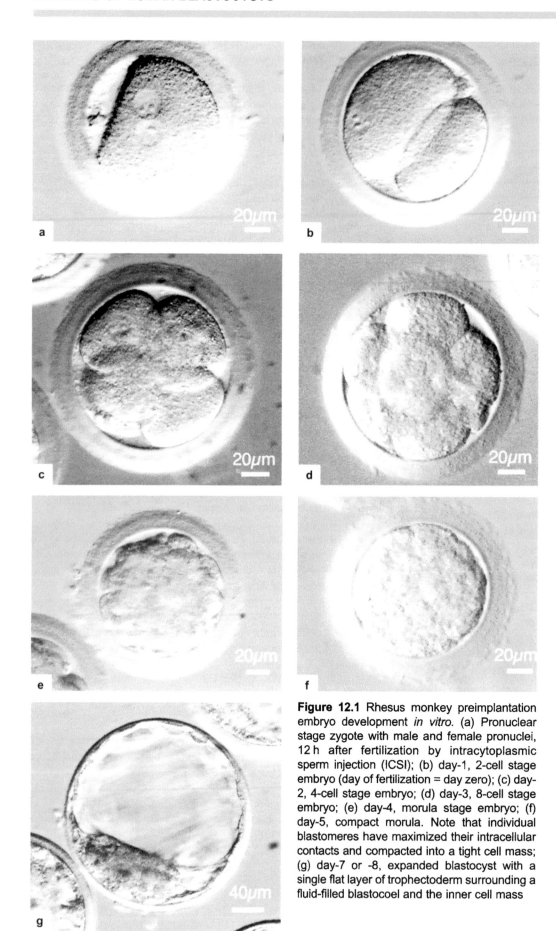

Figure 12.1 Rhesus monkey preimplantation embryo development *in vitro*. (a) Pronuclear stage zygote with male and female pronuclei, 12 h after fertilization by intracytoplasmic sperm injection (ICSI); (b) day-1, 2-cell stage embryo (day of fertilization = day zero); (c) day-2, 4-cell stage embryo; (d) day-3, 8-cell stage embryo; (e) day-4, morula stage embryo; (f) day-5, compact morula. Note that individual blastomeres have maximized their intracellular contacts and compacted into a tight cell mass; (g) day-7 or -8, expanded blastocyst with a single flat layer of trophectoderm surrounding a fluid-filled blastocoel and the inner cell mass

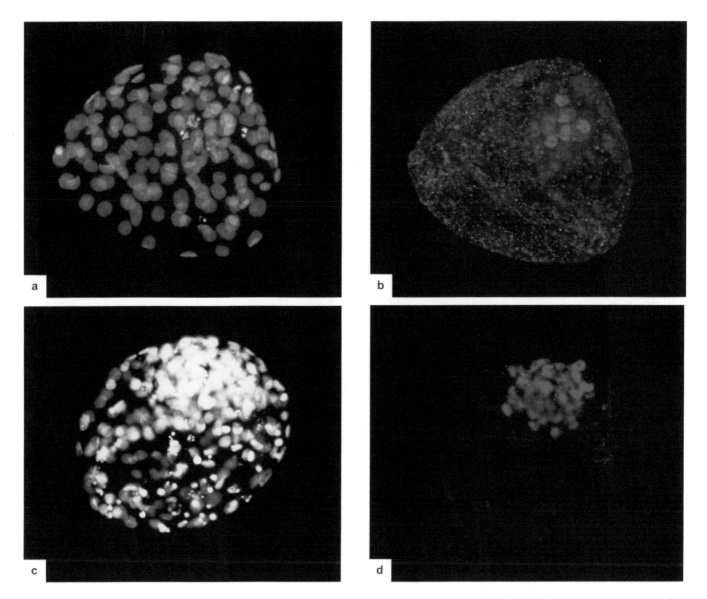

Figure 12.2 *Oct4* expression in rhesus monkey blastocysts. (a) Epifluorescent microscopy of a day-8 rhesus monkey expanded blastocyst stained with the DNA-specific dye, DAPI. (b) The same blastocyst labeled with *Oct4* antibody and secondary antibody conjugated with Cy3. Note the distribution of the immunofluorescence signal in both the ICM and trophectoderm. (c) More advanced day-9 hatched blastocyst. (d) Note the strong expression of *Oct4* in the ICM, with no detectable signal in the TE

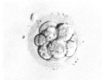

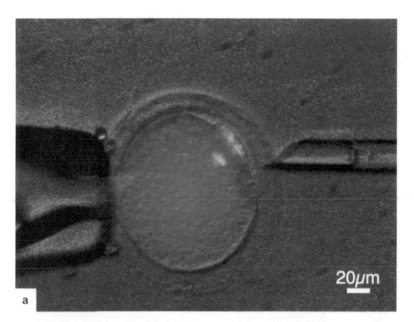

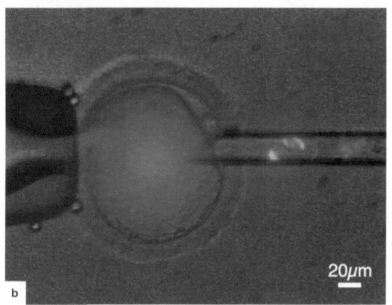

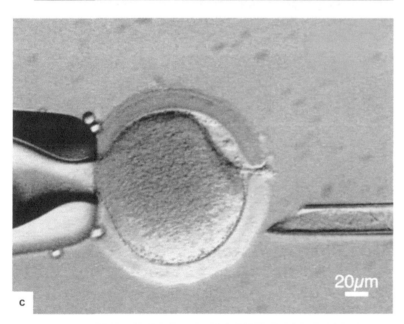

Figure 12.3 Nuclear transfer: preparation of the cytoplast. Enucleation of a metaphase II (MII), rhesus monkey oocyte. (a) Epifluorescence visualization of the metaphase spindle labeled with bisbenzimide. In the freshly matured MII oocyte, the spindle is localized in the cytoplasm/cortex beneath the first polar body. (b) Removal of the first polar body and the metaphase spindle by aspiration into an enucleation pipette. (c) Enucleated oocyte (cytoplast) under Hoffman optics

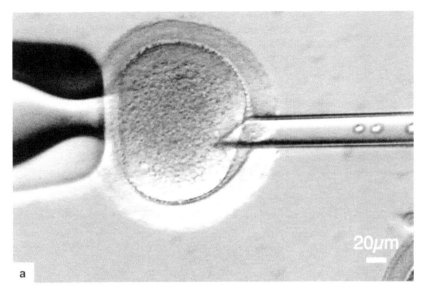

a

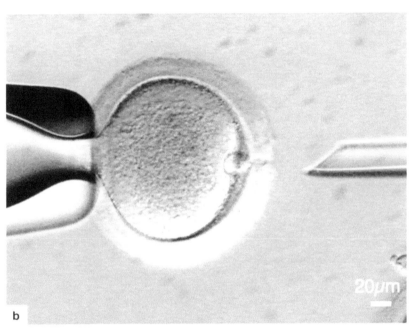

b

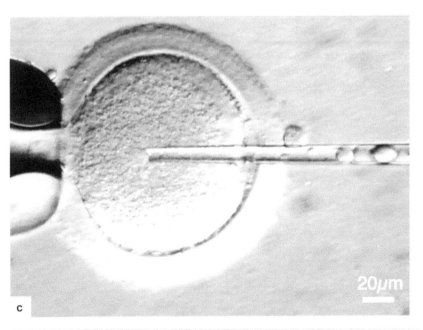

c

Figure 12.4 Nuclear transfer: creation of the fusion pair. Introducing the donor DNA material into the cytoplast. (a, b) Placing the intact donor cell into the perivitelline space with a micropipette. This procedure is followed by electrofusion that induces membrane fusion and incorporation of the entire nuclear donor cell. (c) Direct injection of an isolated nucleus into the cytoplast, similar to sperm transfer in the intracytoplasmic sperm injection (ICSI) procedure, is another method of introducing the donor nucleus.

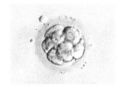

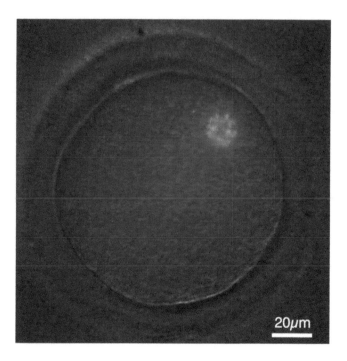

Figure 12.5 Nuclear transfer: cytoplast activation. Premature chromosome condensation. High levels of maturation/meiosis/mitosis-promoting factor (MPF) of the non-activated cytoplast induce rapid nuclear envelope breakdown in the donor nucleus followed by premature chromosome condensation (PCC). Activation is subsequently achieved by exposure to ionophores and general protein synthesis or phosphorylation inhibitors

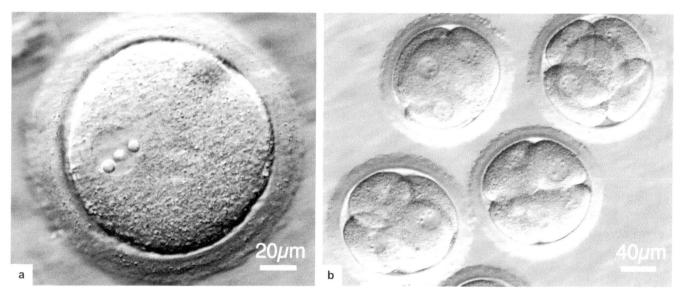

Figure 12.6 Nuclear transfer: embryo development. (a) Pronuclear-stage, rhesus monkey, somatic cell nuclear transfer (NT) embryo 10 h post-activation with a single pronucleus containing multiple nucleoli. (b) Rhesus monkey, somatic cell, NT embryos at the 4–6-cell stage. Note the presence of a clear distinctive nucleus in each blastomere

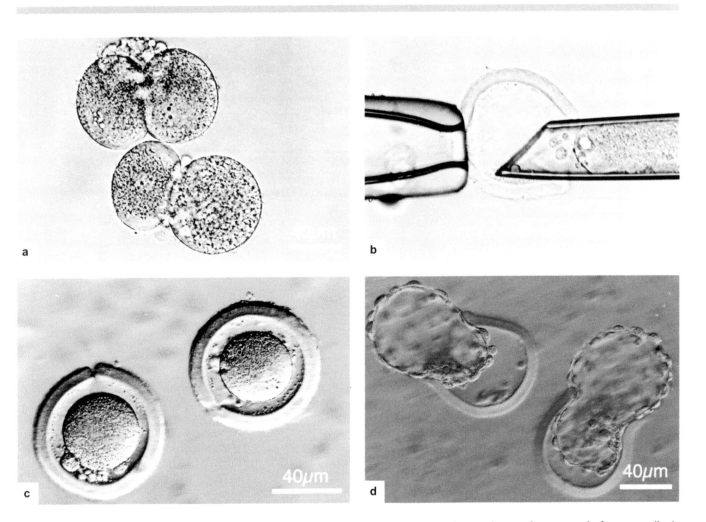

Figure 12.7 Embryo twinning by blastomere separation. (a) 2-cell stage rhesus monkey embryos after removal of zonae pelluci-dae; (b) a single blastomere from a 2-cell embryo in the transfer pipette, positioned for placement inside a surrogate zona pellu-cida which is immobilized on a holding pipette; (c) monozygotic, 1-cell, demi-embryos produced by blastomere separation; (d) hatching, monozygotic, demi-blastocysts after *in vitro* culture for 8 days

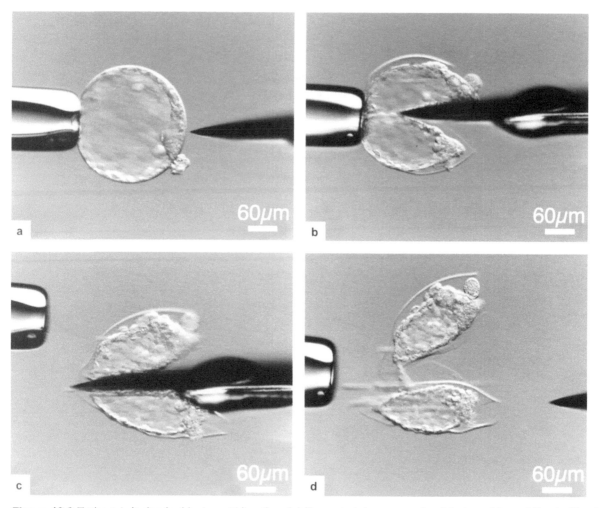

Figure 12.8 Embryo twinning by blastocyst bisection. (a) Expanded rhesus monkey blastocyst immobilized with a holding pipette positioned opposite the inner cell mass (ICM); (b) initial bisection of the ICM with a surgical microblade while holding the blastocyst; (c) completion of the bisection process after release from the holding pipette; (d) monozygotic, demi-blastocyst immediately upon completion of the bisection step

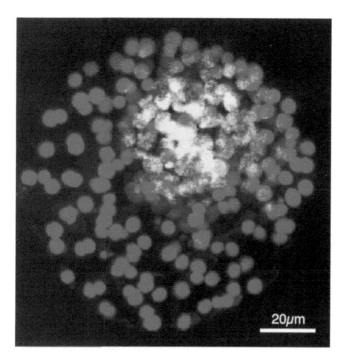

Figure 12.9 Differential staining of a rhesus monkey blastocyst. Inner cell mass (ICM) nuclei labeled with bisbenzimide appear green, while trophectoderm nuclei labeled with both bisbenzimide and propidium iodide appear pink or red. Individual cells can be quantitated by this technique

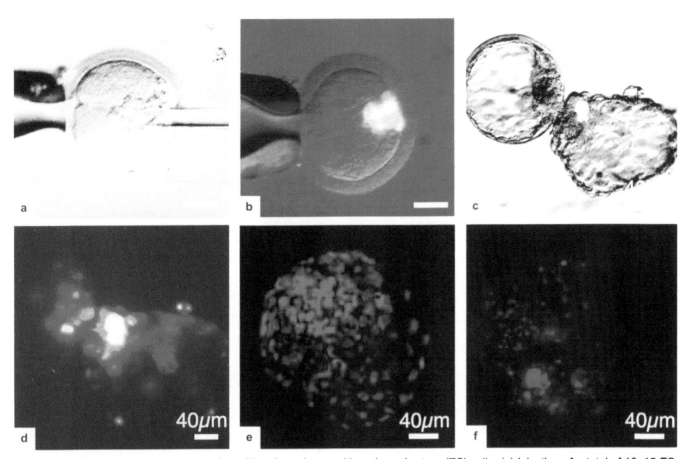

Figure 12.10 Production of rhesus monkey chimeric embryos with embryonic stem (ES) cells. (a) Injection of a total of 10–15 ES cells into the perivitelline space of a 4–8-cell stage embryo (Hoffman optics); (b) epifluorescence microscopy of embryos injected with PKH-26 labeled ES cells; (c) injected embryo cultured to the hatching blastocyst stage; (d) the same blastocyst under epifluorescence microscopy showing colonization of labeled ES cell derivatives in both the inner cell mass (ICM) and trophectoderm. The intensely fluorescent area is thought to arise from degenerating ES cells; (e) epifluorescent microscopy of a day-8, expanded rhesus monkey blastocyst stained with bisbenzimide (blue); (f) the same embryo displaying labeled ES cell contributions (red) to the ICM and trophectoderm

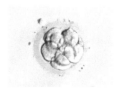

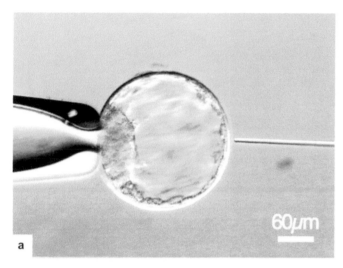

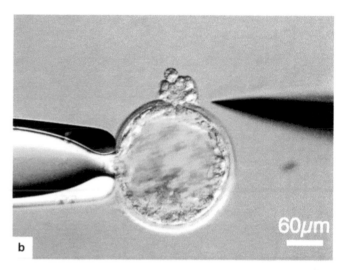

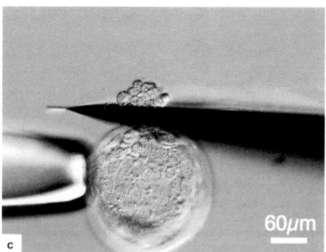

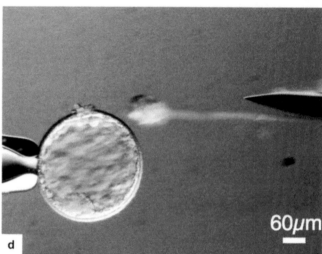

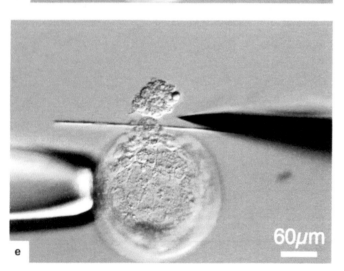

Figure 12.11 Trophectoderm biopsy for preimplantation genetic diagnosis. (a) Expanded rhesus monkey blastocyst immobilized with a holding pipette. The zona drilling pipette filled with acidified Tyrode's solution is positioned opposite the inner cell mass (ICM); (b) hatching of trophectodermal cells after zona drilling and culture for several hours while the ICM remains inside the zona. The extent of hatching can be regulated by the culture interval; (c) initial excision of the hatched trophectodermal cells with a surgical microblade while holding the blastocyst; (d) embryo immediately upon completion of the biopsy step. Note that biopsy did not cause collapse of the blastocyst, indicating minimum damage; (e) biopsy material containing 15–20 trophectodermal cells

13 The moral status of the human blastocyst

Howard W. Jones, Jr

As interest in the human blastocyst waxes not only as a means for improving clinical pregnancy rates with *in vitro* fertilization (IVF) but also in the basic science arena as a source of embryonic stem cells, it is fitting that the ethical/moral status of the blastocyst be examined once more. Here, as an aside, it is perhaps appropriate to comment on the difference between ethics and morality. This was discussed in a chapter by Ernlé Young in *The Human Embryonic Stem Cell Debate*[1]. Young holds that ethics analyzes an action or situation from the point of view of natural reason, whereas morality analyzes an action or situation from the point of view of traditional canon law.

Different views on the moral status of the preembryo (of which the blastocyst is a part) became public issue when IVF was first introduced as a treatment modality to assist in overcoming infertility[2]. At the heart of the matter is determining when, during development, personhood is achieved. Personhood in this context means the achievement of a developmental status that deserves protection by society. From a clinical view this is not important for the blastocyst which, when transferred, implants and develops or which, when transferred, fails to develop, but it is important for those that are not transferred. From the point of view of basic scientists and embryologists, great importance is placed on the moral/ethical status of blastocysts not transferred or those used for experimentation.

The acquisition of personhood or ensoulment has been considered by at least three disciplines of our culture. Note that ensoulment is equated with personhood in this context. It is generally agreed that the soul and person are different entities, i.e. the soul is a somewhat ethereal entity with quite an individual identity, whereas the person can be considered a civil designation with certain social and legal rights and responsibilities. However, if after ensoulment there is the implication that civil protection is required, then the soul and the person are the same in this particular context.

Canon law according to the classical tradition, canon law according to the current tradition, Jewish tradition and law, Islamic tradition and law, American civil law, and natural reason

Canon law: the classical tradition

The classical tradition can be traced to Aristotle and perhaps even before, to Egyptian culture (Figure 13.1). In *De Anima*, Aristotle indicated a belief that the individual acquired three different souls in sequence (approximately 350BC). First came a vegetable soul, then an animal soul and finally at birth a rational soul. Aristotle specified a time sequence. For males, the animal soul was acquired at approximately 40 days of development, while females acquired theirs at closer to 80 days. This concept of multiple souls was adopted by the early church fathers, and is seen in the writings of St Thomas, St Augustine, St Jerome and many others. The monk and teacher, Gratian, then summarized the matter in his influential publication, *Decretum* (AD1140), a cornerstone text of canon law (Figure 13.2). He codified several revisions of law having to do with a variety of ecclesiastical matters, but particularly with regard to abortion. The summary therefore is very relevant and

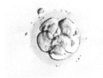

authoritative to the matter at hand. According to Gratian, abortion was not murder if the soul had not been infused. In other words, he accepted the notion that the soul had not been infused until some point during development after implantation. As proof, he offered the following: first, a statement by St Augustine regarding destruction of the non-animated fetus; second, the fact that the body must be formed to accept the soul, as for example in the case of Adam; and third, the statement of St Jerome saying that murder requires a formed fetus.

There can be little doubt that the early church fathers, before and during the Middle Ages, clearly accepted the notion that ensoulment did not occur until some time during development. We can interpret this in modern terms by saying that the preembryo, and probably the embryo, were not considered by these early Christian leaders as being ensouled, i.e. they were not persons and thus did not deserve special protection by society.

Canon law: the current tradition

All Christians have been born and educated in a world in which the tradition of canon law of the Roman Church states that ensoulment occurs with fertilization. This has therefore been referred to as the current traditional concept within that church. This concept of personhood was powerfully underlined by Pope Pius IX who convened the XXth Ecumenical Council of the Roman Church, commonly referred to as Vatican I, which was in session from 1869 to 1870. The approval of the content of several of the popes' encyclicals and other writings by Vatican I had the effect of establishing or modifying canon law, the basic laws of governance of the Roman Church. Our interest here centers on two laws promulgated by Vatican I. The first is 'Pastor Aeternus', which declared that in matters of faith or morals the pope could speak with infallibility, and 'Apostolicus Sedis', in which punishment is outlined for those who commit certain crimes. The highest punishment of excommunication is prescribed for perpetrators of several acts, including those seeking to procure (provide/bring about) abortion if the desired effect ensues. The significant aspect of 'Apostolicus Sedis' is that it no longer recognized a period during embryonic development before which excommunication did not apply. This has generally been interpreted and often cited as the concept that resulted in the modification of canon law to mean that ensoulment, i.e. personhood, was acquired with fertilization. This matter has been thoroughly reviewed in *The Crime of Abortion*

in Canon Law by Father John Huser[3]. Important to recognize is the distinction between church legislation, i.e. canon law, and church practice as annunciated by clergy in good standing. This is especially true at the pastoral level but at other levels as well. This view is clarified in *Health and Medicine in the Catholic Tradition* by Father Richard A. McCormick[4].

It is astonishing to realize that it was as recent as 1869 and after 18 centuries of the classical tradition that canon law concerning punishment for abortion was altered from the Aristotelian teaching, which was adopted by the early church fathers, to what we now regard as the traditional view of the Roman Catholic Church and several other religious traditions.

Jewish tradition and law

According to Jewish tradition and law, the unborn fetus is not considered a person until it has been born[5]. Up to 40 days after fertilization, the preembryo is considered as 'mere fluid' or 'water', and regarded as part of the mother's body. These facts form the basis for the Jewish legal view on abortion, allowing it to be carried out under certain circumstances. Abortion on demand, however, is repulsive to the ethics of the Talmudic Halakha, although there are many situations for which a pregnancy might be terminated, including saving the mother's life. Furthermore, the creation of a preembryo for research purposes might be allowed if there is a true opportunity for the sperm owner to benefit in having a child as a result of the research. Interestingly, Jewish law forbids the destruction of a preembryo if it possesses the potential for implantation, but one already hatched from its zona pellucida is regarded as having lost this potential, thus becoming acceptable for use in approved research[5].

Islamic tradition and law

It is relevant to note that the understanding of classical Greece can also be found in the Islamic tradition, as well as others, either stemming from Greek philosophy or borne of independent origin. These derivations are wonderfully summarized in 'The human embryo: Aristotle and the Arabic and European traditions'[6] by Father Gordon Dunstan, Professor Emeritus of Moral Social Theology at the University of London and research fellow at the University of Exeter, as well as by others. Dunstan stated the 'Quran left us no doubt that the fetus undergoes a series of transformations before becoming human.'

Islamic views generally place ensoulment on or after the 120th day, after three 40-day periods of development[7]. The preembryo itself has no precisely defined moral status. According to a publication from the National Bioethics Advisory Commission, research on preembryos and stem cells is regarded as 'an act of faith in the ultimate will of God as the Giver of all life, as long as such an intervention is undertaken with the purpose of improving human health'[8].

American civil law

Generally speaking, American civil law has not recognized the early conceptus as a person entitled to rights associated with personhood. Before medical technology introduced the possibility of extracorporeal preembryos, American jurisprudents addressed rights-related issues pertaining to a conceptus or fetus largely in the context of procreative or abortion-related privacy rights of the adult seeking to create or not create a child. As a long line of United States Supreme Court cases made clear, the 'law affords constitutional protection to personal decisions relating to marriage, procreation, contraception, family relationships, child rearing, and education' (*Planned Parenthood of Southeast Pennsylvania v. Casey* (1992)). The Supreme Court ruling in *Roe v. Wade* clearly established the pre-eminent right of women to terminate a pregnancy up to the point of viability. At the same time, the Court acknowledged that the state had an 'important and legitimate interest in protecting the potentiality of human life' (1973).

The status of preembryos has been the subject of only a handful of lawsuits, all civil suits involving the disposition those cryopreserved after social or marital circumstances changed for the adults involved. The three earliest cases were *York v. Jones* (1989), *Davis v. Davis* (1992), and *Kass v. Kass* (1998). Since then, a growing number of courts have been confronted with these issues. In *York v. Jones*, the case involved transporting a preembryo from one clinic to another. The court ultimately considered the preembryo to be personal property belonging to the parents, and refused rights of protectorship requested by the clinic performing the freezing of and caring for the preembryo during cryostorage. In the second case, *Davis v. Davis*, a divorcing couple was unable to agree whether cryopreserved preembryos should be given to the wife for future attempts at motherhood or to the husband for destruction because of his desire to avoid parenthood. In this case, the trial court considered the preembryos as persons and awarded 'custody' to the wife. Nonetheless,

the Supreme Court of Tennessee reversed the decision and squarely rejected any characterization of the preembryos as persons, either under state or federal law, and concluded that they must occupy an interim position which entitles them to another form of respect because of their potential for human life. Finally, in *Kass v. Kass*, a New York court concluded that a divorced couple's previous wishes in this 'quintessentially personal private decision', wishes evidenced in a signed cryopreservation agreement, should rule. Although the courts differ somewhat both in the characterization of preembryos and over who should have the right to control them, no court has ultimately recognized the preembryo as a person or entity entitled to the full panoply of rights associated with personhood, or even to the more limited rights associated with fetal viability.

Natural reason

Natural reason accepts that biology is unable to identify a point in the development of an individual that signifies the acquisition of what we define as personhood. It furthermore rejects the external infusion of an element which can be defined as personhood. Personhood, therefore, according to natural reason, develops in a Darwinian sense, i.e. slowly and through biological development. This concept recognizes that, for practical purposes, it is necessary for society to set certain arbitrary times as to when a preembryo, embryo, fetus or living person may acquire various rights as provided under civil law. Underscoring this is the belief that an ideal society expresses the will of the people and does so in a democratically organized manner. This point of view is eloquently set forth in *Darwin's Dangerous Idea: Evolution and the Meanings of Life* by Daniel Dennett[9].

Blastocysts and research

Why is this important at this time? It has to do with stem cells. The public is concerned about, and wants to be informed about, the exact stage of development from which stem cells are obtained. The concern is that, if the removal of pluripotent stem cells results in the cessation of development, then that stage acquires significance in terms of whether or not it is beyond a trigger point that designates protection by society.

To be sure, the processes of spermatogenesis, oogenesis, fertilization and development are a continuum. Nevertheless, there are milestones, i.e. clear marker events, which conveniently segment various stages of

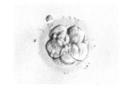

development, e.g. beginning of the embryonic period, beginning of the fetal period (Figure 13.3). The events of the first few days of development are so biologically unique that they deserve to be described and segregated. This is the preembryonic period previously described[10]. This turbulent period has the following characteristics:

(1) Large numbers of abnormalities occur. Estimates vary as to the extent of these abnormalities which cause loss, but a conservative estimate is that at least two-thirds of the products of oocyte and sperm interaction are in some way defective, either chromosomally or at a molecular level. The carrier of these abnormalities is so abnormal that it never implants, or, if it does implant, it usually perishes very early in development.

(2) During this early phase of development, most of the developing structures will be devoted to nourishing the subsequent embryo. The trophectoderm predominates and is the predecessor of the placenta and extraembryonic membranes that will be discarded at the time of birth. While the inner cell mass is recognizable during the blastocyst stage, it consists of only a few cells, rudiments of the actual embryo that will form. It is from these cells that stem cells may be obtained.

(3) Before the actual embryo forms with its neural groove, twinning may occur. There is no guarantee that there will be a single individual until the end of the preembryonic period, i.e. until a single primitive streak develops (Figure 13.4).

(4) An individual may not develop at all. As a result of fertilization, the products of fertilization may end up as a tumor, a hydatidiform mole or, even worse, a chorioepithelioma that may ultimately destroy the host.

(5) The lack of specificity of individual development is illustrated by the fact that, during this interval, fusion of two preembryos can occur and result in the development of a single fetus. This is well established in the human where fusion occasionally takes place with preembryos of different sexes. The presumption must be that, if this is possible, there should be at least an equal number of instances where fusion occurs between two XX preembryos or between two XY preembryos. Thus, the primitive streak guarantees biological individuation and terminates the preembryonic period.

Stem cells seem best obtained from the pluripotential cells of the inner cell mass of the blastocyst, a stage

occurring during the preembryonic interval (Figure 13.5). For those who place the acquisition of personhood beyond this stage, using pluripotent cells from donated (and, otherwise, discarded) preembryos is carried out with a clear conscience. The recent discussions about stem cells through print, visual and audible media, and by both the general public and the scientific community, have indicated that there is considerable variation in the concepts of the stages of development and the significance thereof.

The concept of a preembryonic stage occurring earlier than an embryonic one was introduced in 1986 by the American Fertility Society, now the American Society for Reproductive Medicine, through its Ethics Committee, with the issuance of the report of that committee[11]. At the same time, the term *preembryo* was also introduced independently by the Volunteer Licensing Authority, an arm of the Royal College of Obstetricians and Gynaecologists and the British Medical Research Council. The preembryonic stage was identified as the interval up to the appearance of the primitive streak, a stage which guarantees biological individualization at about 14 days. It is of some significance that, quite independently, the Ethics Advisory Board of the Department of Health, Education and Welfare in its report in 1979 designated the period up to 14 days as having attained special moral status. This period approved for research by certain ethical committees is not recognized under Jewish law[5].

A final thought

Surely there is controversy about almost every point in this discussion. This controversy whirls in the heads of patients, doctors, nurses and medical support staff, and in the heads of religious counsellors, ethicists, philosophers, teachers, legislators, lawyers, judges and all those who address these issues, including prospective parents.

An examination of the roots of our belief systems may help in converting controversy to consensus. One thing seems clear: medical care-givers at all levels must understand why they believe what they do, so that they are capable of intelligent discussion of these issues with patients. Only through an ordered and rational thought process may we genuinely assist couples in becoming comfortable with the difficult decisions they may be forced to make in today's new era of reproductive options.

References

1. Young E. Ethical issues: a secular perspective. In Holland S, Lebacqz K, Zoloth L, eds. *The Human Embryonic Stem Cell Debate: Science, Ethics, and Public Policy. Basic Bioethics.* Cambridge, MA: MIT Press, 2001;163–74

2. Jones HW, Crockin SL. On assisted reproduction, religion, and civil law. *Fertil Steril* 2000;73:447–52

3. Huser RJ. *The Crime of Abortion in Canon Law: An Historical Synopsis and Commentary.* Washington, DC: The Catholic University of America Press, 1942

4. McCormick RA. *Health and Medicine in the Catholic Tradition: Tradition in Transition.* New York: Crossroad, 1984

5. Schenker JG. Infertility evaluation and treatment according to Jewish law. *Eur J Obstet Gynecol Reprod Biol* 1997;71:113–21

6. Dunstan GR, Seller MJ. The human embryo: Aristotle and the Arabic and European traditions. In Dunstan GR, ed. *The Status of the Human Embryo: Perspectives from Moral Tradition.* London: King Edward's Hospital Fund for London, 1988:38

7. Wertz DC. Embryo and stem cell research in the United States: history and politics. *Gene Ther* 2002;9:674–8

8. Sachedina A. Islamic perspectives on research with human embryonic stem cells. In *Ethical Issues in Human Stem Cell Research, Vol III, Religious Perspectives.* Rockville, MD: National Bioethics Advisory Commission, US Government Printing Office, 2000:G1–6

9. Dennett DC. *Darwin's Dangerous Idea: Evolution and the Meanings of Life.* New York: Simon & Schuster, 1995

10. Jones HW Jr, Schrader C. And just what is a preembryo? *Fertil Steril* 1989;52:189–91

11. Ethics Committee of the American Fertility Society. Ethical considerations of the new reproductive technologies. *Fertil Steril* 1986;46 (Suppl 1):1S–94S

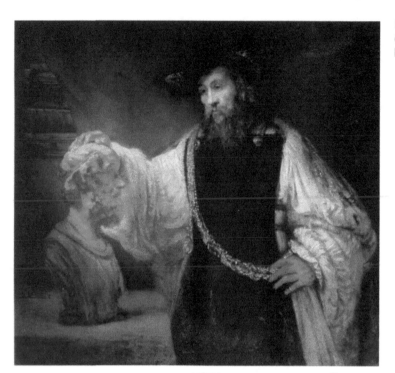

Figure 13.1 Aristotle contemplating the bust of Homer (1653), by Rembrandt van Rijn. (New York Metropolitan Museum of Art)

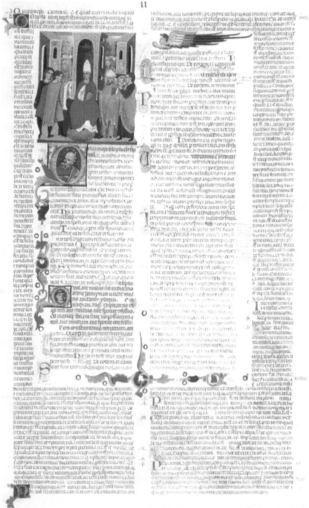

Figure 13.2 Gratian's Decretum

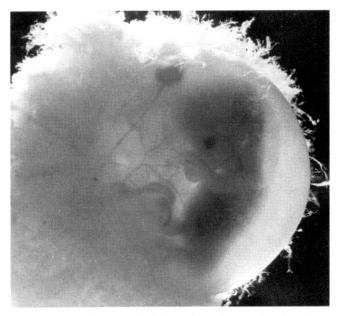

Figure 13.3 Eight-week fetus, 4 cm in length. Courtesy Lennart Nilsson, *A Child is Born*, 1990, Delacorte Press, p. 91. The early fetus is suspended in the amniotic fluid

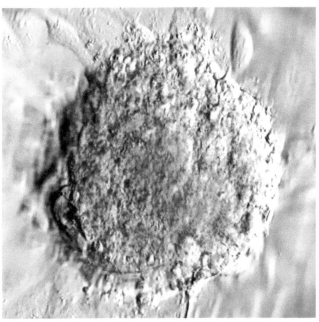

Figure 13.5 High magnification of the inner cell mass of a developing blastocyst. Photograph courtesy of L. Veeck

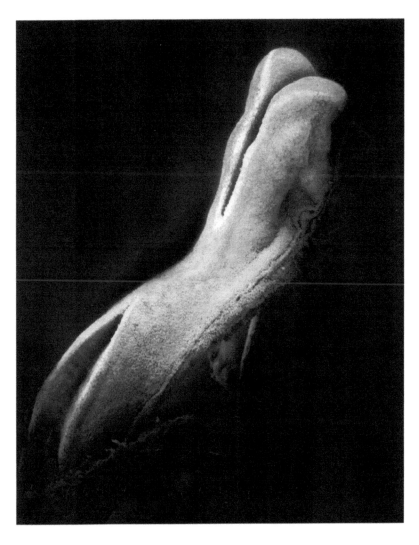

Figure 13.4 Neural tube, 2 mm in length. Courtesy Lennart Nilsson, *A Child is Born*, 1990, Delacorte Press, p. 77. The outer layer, the skin, is cleft by the groove of the neural tube. The swelling above is the rudimentary forebrain

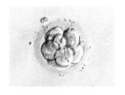

Glossary of terms

Abembryonic

Away from the embryo or away from the inner cell mass

Acrosome reaction

A reaction that occurs when a spermatozoon contacts the zona pellucida in mammals; the acrosome reaction involves a sequence of structural changes in the sperm acrosome, including the liberation of enzymes which are thought to assist sperm penetration through the zona pellucida

Activation (oocyte activation)

The process through which a secondary oocyte is stimulated to resume meiosis. This can occur by a penetrating spermatozoon or an artificial substitute

Adherens junctions

Junctions which provide strong mechanical attachments between adjacent cells, built from *cadherins* and *catenins*

Adhesion molecules

Surface ligands, usually glycoproteins, that mediate cell-to-cell adhesion. Their functions include the assembly and interconnection of various vertebrate systems, as well as maintenance of tissue integration, wound healing, morphogenic movements, cellular migrations and metastasis

AHA or assisted hatching

Assisted hatching; a procedure undertaken in *in vitro* fertilization (IVF) laboratories where a small hole is made in the zona pellucida of a preembryo to facilitate natural hatching

Amnion

The innermost membrane enclosing the embryo or fetus

Aneuploidy

Any deviation from an exact multiple of the haploid number of chromosomes, whether fewer or more

Animal pole/vegetal pole

In an oocyte, the animal pole represents the region from which the polar bodies arise. The vegetal pole is opposite the animal pole

Apoptosis

A form of cell death in which a programmed sequence of events leads to the elimination of cells without releasing harmful substances into the surrounding area. Apoptosis is also called programmed cell death or cell suicide. Apoptosis plays a crucial role in developing and maintaining health by eliminating old cells, unnecessary cells and unhealthy cells

ART

Assisted reproductive technology

Aspermia

Failure to form or produce an ejaculate

Asthenozoospermia

Production of an ejaculate with very poor motility

Azoospermia

Production of an ejaculate devoid of spermatozoa

Biopsy

A procedure where small pieces of tissue or individual cells are taken for microscopic study, preimplantation genetic diagnosis, use in reproductive techniques or tissue culture

Blastocoel

The fluid-filled cavity of the blastocyst

Blastocyst

The mammalian conceptus in the postmorula stage. The cells of the blastocyst form a spherical shell enclosing the blastocoel, with one pole distinguished by the *inner cell mass* from which the embryo forms. The outer cell layer forms the first differentiated epithelial-like cell line, the *trophectoderm*

Blastomere

One of the cells produced by the cleavage of a fertilized oocyte; a cleavage cell

Cadherins

Membrane-bound proteins that mediate the binding of like tissues. Neural tissues express N-cadherins while surface ectoderm expresses E-cadherins

Cavitation

The process involving formation of the fluid-filled extracellular cavity within a compacted preembryo; this cavity increases in size to form the blastocoel

Cell allocation

The movement of cells to different regions or their assignment of different functions or purposes within an organism

Centriole

One of a pair of cellular organelles that are adjacent to the nucleus, function in the formation of the mitotic apparatus and consist of a cylinder with nine microtubules arranged peripherally in a circle

Chorion

The outermost fetal membrane that encloses the amnion, closest to the wall of the uterus

Chromosome

The structures in the cell that carry the genetic material (genes); the genetic messengers of inheritance. The human has 46 chromosomes, 23 coming from the oocyte and 23 coming from the spermatozoon

Cleavage

A series of cell divisions that occur early in development to divide the 1-cell zygote into a large number of blastomeres

Cloning

The production of identical copies of a living organism

Coculture

A laboratory technique that involves growing a specimen (in IVF, a fertilized oocyte or preembryo) on a monolayer of feeder cells (e.g. epithelial cells) or medium that has been conditioned with such cells. These feeder cells are thought to enhance properties of the culture medium by absorbing toxins or releasing favorable growth factors

Colchicine

A chemical that disrupts microtubule formation

Compaction

A process through which a cleaving preembryo changes from a collection of individual cells into a solid mass with indistinguishable cell membranes. Compaction results from the formation of tight intercellular junctions which cause blastomeres to become closely apposed

Conceptus

The derivatives of a fertilized oocyte at any stage of development from fertilization to birth; includes extraembryonic membranes, as well as the preembryo, embryo or fetus. The products of conception; all structures that develop from the zygote, both embryonic and extraembryonic. A term commonly interchanged with the term *preembryo* during IVF treatment

Corona radiata

A closely apposed layer of follicle cells which surrounds the mature oocyte

Corticosteroids

Synthetic steroid hormones; may be used clinically in a prophylactic manner to suppress the immune response

Crossing-over

A process occurring during synapsis in which pairs of homologous chromosomes bearing linked genes mutually exchange corresponding parts

Cryopreservation

Freezing of cells or tissues in order to maintain viability with storage at very low temperatures

Culture medium

A substance or preparation used for the cultivation of living cells

Cumulus oophorus

A multilayered mass of follicular cells surrounding the oocyte. Cells of the cumulus are instrumental, via gap junctions, in nurturing the oocyte during growth and possibly in passing inhibiting factors necessary for deterring the resumption of meiosis. The innermost layer of cells is called the *corona* or *coronal layer*. This layer expands and presents a radiant pattern as oocytes mature in response to exogenous human chorionic gonadotropin (hCG) or a mid-cycle surge of luteinizing hormone (LH). Near ovulation, as they loosen and expand, cumulus cells are observed to retract from the zona pellucida of the oocyte, presumably cutting off the previously important cellular–oocyte communication

Cytokinesis

A phase in mitosis or meiosis which involves the division of the cytoplasm

Cytoplasmic fragmentation

Disorganized fractioning of the cytoplasm, often in a manner that superficially resembles cleavage. Fragments may contain DNA, but they are more likely to contain no nuclear material at all

Cytotrophoblast

The thin inner layer of the trophoblast

Desmosomes

A type of junction that attaches one cell to its neighbor; one of a number of differentiated regions which occur, for example, where the cytoplasmic membranes of adjacent epithelial cells are closely apposed; consists of a circular region of each membrane together with associated intercellular microfilaments and an intercellular material

Diandry

Triploidy in which the extra haploid set is of paternal origin

Differentiation

The process of acquiring completely individual functions or characteristics, as occurs in the progressive diversification of cells and tissues of the developing embryo; the process by which a single pluripotent cell gives rise to a variety of different, more specialized cells

Digyny

Triploidy in which the extra haploid set is of maternal origin

Dizygotic

Pertaining to or derived from two separate zygotes, as in dizygotic (fraternal) twins

DNA

Abbreviation for *deoxyribonucleic acid*, a nucleic acid that is the carrier of genetic information for all organisms except the RNA viruses; DNA is found in all living cells

Donor oocyte cycle

A procedure of ART where a preembryo is formed from the oocyte of one woman (the donor) and transferred to another woman (the recipient) for purposes of establishing pregnancy

Down's syndrome (trisomy 21)

A condition marked by an extra chromosome 21 or extra part of chromosome 21. Individuals are characterized by a small, anteroposteriorly flattened skull, short, flat-bridged nose, epicanthal folds, short phalanges, widened space between the first and second digits of hands and feet, or variations in these stigmata, including moderate to severe mental retardation

Ectoderm

The outermost of the three primary germ layers of the embryo; cells of this layer will go on to form the epidermis and epidermal tissues (such as hair, nails, glands of the skin), external sense organs (ear, eye), some mucous membranes and nervous system of the adult

Ectopic pregnancy

A pregnancy in which the fertilized oocyte implants in a location outside the uterus, usually in the Fallopian tube, the ovary or the abdominal cavity

Egg

A term best reserved for a nutritive object frequently seen on the breakfast table; in humans, an oocyte

Embryo

The stage of the organism after development of the primitive streak; persists until major organs are developed. Once the neural groove and the first somites are present, the embryo is considered formed. In the human, the embryonic stage begins at approximately 14 days after fertilization and encompasses the period when organs and organ systems are coming into existence

Embryogenesis

The developmental process by which the embryo is formed

Embryologist

Scientist with training and skills in handling spermatozoa, oocytes and preembryos in the laboratory; a scientist with specialized training in embryology

Embryonic disc

A structure in the stage of embryo development marked by the formation of ectoderm, mesoderm and endoderm

Endocrinologist

A medical doctor or scientist who specializes in disorders of the endocrine glands and the study of hormones

Endoderm

The innermost of the three primary germ layers of the embryo; cells of this layer will go on to form the digestive tract, epithelium of the pharynx, respiratory tract (except nose), bladder, urethra, lungs, etc. of the adult

Endometrium

The inner mucous membrane of the uterus, the thickness and structure of which vary with the phase of the menstrual cycle. It is functionally divisible into three layers: the stratum basale, stratum spongiosum and stratum compactum, the last two layers together forming the stratum functionale. The implanting human conceptus invades the endometrium

Endoplasmic reticulum

A cell organelle consisting of a complicated network of fine, branching and anastomosing tubules or spaces (cisternae) or isolated vesicles present in the cytoplasm of most cells. Endoplasmic reticulum forms a structural framework for the cells and a circulation pathway between the plasma membrane and nuclear membrane. Its surface may bear ribosomes, the site of protein synthesis

Epididymis

The elongated cordlike structure along the posterior border of the testis, whose elongated coiled duct provides for storage, transit, and maturation of spermatozoa and is continuous with the ductus deferens. It consists of a head (caput epididymis), body (corpus epididymis), and tail (cauda epididymis).

Estrogen

A female sex hormone responsible for secondary sex characteristics, the menstrual cycle and pregnancy

Fallopian tube

The oviduct; the tube leading from the ovary that is responsible for transporting the oocyte or fertilized oocyte to the uterus

Fertilization

The union of male and female gametes leading to the formation of a unique zygote

Fetus

The developing conceptus after the embryonic stage; the fetal period begins at the end of the eighth post-ovulatory week when greater than 90% of the more than 4500 named structures of the adult body have appeared. The fetal period persists until birth

Follicle

A structure in the ovaries that contains the oocyte and other cells

Follicle stimulating hormone

FSH; a hormone released by the pituitary gland that stimulates the growth of the follicle and spermatogenesis

Gamete

The oocyte or the spermatozoon; a mature haploid reproductive cell; any cell which, upon union with another cell, results in the development of a new individual

Gametogenesis

The developmental process by which gametes are formed. In females the process is known more specifically as oogenesis; in males it is known as *spermatogenesis*

Gap junctions

Connections between cells which allow passage of small molecules and electric current. Gap junctions were first described anatomically as regions of close apposition between cells with a narrow (1–2 nm) gap between cell membranes. The variety in the properties of gap junctions is reflected in the number of connexins, the family of proteins which form the junctions

Gene

The functional unit of heredity which is a segment of DNA located at a specific site on a chromosome. A gene directs the formation of an enzyme or other protein

Gene expression

The full use of the information in a gene via transcription and translation leading to production of a protein and hence the appearance of the phenotype determined by that gene. Gene expression is assumed to be controlled at various points in the sequence leading to protein synthesis and this control is thought to be the major determinant of cellular differentiation in eukaryotes

Genetics

The science dealing with the passing of physical and chemical characteristics from parents to offspring and the impact of the environment on genes and genetic expression

Genome activation (preembryonic)

Transition of preembryonic development from control by maternally coded and stored messenger RNA from the oocyte to newly formed products of the preembryonic genome, including the paternally derived component. Genomic activation occurs at the 4–8-cell stage in human preembryos

Germ cell

In the male the testicular cell that divides ultimately to produce the spermatozoon; in the woman the ovarian cell that divides ultimately to form the oocyte

Gestation

The period of time from conception to birth

Gestational carrier

A woman who enters into a social arrangement where she will carry a child created from another couple's gametes with the expectation of relinquishing the child at birth (*see Surrogacy* for a similar arrangement involving carrying and giving birth to a genetically related child)

Gestational sac

A fluid-filled structure that develops within the uterus early in pregnancy. In a normal pregnancy, a gestational sac contains a developing embryo and, subsequently, the fetus

Golgi apparatus, Golgi complex, Golgi system

A cytoplasmic organelle especially well developed in neurons and secretory cells, thought to play a role in the process of secretion. Golgi bodies can be considered the final packaging location for proteins and lipids. Each Golgi body consists of flattened membrane sacs. It is within the flattened membrane sacs that enzymes ready these proteins and lipids for shipment to specific locations. Vesicles form at the final region of a Golgi body when parts of the membrane begin to bulge. These vesicles then break away, via exocytosis, for the transport of these proteins and lipids to their final destination

Gonadotropin

Any hormone having a stimulating effect on the gonads. FSH and LH are two such hormones secreted by the anterior pituitary

Gonadotropin-releasing factor

A substance causing the pituitary gland to release LH and FSH

Granulosa cells; membrana granulosa cells

Cells of the membrana granulosa lining the vesicular ovarian follicle which become luteal cells after ovulation; the layer of small cells that forms the wall of an ovarian follicle

Haploid

Possessing half the diploid or somatic number of chromosomes

Hatched

The end result of the hatching process where the blastocyst is completely removed from the zona pellucida

Hatching

The process by which the expanded blastocyst breaches and escapes through the zona pellucida; hatching must occur before implantation is possible

HOMP

High-order multiple pregnancy; more than two fetal hearts by ultrasound

Human chorionic gonadotropin

hCG; a hormone produced by the chorionic villi of the implanted/implanting conceptus; triggers the release of estrogen and progesterone

Human menopausal gonadotropin

A fertility hormone (drug) which is administered to promote follicular growth

ICSI

Intracytoplasmic sperm injection. A procedure performed in IVF laboratories where a single sperm is injected into the cytoplasm of an oocyte to assist the fertilization process

Immature oocyte

An oocyte with chromosomes at prophase I (PI), a germinal vesicle-bearing oocyte

Implantation

The process involving attachment of the human blastocyst to the luminal epithelium of the uterus, its penetration through, and embedding within, the endometrium; in humans, this occurs 6–8 days after fertilization

Implantation rate

The proportion of gestational sacs by ultrasound divided by the number of conceptuses transferred to the uterus; given as a percentage

Inner cell mass

The cluster of pluripotent cells located at one point on the inner surface of the trophectoderm; these cells will form the body of the embryo after implantation

Intermediate oocyte

An oocyte with chromosomes at metaphase I (MI), characterized by the absence of both a first polar body and a germinal vesicle

Intrauterine transfer; transfer; replacement

The transfer of conceptuses to the uterine cavity for the purposes of establishing pregnancy

IVF

In vitro fertilization. A procedure wherein oocytes are fertilized and cultured outside the body

Klinefelter's syndrome

A syndrome typically marked by a karyotype of 47,XXY (or XXYY, XXXY or XXXXY), or varying forms of mosaicism involving 46,XX and 46,XY cell lines. Individuals with Klinefelter's syndrome experience infertility and usually exhibit variable degrees of masculinization, small testes and, sometimes, gynecomastia

Leydig cells

Cells of the testes that produce the male hormone testosterone

Live birth

The delivery of one or more living babies

Luteinization

The process by which a post-ovulatory ovarian follicle transforms into a corpus luteum through vascularization, follicular cell hypertrophy and lipid accumulation

Luteinizing hormone

LH; a hormone produced by the pituitary gland

Male factor infertility

Any cause of infertility due to low sperm count, motility, morphology or sperm function that makes it difficult for a sperm to fertilize an oocyte under normal conditions

Mature oocyte

An oocyte with chromosomes at metaphase II (MII), characterized by the presence of a first polar body

Meiosis

A specialized form of nuclear division in which there two successive nuclear divisions (meiosis I and II) without any chromosome replication between. Each division can be divided into four stages similar to those of mitosis (prophase, metaphase, anaphase and telophase). Meiosis reduces the starting number of 4n chromosomes in the parent cell to n in each of the four daughter cells. Each cell receives only one of each homologous chromosome pair, with the maternal and paternal chromosomes being distributed randomly between the cells. This is vital for the segregation of genes. During prophase of meiosis I (classically divided into stages: leptotene, zygotene, pachytene, diplotene and diakinesis), homologous chromosomes pair to form bivalents, thus allowing crossing over, the physical exchange of chromatid segments. This results in the recombination of genes. Meiosis occurs during the formation of gametes in animals, which are thus haploid; fertilization gives rise to a diploid oocyte

Menopause

The 'change of life' or time when menstruation ceases, usually between the ages of 45 and 55 years

Menstrual cycle

Follicular phase The 12–14-day preovulatory phase of a woman's menstrual cycle during which time a follicle grows

Periovulatory   Around the time of ovulation

Luteal phase   Post-ovulatory phase of a woman's menstrual cycle. The corpus luteum produces progesterone, which causes the uterine lining to thicken to support implantation

Menstruation   The cyclic (monthly) shedding of the uterine lining in response to stimulation from estrogen and progesterone

MESA

Microsurgical epididymal sperm aspiration; surgical harvest of spermatozoa from the epididymis

Mesoderm

The middle layer of the three germ layers; cells of this layer will go on to form blood, blood vessels, lymphatics and lymphoid organs, gonads, peritoneum, notochord, pleura, pericardium, heart, kidneys, muscle, bone, cartilage, connective tissue, etc. of the adult

Metaphase I oocyte

An oocyte with chromosomes at metaphase I of maturation, characterized by the absence of both a first polar body and a germinal vesicle. An oocyte at an intermediate stage of maturation

Metaphase II oocyte

An oocyte with chromosomes at metaphase II of maturation, characterized by the presence of a first polar body. A fully mature oocyte. A secondary oocyte

Miscarriage

The loss of the products of conception from the uterus after a clinical pregnancy is established, but before the fetus is viable; spontaneous abortion

Mitochondria

One of the minute, spherical rod-shaped or filamentous organelles present in all cells. They contain many enzymes of the Kreb's citric acid cycle and the electron transport systems, hence are of primary importance in the metabolic activities of cells; mitochondria are the principal sites for the generation of energy and the only organelles other than the nucleus to possess DNA (mtDNA)

Mitosis

Division of a cell in which the two daughter nuclei normally receive identical complements of the number of chromosomes characteristic of the somatic cells of the species. Mitosis, the process by which the body grows and replaces cells, is divided into four phases:

Prophase Formation of paired chromosomes, disappearance of nuclear membrane, appearance of the achromatic spindle, formation of polar bodies

Metaphase Arrangement of chromosomes in the equatorial plane of the central spindle to form the monaster. Chromosomes separate into exactly similar halves

Anaphas The two groups of daughter chromosomes separate and move along the fibers of the central spindle, each towards one of the asters, forming the diaster

Telophase The daughter chromosomes resolve themselves into a reticulum and the daughter nuclei are formed, the cytoplasm divides, forming two complete daughter cells

The term mitosis is used interchangeably with cell division, but strictly speaking it refers to nuclear division, whereas cytokinesis refers to division of the cytoplasm

Monosomy

A condition characterized by one less than the normal diploid number of chromosomes $(2n - 1)$

Monozygotic

Pertaining to or derived from one fertilized oocyte or zygote, as in identical twins

Morula

Generally, the 8–16-cell stage when compaction commences until blastocyst formation; the stage commonly observed between 72 and 96 h after insemination. Some authors believe that the term morula is historically inappropriate for mammals

Mosaicism

A condition in which a conceptus or individual possesses two separate and distinct chromosome lines

Multinucleation

A state where cells possess more than one nucleus. Multinucleated blastomeres contain more than a single nucleus and are associated with preembryos demonstrating a reduced implantation potential

Natural cycle

Menstrual cycle that is not controlled or stimulated by exogenous drugs

Natural selection

The Darwinian principle that individuals or organisms with characteristics best suited to survival in a particular environment become a greater proportion of their species within that environment with each generation

Neural tube

The structure that forms from ectoderm on the dorsal side of a vertebrate that has been induced to form neural tissue. The neural tube goes on to form the spinal chord and brain

Nondisjunction

The failure of a pair of homologous chromosomes to separate during the reduction division

Notochord

A tube of cells joined in the embryo foreshadowing the spine

Nucleolus

A rounded refractile body present in the nucleus of most cells which is the site of the synthesis of ribosomal RNA; the nucleolus becomes enlarged during periods of synthesis and atrophied during quiescent periods

Nucleus

The spheroid mass, enclosed in a thin membrane, which is the center for the synthesis of specific cellular proteins and the transmission of heredity traits; contains a nucleolus or several nucleoli, a diffuse nucleoplasm and DNA

Oct4

A transcription factor essential for the maintenance of germ cell totipotence; *Oct4* prevents germ cells from differentiating

Oligozoospermia

Production of an ejaculate with few sperm

Oocyte

The female gamete from inception of the first meiotic division until fertilization. In oogenesis, a cell which develops from an oogonium

Oogonium

The cell that gives rise to the primary oocyte during oogenesis. Oogonia proliferate by mitotic division during early fetal life

Oolemma

Plasma membrane of an oocyte

Ooplasm

Cytoplasm of the oocyte

Ooplasm/cytoplasm descriptions

Degenerative	Non-viable
Fragmented blebs	Exhibiting extracytoplasmic fragments or
Granular	Exhibiting dense granules of darkish color
Mottled 'spotted'	Exhibiting 'orange-peel' granularity;
Vacuolated	Exhibiting spaces or small cavities within the cytoplasm of an oocyte or blastomere; may be the result of an aberrant endocytosis caused by oolemma instability

Ootid

The prezyote; the pronuclear stage oocyte before entrance into syngamy; the stage at which pronuclei are visible

Ovarian stimulation

The use of drugs (oral or injected) to stimulate the ovaries to develop follicles and ooctyes

Ovary

The female gonad; either of the two sexual glands in which oocytes are formed

Ovulation

The periodic production and discharge of an oocyte by the ovary

Ovum

A female gamete or germ cell; an oocyte. The term *ovum*, which has been used for such disparate structures as an oocyte and a 3-week embryo, has no scientific usefulness

Parthenogenesis

The activation and subsequent development of a oocyte without fertilization; may occur naturally or through artificial stimulation

Penetrated oocyte

An oocyte that has been penetrated by a spermatozoon; strictly, one in which gamete plasma membranes have become confluent. The stage before pronuclei are formed. Penetration of the oocyte usually occurs within 3 h of insemination

Perivitelline space

Space surrounding the vitellus (technically, yolk; in this sense, the oocyte); the space between the oocyte and the zona pellucida; subzonal space. This space may possess the first and second polar bodies or extracellular fragments

PESA

Percutaneous epdidymal sperm aspiration; harvest of spermatozoa from the epdidymis without open surgery

PGD

Preimplantation genetic diagnosis. The procedure involving the removal of a blastomere or blastomeres from the developing preembryo for purposes of genetic analysis

Pituitary gland

The hypophysis; a small, oval endocrine gland lodged at the base of the brain that affects other endocrine glands

Placenta

A temporary organ which exchanges nutrients and wastes between mother and fetus and produces hormones needed to maintain pregnancy

Pluripotent

Cells capable of forming most tissues, i.e. cells of the inner mass (ICM). Although cells of the ICM can form every type of cell found in the human body, they cannot form an organism because they are unable to give rise to the placenta and supporting tissues necessary for development in the human uterus. These ICM cells are therefore 'pluripotent'. Pluripotent stem cells undergo further specialization into stem cells that are committed to give rise to cells that have a particular function. Examples of this include blood stem cells which give rise to red blood cells, white blood cells and platelets; and skin stem cells that give rise to the various types of skin cells. These more specialized stem cells are called *multipotent*

Polar body

First polar body The structure extruded into the perivitelline space at the end of telophase I. Human chromosomes are divided between the oocyte and the first polar body (23 chromosomes, 46 chromatids, $2n$ DNA in each), those in the oocyte being attached to spindle microtubules. For a while after its formation, the first polar body remains connected to the oocyte by the meiotic spindle, forming a cytoplasmic bridge. Chromosomes within the first polar body may remain clumped together, may undergo a second meiotic division or may scatter within the cytoplasm; generally a nucleus is not formed. The first polar body contains cortical granules because of its extrusion before sperm penetration and cortical granule release

Second polar body The structure extruded into the perivitelline space after sperm penetration; contains 23 single-stranded chromosomes ($1n$ DNA) after telophase II and may be nucleated

Polarized; polarity

The state or condition of having poles or possessing parts or regions of opposite or contrasting effects; cells that are polarized organize themselves or migrate to given poles, i.e. polar versus mural regions or inner cell mass versus trophectoderm, etc.

Polar trophectoderm; mural trophectoderm

Cells making up the trophectoderm of a blastocyst which are either polar (nearest or coming into contact with the inner cell mass), or mural (opposite or making no contact with the inner cell mass)

Polyploidy

A condition in which a conceptus or individual possesses one or more sets of homologous chromosomes in excess of the normal diploid set, as in triploidy ($3n$), tetraploidy ($4n$), hexaploidy ($6n$) or octoploidy ($8n$)

Polyspermy

The condition that occurs when an oocyte is penetrated by more than one fertilizing spermatozoon

Post-transfer observation period

The 1–3 days following intrauterine transfer when preembryos not frozen or replaced are evaluated daily to determine their suitability for freezing; also called the 'post ob' period

Preembryo

The conceptus during early cleavage stages until development of the embryo. The preembryonic period ends at approximately 14 days after fertilization with development of the primitive streak

Pregnancy

Clinical A pregnancy documented by ultrasonic investigation that shows a gestational sac in the uterus and requires dilatation and curettage (D&C) if miscarried

Preclinical A pregnancy does not develop to the clinical stage despite initial positive testing

Prezygote

The pronuclear oocyte. The stage of development before syngamy, when the term *zygote* becomes appropriate. Some authors refer to this stage as an *ootid*. Prezygotes are commonly observed 6–20 h after insemination or injection

Primary oocyte

The oocyte formed in the ovary before birth. Primary oocytes begin the first meiotic division before birth, but completion of prophase does not occur until after puberty

Primitive streak

A thick, opaque groove in the ectoderm that accompanies the emergence of the mesoderm and notochord

Primordia

The forerunners of organs or other structures in the embryo

Primordial follicle

An ovarian structure consisting of an oocyte surrounded by a single layer of granulosa cells

Progesterone

A hormone produced by the corpus luteum and placenta that readies the endometrium for implantation and breasts for lactation, and maintains pregnancy

Pronuclei

Structures formed during fertilization from sperm and oocyte chromatin. Normal pronuclei are approximately 30 μm in diameter. *See Prezygote*

Prophase I oocyte

An oocyte with chromosomes at prophase I of maturation, characterized by a germinal vesicle

Reactive oxygen species (ROS)

Highly reactive substrates that sometimes form as byproducts of metabolism and are thought to cause permanent irreparable damage to the organism (preembryo, embryo or body)

Recombinant DNA

DNA artificially drawn from one species, combined with DNA from the same or a different species, and transplanted to the original or another species

Refractile body

An aggregation of lipid material and dense granules in the oocyte of approximately 10 μm size; associated with poor fertilization

Secondary oocyte

The oocyte after completion of the first meiotic division and arrest at metaphase of the second meiotic division. Also called a *mature oocyte or metaphase II oocyte*, this is the stage commonly associated with ovulated specimens or those collected from mature follicles for IVF. The secondary oocyte is characterized by a first polar body and no nucleus

Seeding

During cryopreservation, the process of introducing an ice crystal to the freezing solution in a controlled manner to prevent supercooling

Selective reduction; multifetal pregnancy reduction

A procedure used to decrease the number of fetuses a woman carries in order to improve the chances that the remaining fetus(es) will develop into a healthy infant(s). Reductions that occur naturally are referred to as spontaneous reductions

Seminiferous tubules

The small tubes of the testicles that produce spermatozoa

Sertoli cells

Cells in the seminiferous tubules that nurture developing spermatozoa

Sex ratio, liveborn

An expression of the number of live-born males in a population to the number of live-born females, usually stated as the number of males per 100 females

Somites

Somites form from the lateral mesoderm. They are the precursors to the vertebrae and their associated muscles

Spermatids

The cells formed after the second phase of meiotic division (meiosis II) of the secondary spermatocytes

Spermatogonium

A primordial germ cell that gives rise to a primary spermatocyte

Spermatozoon

A mature germ cell, the specific output of the testes. The generative element of the semen which serves to fertilize the oocyte, it consists of a head, neck, midpiece, and tail

Spermiogenesis

The transformation of a spermatid into a mature spermatozoon

SSEAs

Stage-specific embryonic (surface) antigens; carbohydrates associated with cell surface glycolipids, glycoproteins and proteoglycans. These antigens may be used as markers of cell differentiation and show species-specific expression

Stem cells (embryonic stem cells)

Cells with the ability to divide for indefinite periods in culture and give rise to specialized cells; pluripotent cells generated from the inner cell mass

Stillbirth

The birth of an infant with no signs of life after 20 or more weeks of gestation

Subnuclei

Nuclear or pronuclear fragments containing scattered, membrane-bound chromatin

Supercooling

During cryopreservation, the process of cooling to well below the freezing point without extracellular ice formation; when solutions supercool, cells do not dehydrate appropriately

Surrogacy

A social arrangement where one woman carries a child created from her own oocyte and donated semen for another woman (anonymous semen donor), man (directed semen donor) or couple (husband semen donor) with the expectation of relinquishing it at birth (see Gestational carrier for a similar arrangement involving carrying and giving birth to a genetically unrelated child)

Synapsis

The coming together in pairs of homologous chromosomes during meiosis

Syncytiotrophoblast

The outer layer of the trophoblast that invades the endometrium during implantation

Syngamy

The active union of two gametes in fertilization to form a zygote; the process of reorganization and pairing of maternal and paternal chromosomes in the zygote after pronuclear membrane breakdown

Teratozoospermia

Production of an ejaculate with a high percentage of abnormal forms (abnormal shapes)

TESE

Testicular sperm extraction; microsurgical extraction of spermatozoa from the testis

Testis (plural: testes)

The male gonad; either of the pear-shaped glands normally situated in the scrotum

Testosterone

The principal steroid hormone produced in men, responsible for secondary sex characteristics

Tight junctions

Cell–cell junctions that seal adjacent epithelial cells (or epithelial-like trophectoderm cells) together, preventing the passage of most dissolved molecules from one side of the epithelial sheet to the other

Totipotent

Having unlimited capability to produce any type of cell. Totipotent cells have the capability to turn into (to 'specialize' or 'differentiate' into) the tissues surrounding the developing embryo, the embryo itself, and all of the tissues and organs that are present in the developed organism. The fertilized oocyte is totipotent until, perhaps, the 8-cell stage, meaning that its potential is total

Translocation, chromosomal

Interchange of chromatin between two or more chromosomes

Triploidy

A condition in which a conceptus or individual possesses three times the haploid number of chromosomes ($3n$)

Trisomy

A condition characterized by having one more than the diploid set of chromosomes ($2n + 1$). Common trisomies have been given the names of those individuals first describing them: trisomy 13 (*Patau's syndrome*), trisomy 18 (*Edward's syndrome*); trisomy 21 (*Down's syndrome*)

Trophectoderm

An outer, single layer of differentiated, polarized, epithelial-like cells forming the blastocyst; these cells ultimately give rise to the placenta and extraembryonic tissues after implantation.

Polar trophectoderm Region of the trophectoderm in mammals that makes direct contact with the inner cell mass

Mural trophectoderm Region of the trophectoderm in mammals not making contact with the inner cell mass

Turner's syndrome

A syndrome marked by a karyotype of 45,X or varying forms of mosaicism involving 46,XX and 46,XY cell lines. Individuals with Turner's syndrome experience ovarian failure and usually exhibit short stature and other somatic stigmata as described by Henry Turner

Ultrasound

A technique used in ART for visualizing the follicles in the ovary, the gestational sac or the fetus

Varicocele (male)

A varicose condition of the veins of the pampiniform plexus, forming a swelling that appears bluish through the skin of the scrotum, and accompanied by a constant pulling, dragging, or dull pain

Vegetal pole/animal pole

In an oocyte, the vegetal pole is opposite the animal pole. In contrast, the animal pole represents the region from which the polar bodies arise

Zona pellucida

The covering that surrounds the oocyte; believed to be produced largely by the surrounding follicular cells. In the human, the oocyte measures about 115 μm and the thickness of the zona measures between 12 and 20 μm. The zona pellucida is covered externally by the corona radiata, which is a loose investment of granulosa cells from the ovarian follicle

Zona reaction

A process usually occurring during fertilization in which the chemistry and composition of the zona pellucida change to render it impermeable by other spermatozoa

ZP1, ZP2, ZP3

Acidic glycoproteins localized in the zona pellucida of mammals; ZP3 is believed to be the major spermatozoon-binding protein and inducer of the acrosome reaction

Zygote

The 1-cell stage after pronuclear membrane breakdown and before the first cleavage. This stage is characterized by maternal and paternal chromosomes assuming positions on the first cleavage spindle and, thus, lacks a nucleus. Commonly observed 18–24 h after insemination or injection

Abbreviations and symbols used for embryology documentation

Abbreviations

abn	abnormal
c–c	cell–cell contact (noted just before compaction, as blastomeres become closely apposed)
clp	clear areas at periphery of cells
cont	contracted
deg	degenerative
dk, dksh	dark, darkish
f	faint
fert	fertilization
frag	fragmented
fz	fractured or broken zona pellucida
lg, med, sm	large, medium, small
m	many
mnb	multinucleated blastomeres
oval	oval shape
POB	post-transfer observation period
pb	polar body
pn	pronucleus/pronuclei
pvd	perivitelline debris
pvs	perivitelline space
rb	refractile body
sl	slight or slightly
subnuc	subnuclei
thk, thn	thick, thin
v	very
vacs	vacuoles
zf	zona-free
zp	zona pellucida

Symbols

Δ	irregular shape (relates to shape of oocyte or blastomere)
$\equiv$	even (equivalent) sized blastomeres (relates to size)
$\approx$	approximately even (approximately equal) sized blastomeres
$\neq$	uneven (not equivalent) sized blastomeres
$\div$	cleaving (in the process of dividing)
⊕ing	compacting
⊕ed	compacted
⊙	large pvs
℧	zona artifact
ô	bilayered zona
ö	porous zona
ō	dark zona
Ⓜ	mottled cytoplasm
Ⓖ	granular cytoplasm
√	good morphology
√√	excellent morphology
⊗	very poor morphology

References

Dorland's Illustrated Medical Dictionary, 26th edn. Philadelphia: WB Saunders, 1981

Moore KL. *The Developing Human*, 3rd edn. Philadelphia: WB Saunders, 1982

O'Rahilly R, Muller F. *Developmental Stages in Human Embryos*. Washington, DC: Carnegie Institution of Washington, Publication 637, 1987

Society for Assisted Reproductive Technology/ Centers for Disease Control and Prevention. *Assisted Reproductive Success Rates* (http://www.cdc.gov)

Stedman's Medical Dictionary, 25th edn. Baltimore: Williams & Wilkins, 1990

Steen EB. *Dictionary of Biology*. Savage, MD: Barnes and Noble Books, 1971

Veeck LL. *Atlas of the Human Oocyte and Early Conceptus*. Baltimore: Williams & Wilkins, 1986

Index

9780367395285

T - #0571 - 071024 - C288 - 297/210/14 - PB - 9780367395285 - Gloss Lamination